Breastfeeding Handbook for Physicians

2nd Edition

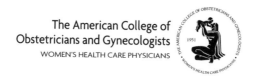

The American College of
Obstetricians and Gynecologists
WOMEN'S HEALTH CARE PHYSICIANS

American Academy
of Pediatrics

DEDICATED TO THE HEALTH OF ALL CHILDREN™

American Academy of Pediatrics Department of Marketing and Publications

Maureen DeRosa, MPA, Director, Department of Marketing and Publications

Mark Grimes, Director, Division of Product Development

Alain Park, Senior Product Development Editor

Sandi King, MS, Director, Division of Publishing and Production Services

Theresa Wiener, Manager, Publications Production and Manufacturing

Jason Crase, Manager, Editorial Services

Linda Diamond, Manager, Art Direction and Production

Julia Lee, Director, Division of Marketing and Sales

Linda Smessaert, MSIMC, Brand Manager, Clinical and Professional Publications

Library of Congress Control Number: 2013949402
ISBN 978-1-58110-804-0
eISBN 978-1-58110-805-7
MA0670

American Academy of Pediatrics
141 Northwest Point Blvd
Elk Grove Village, IL 60007-1019

The American College of Obstetricians and Gynecologists
409 12th St SW
PO Box 96920
Washington, DC 20090-6920

Illustrations by Anthony Alex LeTourneau

The recommendations in this publication do not indicate an exclusive course of treatment or serve as a standard of care. Variations, taking into account individual circumstances, may be appropriate.

This book has been developed by the American Academy of Pediatrics and The American College of Obstetricians and Gynecologists. The authors, editors, and contributors are expert authorities in the field of pediatrics. No commercial involvement of any kind has been solicited or accepted in the development of the content of this publication.

Products are mentioned for informational puporses only. Inclusion in the publication does not imply endorsement by the American Academy of Pediatrics and The American College of Obstetricians and Gynecologists.

The publishers have made every effort to trace the copyright holders for borrowed material. If they have inadvertently overlooked any, they will be pleased to make the necessary arrangements at first opportunity.

4-97/0913

1 2 3 4 5 6 7 8 9 10

AAP Section on Breastfeeding Executive Committee

2012–2013

Richard J. Schanler, MD, FAAP (Chair)
Margreete Johnston, MD, FAAP
Susan Landers, MD, FAAP
Lawrence Noble, MD, FAAP
Kinga Szucs, MD, FAAP
Laura Viehmann, MD, FAAP

Subcommittee Chairpersons

Lori Feldman-Winter, MD, FAAP
Ruth A. Lawrence, MD, FAAP
Joan Younger Meek, MD, FAAP
Sandra Sullivan, MD, FAAP
Jennifer Thomas, MD, FAAP

2013–2014

Richard J. Schanler, MD, FAAP (Chair)
Margreete Johnston, MD, FAAP
Susan Landers, MD, FAAP
Mary O'Connor, MD, FAAP
Joan Meek, MD, FAAP
Kinga Szucs, MD, FAAP

Subcommittee Chairpersons

Lori Feldman-Winter, MD, FAAP
Ruth A. Lawrence, MD, FAAP
Natasha Sriraman, MD, FAAP
Sandra Sullivan, MD, FAAP
Jennifer Thomas, MD, FAAP

ACOG Committee on Obstetric Practice

Members, 2012–2013

George A. Macones, MD, FACOG (Chair)

Jeffrey L. Ecker, MD, FACOG (Vice Chair)

Richard H. Beigi, MD, FACOG

Aaron B. Caughey, MD, FACOG

Lorraine Dugoff, MD, FACOG

James D. Goldberg, MD, FACOG

Rebecca Jackson, MD, FACOG

Denise J. Jamieson, MD, MPH, FACOG

Howard L. Minkoff, MD, FACOG

Karla W. Nacion, PhD, CNM

Michelle Y. Owens, MD, FACOG

Christian Michael Pettker, MD, FACOG

Eva K. Pressman, MD, FACOG

Raymond L. Cox, Jr, MD, MBA, FACOG (Ex Officio)

Neil S. Silverman, MD, FACOG (Ex Officio)

Cathy Whittlesey, (Ex Officio)

Liaison Representatives

Vincenzo Berghella, MD, FACOG

Debra Bingham, PhD

William M. Callaghan, MD, FACOG

Julia Carey-Corrado, MD, FACOG

Beth Choby, MD, FAAFP

Joshua M. Copel, MD, FACOG

Craig M. Palmer, MD

Lu-Ann Papile, MD, FAAP

Phillip Price, MD, FACOG

Uma M. Reddy, MD, MPH, FACOG

Members, 2013–2014

Jeffrey L. Ecker, MD, FACOG (Chair)

James D. Goldberg, MD, FACOG (Vice-Chair)

Richard H. Beigi, MD, FACOG

Aaron B. Caughey, MD, FACOG

Lorraine Dugoff, MD, FACOG

Yasser Yehia El-Sayed, MD, FACOG

Rebecca Jackson, MD, FACOG

Denise J. Jamieson, MD, MPH, FACOG

Howard L. Minkoff, MD, FACOG

Karla W. Nacion, PhD, CNM

Christian Michael Pettker, MD, FACOG

Alison M. Stuebe, MD, FACOG

Methodius G. Tuuli, MD, FACOG

Joseph R. Wax, MD, FACOG

Tina Clark-Samazan Foster, MD FACOG (Ex Officio)

William A. Grobman, MD, FACOG (Ex Officio)

Cathy Whittlesey (Ex Officio)

Liaison Representatives

Vincenzo Berghella, MD, FACOG

Debra Bingham, PhD

William M. Callaghan, MD, FACOG

Julia Carey-Corrado, MD, FACOG

Beth Choby, MD, FAAFP

Joshua Copel, MD, FACOG

Rhonda Hearns-Stokes, MD, FACOG

Craig M. Palmer, MD

Uma M. Reddy, MD, MPH, FACOG

Kristi L. Watterberg, MD, FAAP

Contributors

The following individuals have provided valuable advice and skill in preparation of this revision of the *Breastfeeding Handbook for Physicians*.

Philip O. Anderson, PharmD, FASHP
University of California San Diego, La Jolla, CA

Michelle G. Brenner, MD, IBCLC, FAAP
Eastern Virginia Medical School/Children's Hospital of
The King's Daughters, Norfolk, VA

Lori Feldman-Winter, MD, MPH, FAAP
Cooper Medical School of Rowan University, Division of Adolescent
Medicine, Children's Regional Hospital at Cooper, Camden, NJ

Margreete Johnston, MD, MPH, FAAP
Meharry Medical College and Vanderbilt University, Department
of Pediatrics, Children's Clinic East, Nashville, TN

Nancy Krebs, MD, MS, FAAP
University of Colorado School of Medicine, Aurora, CO

Susan Landers, MD, FAAP, FABM
Pediatrix Medical Group, Seton Healthcare Family, Austin, TX

Ruth A. Lawrence, MD, FAAP, FABM
University of Rochester School of Medicine, Rochester, NY

Sharon Mass, MD, FACOG
Morristown Memorial Hospital, Morristown, NJ

Joan Younger Meek, MD, MS, RD, FAAP, FABM, IBCLC
The Florida State University College of Medicine, Orlando, FL

Lawrence Noble, MD, FAAP
Mount Sinai School of Medicine, New York, NY

Richard J. Schanler, MD, FAAP, FABM
Cohen Children's Medical Center of New York and
Hofstra North Shore-LIJ School of Medicine, Hempstead, NY

Kinga A. Szucs, MD, FAAP
Indiana University School of Medicine, Indianapolis, IN

Jennifer Thomas, MD, MPH, IBCLC, FAAP, FABM
Lakeshore Medical Clinic, Franklin, WI, and
Medical College of Wisconsin, Milwaukee, WI

Laura Viehmann, MD, FAAP
Warren Alpert Medical School of Brown University, Providence, RI

Todd Wolynn, MD, MMM, IBCLC, FAAP
Kids Plus Pediatrics, Pittsburgh, PA

The editors would also like to acknowledge the work done by the contributors of the previous edition.

Pamela D. Berens, MD, FACOG, FABM
Lori Berkowitz, MD, FACOG
Cheston M. Berlin Jr, MD, FAAP
Linda S. Black, MD, FAAP
Keith R. Brill, MD, FACOG, FACS
Margarett K. Davis, MD, MPH
Sharon L. Dooley, MD, MPH, FACOG
Arthur I. Eidelman, MD, FAAP
Lori Feldman-Winter, MD, MPH, FAAP
Lawrence M. Gartner, MD, FAAP
Madeline H. Gartner, MD, FACS
M. Jane Heinig, PhD
Nancy Krebs, MD, MS, FAAP
Susan Landers, MD, FAAP, FABM
Ruth A. Lawrence, MD, FAAP, FABM
Sharon Mass, MD, FACOG
Joan Y. Meek, MD, MS, RD, FAAP, FABM, IBCLC
Margaret C. (Peggy) Neville, PhD
Edward R. Newton, MD, FACOG, FABM
Victoria Nichols-Johnson, MD, FACOG
Barbara L. Philipp, MD, FAAP, FABM
Larry Pickering, MD, FAAP
Nancy G. Powers, MD, FAAP, FABM
Richard J. Schanler, MD, FAAP, FABM
Wendelin Slusser, MD, MS, FAAP
Carol L. Wagner, MD, FAAP, FABM, FASCN
Nancy E. Wight, MD, FAAP, FABM

Contents

Preface

Breastfeeding Handbook for Physicians was written with the goal of providing physicians in all specialties with a concise reference and teaching aid on breastfeeding and human lactation. The hope for this book is that with enhanced knowledge of breastfeeding, from physiology to clinical practice, the physician will be in a far better position to comfortably promote and support breastfeeding and lead the team of collaborating health care providers.

This handbook represents the collaborative efforts of the American Academy of Pediatrics and the American College of Obstetricians and Gynecologists. As befits a book written jointly by different specialties, it addresses collaboration among physicians and between physicians and other health care professionals, especially lactation specialists. We recognize and acknowledge that the physician is at the center of a larger health care team of professionals involved with the medical care of the infant and mother. As such, the concept of the medical home for both infant and mother is stressed, and it is therefore also understandable that all physicians should receive appropriate education in breastfeeding and human lactation.

Nonetheless, even though this book is designed primarily for physicians, use by other health professionals is welcomed, including nurses and nurse practitioners, midwives, dietitians, and lactation specialists. This handbook serves as a bridge between all health care professionals interested in achieving coordinated and optimal care for infants and mothers.

This revision also comes at an important time in the United States when there is an increased national interest in supporting breastfeeding and human lactation. As reported by the Centers for Disease Control and Prevention (CDC), US breastfeeding rates are increasing, with 77% initiation and 26% as the rate for any breastfeeding at 12 months. However, there is still room for improvement, with the rate of exclusive breastfeeding at 6 months being 16%, only 6% of births occurring at Baby-Friendly facilities, and 25% of all newborns routinely receiving formula in the first 48 hours! The CDC reports these yearly statistical updates on breastfeeding, cultural diversity issues, and hospital practice assessments; implements research in the field of human milk and lactation (see Appendix); and now includes exclusive breastfeeding rates through 1 year, workplace accommodations for lactation, and births in Baby-Friendly hospitals. The Joint Commission now assesses exclusive breastfeeding rates in birth hospitals.

Other national initiatives with a focus on breastfeeding include the multifaceted 2011 *Surgeon General's Call to Action to Support Breastfeeding,* updated Healthy People 2020 targets for breastfeeding, the Maternal and Child Health Bureau's publication of the *Business Case for Breastfeeding,* changes to the Women, Infants, and Children (WIC) program, and many provisions in the 2010 Patient Protection and Affordable Care Act, which promote and support breastfeeding, and all of which are discussed in this edition.

The American Academy of Pediatrics has also recently revised and published its policy statement, *Breastfeeding and the Use of Human Milk* (see Appendix), which updates our knowledge and supports global breastfeeding practices. The AAP advocates breastfeeding as a public health issue for infants and mothers. Exclusive breastfeeding is the goal for about 6 months, followed by continued breastfeeding while complementary foods are introduced. While this remains the goal, providers should remember that breastfeeding is a personal choice for each woman. Virtually all mothers who are initially undecided or hesitant to breastfeed can do so successfully with appropriate counseling, education, and knowledgeable support. Formula feeding should not be portrayed as equivalent to human milk feeding. However, if the mother chooses not to breastfeed after these interventions have been implemented, she should be supported in her decision.

Not only did we include in this edition the above efforts and other updates on many areas from the first edition, but we have made important changes as well. The chapter on benefits has been expanded and the concept of dose dependency addressed. The unique benefit of breastfeeding and human milk to preterm infants is discussed in detail as its own chapter and the chapter on creating a breastfeeding-friendly office practice has been expanded. Preventive health care visit checklists have been revised to reflect the magnitude of breastfeeding, and there is a new chapter devoted to breastfeeding issues during a disaster.

We hope that the revised *Breastfeeding Handbook for Physicians* can be used as a guide to teaching lactation theory and breastfeeding practice to medical students, residents, and fellows. Similarly, postgraduate continuing medical education programs can be built around its contents. It is hoped that this handbook will encourage physicians to become teachers of breastfeeding and lactation medicine, and that it may provide a framework on which to build hospital and office policies.

The development of *Breastfeeding Handbook for Physicians* is the product of numerous experts in the field of breastfeeding and human lactation. It is our hope that you will find this reference useful for breastfeeding education and support in many arenas.

The Editors

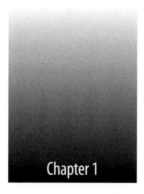

Chapter 1

The Scope of Breastfeeding

Breastfeeding is the normative standard for infant feeding and nutrition and as such should be considered a national and international public health priority and not only a lifestyle choice. Physicians of all specialties benefit by understanding the biology and physiology of breastfeeding, as well as the prevalence and social behaviors associated with breastfeeding. The American Academy of Pediatrics (AAP) and the American College of Obstetricians and Gynecologists (ACOG) recommend all mothers and infants, with rare exceptions, breastfeed exclusively for about the first 6 months. The AAP recommends those 6 months be followed by continued breastfeeding after the addition of complementary foods for at least a year or until mutually desired by mother and child. The United States has been tracking rates of breastfeeding among different populations and uses these data to set national goals for breastfeeding. The United States also tracks multiple process indicators for breastfeeding protection, promotion, and support. These indicators help health care professionals design interventions to overcome persistent disparities in breastfeeding within the United States.

Successful breastfeeding requires education, support, and an environment that values and understands breastfeeding. This need for support may derive from the fact that our modern culture has evolved a series of messages that inhibit automatic and natural behaviors related to breastfeeding. Because breastfeeding is rarely observed in our society, health care professionals must supply the appropriate education, support, and encouragement necessary for breastfeeding to occur and to help mothers meet their breastfeeding goals. In addition, there is a growing database defining the beneficial effects of the use of human milk for preterm infants. These will be reviewed in chapters 2 and 14.

Categories of Breastfeeding

Breastfeeding *intensity* (exclusivity) has been categorized in various ways, and clarity in regard to these terms can facilitate teaching, research, and clinical evaluation (Box 1-1). The term *any* breastfeeding may be confusing, although it is often used to describe a population that includes both those exclusively breastfeeding and those combining formula feeding and breast-feeding. Furthermore, the actual prevalence of exclusive breastfeeding for 6 months in the United States is low and accounts for the difficulties in inter-preting health outcomes that are tied to exclusivity of human milk (absence of any other food or fluid). Many women may be exclusively breastfeeding for some or even most of the first 6 months, although there may be temporary interruptions when formula or food is given. Yet, these mothers may report at any time point that they are exclusively breastfeeding, thereby confusing the actual prevalence of exclusive breastfeeding and rendering the health research outcomes difficult to interpret.

The *duration* of breastfeeding is also important to define to best understand health outcomes, as well as to fully describe the experience of the mother and

Box 1-1. Breastfeeding Categories

Exclusive: Human milk is the only food provided. Medicines, minerals, and vitamins may also be given under this category, but no water, juice, or other preparations. Infants fed expressed human milk from their own mothers or from a milk bank by gavage tube, cup, or bottle also can be included in this category if they have had no nonhuman milk or foods.

Almost/Predominantly Exclusive: Human milk is the predominant food provided with rare feeding of other milk or food. The infant may have been given 1 or 2 formula bottles during the first few days of life, but none after that.

Partial or Mixed: This may vary from mostly human milk with small amounts or infre-quent feedings of nonhuman milk or food (*high partial*) to infants receiving significant amounts of nonhuman milk or food as well as human milk (*medium partial*) to infants receiving predominantly nonhuman milk or food with some human milk (*low partial*).

Token: The infant is fed almost entirely with nonhuman milk and food, but either had some breastfeeds shortly after birth or continues to have occasional breastfeeds. This type of breastfeeding may be seen late in the weaning process.

Any Breastfeeding: The category includes all of the above.

Never Breastfed: This infant has *never* received *any* human milk, either by direct breastfeeding or expressed milk with artificial means of delivery.

infant. Other factors, such as the number of feeds in a 24-hour period, help identify the adequacy of feeding schedules and support the analysis of weight patterns in the newborn. There has been a shift away from describing the frequency of feeding (such as every so many hours) and the length of feeds at each breast to support the concept that babies feed in irregular patterns and are best supported by cue-based, or "on-demand," feeding. Some feeds may be very short and others long, and this variable pattern is unique to the behaviors and needs of the infant, and also reflects the variability in mothers' milk production throughout the day, week, or months of lactation.

Breastfeeding in the United States

Beginning in July 2001, the United States began tracking breastfeeding rates using the National Immunization Survey, a national surveillance system of the Centers for Disease Control and Prevention's (CDC's) National Immunization Program, in partnership with the CDC's National Center for Health Statistics. The National Immunization Survey uses random-digit dialing to survey those households with children aged 19 to 35 months about breastfeeding. Mothers are asked a series of retrospective questions that include whether the child was ever breastfed or fed human milk, when the child stopped breastfeeding or being fed human milk, and the age when formula was first fed.

In 2008, 74.6% of all US women initiated breastfeeding, meeting the Healthy People 2010 target of 75% initiation, but not yet reaching targets set for 2020 (Table 1-2). Healthy People targets for 2020 include outcome measures such

Table 1-2. Healthy People 2020 Goals

Healthy People 2020 Objective		
MICH-21: Increase the proportion of infants who are breastfed,		
MICH-21.1	Ever	81.9%
MICH-21.2	At 6 months	60.6%
MICH-21.3	At 1 year	34.1%
MICH-21.4	Exclusively through 3 months	46.2%
MICH-21.5	Exclusively through 6 months	25.5%
MICH-22: Increase the proportion of employers that have worksite lactation support programs.		38%
MICH-23: Reduce the proportion of breastfed newborns who receive formula supplementation within the first 2 days of life.		14.2%
MICH-24: Increase the proportion of live births that occur in facilities that provide recommended care for lactating mothers and their babies.		8.1%

as rates of breastfeeding at initiation (6 months and 1 year), exclusive breast-feeding (at 3 and 6 months), as well as process indicators including rates of supplementation in the first 2 days, number of births occurring in facilities designated as Baby-Friendly, and workplace support. The rate of supplementation in the first 2 days is 24% (in 2006) and rising, with the goal for 2020 set at 14%. Being born in a Baby-Friendly designated hospital provides the best opportunity to decrease early formula supplementation, yet only 3% of births occurred in such facilities in 2009, with the 2020 goal being set at 8%. Following the newborn period, mothers need support on return to the workforce. The Healthy People goal for 2020 is for 38% of employers to have lactation support programs, yet in 2009, merely 25% had such programs.

The rates of breastfeeding have increased for *any* breastfeeding and *exclusive* breastfeeding at 3 and 6 months (Figure 1-1); however, initiation of exclusive breastfeeding continues to be a challenge, and most data suggest there has been a decline in exclusivity early on in the newborn period. Compared with 2003 when 62.5% of US newborns were exclusively breastfed at 7 days,

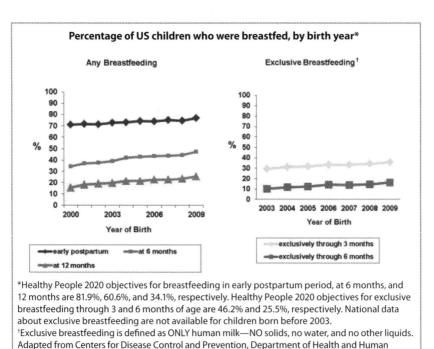

*Healthy People 2020 objectives for breastfeeding in early postpartum period, at 6 months, and 12 months are 81.9%, 60.6%, and 34.1%, respectively. Healthy People 2020 objectives for exclusive breastfeeding through 3 and 6 months of age are 46.2% and 25.5%, respectively. National data about exclusive breastfeeding are not available for children born before 2003.
†Exclusive breastfeeding is defined as ONLY human milk—NO solids, no water, and no other liquids. Adapted from Centers for Disease Control and Prevention, Department of Health and Human Services. 2009 National Immunization Survey. http://www.cdc.gov/breastfeeding/data/NIS_data/index.htm.

Figure 1-1. Breastfeeding Among US Children Born 2000–2009, Centers for Disease Control and Prevention National Immunization Survey

currently, only 53.9% are exclusively breastfeeding at 7 days (Table 1-3, Figure 1-2). Furthermore, the continuation of breastfeeding in the United States is problematic. Whereas the Healthy People goal for 2010 was 25% and the 2020 goal is 34.1% at 12 months, only 25.5% of US mothers report any breastfeeding of their 1-year-old children, and even fewer reach 18 months (Table 1-3). Yet this is better than 2003, when 17.2% breastfed at 12 months and 5.7% breastfed at 18 months. The CDC continually updates its Web site for most recent breastfeeding data (http://www.cdc.gov/breastfeeding/data/NIS_data/index.htm).

Table 1-3. Any and Exclusive Breastfeeding Rates by Age, Among Children Born in 2009 (percent ± half 95% confidence interval)

US National Breastfeeding Rates, 2009		
Child Age	**Breastfeeding (n = 13,757)**	**Exclusive Breastfeeding (n = 13,514)***
At birth	76.9 ± 1.2	
7 days	76.1 ± 1.2	53.9 ± 1.5
14 days	75.3 ± 1.2	51.7 ± 1.5
21 days	73.5 ± 1.3	49.4 ± 1.5
28 days	72.5 ± 1.3	48.4 ± 1.5
42 days	68.4 ± 1.4	43.1 ± 1.5
1 month	72.0 ± 1.3	47.7 ± 1.5
2 months	66.5 ± 1.4	41.8 ± 1.5
3 months	61.3 ± 1.5	36.0 ± 1.5
4 months	54.2 ± 1.5	28.8 ± 1.4
5 months	50.0 ± 1.5	21.0 ± 1.3
6 months	47.2 ± 1.5	16.3 ± 1.2
9 months	33.7 ± 1.4	
12 months	25.5 ± 1.3	
18 months	9.0 ± 0.9	

Interviews with caregivers of children born in 2009 continued through December 2012; provisional rates should be updated with final estimates once data become available in August 2013.
*Exclusive breastfeeding is defined as ONLY human milk—NO solids, no water, and no other liquids. Adapted from Centers for Disease Control and Prevention, Department of Health and Human Services. 2009 National Immunization Survey. Available at: http://www.cdc.gov/breastfeeding/data/NIS_data/index.htm. Sample sizes appearing in the National Immunization Survey (NIS) breastfeeding tables are slightly smaller than the numbers published in other NIS publications because of the fact that in the Division of Nutrition, Physical Activity, and Obesity breastfeeding analyses, the sample was limited to records with valid responses to the breastfeeding questions.

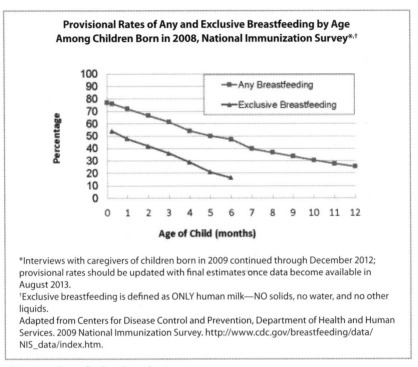

Figure 1-2. Breastfeeding Rates by Age

Disparities in Breastfeeding

Despite the seemingly impressive increase in breastfeeding in the United States, there are still considerable disparities in breastfeeding among racial and ethnic groups, as well as several other important sociodemographic variables. The breastfeeding initiation rate for the Hispanic or Latino population in 2008 was 80.6%, but for the non-Hispanic black or African American population, it was 58.1%. Among low-income mothers (participants in the Special Supplemental Nutrition Program for Women, Infants, and Children [WIC]), the breastfeeding initiation rate was 67.5%, but in those with a higher income ineligible for WIC, it was 84.6%. The breastfeeding initiation rate was merely 37% for low-income non-Hispanic black mothers. Similar disparities are age related, because mothers younger than 20 years initiated breastfeeding at a rate of 59.7% as compared with the rate of 79.3% in mothers older than 30 years. The lowest rates of initiation were seen among non-Hispanic black mothers younger than 20 years, in whom the breastfeeding initiation rate was 30% (Table 1-4).

Table 1-4. Any and Exclusive Breastfeeding Rates by Sociodemographic Factors, Among Children Born in 2007 (percent ± half 95% confidence interval)

Sociodemographic Factors	n	Ever Breastfeeding	Breastfeeding* at 6 Months	Breastfeeding* at 12 Months	n	Exclusive Breastfeeding† Through 3 Months	Exclusive Breastfeeding† Through 6 Months
US national	16,629	75.0 ± 1.2	43.0 ± 1.3	22.4 ± 1.1	16,336	33.0 ± 1.2	13.3 ± 0.9
Sex							
Male	8,538	75.4 ± 1.6	42.6 ± 1.8	22.0 ± 1.5	8,393	33.1 ± 1.7	12.9 ± 1.2
Female	8,091	74.6 ± 1.7	43.5 ± 1.9	22.8 ± 1.7	7,943	32.9 ± 1.8	13.7 ± 1.3
Race/Ethnicity							
American Indian or Alaska Native	552	73.8 ± 6.9	42.4 ± 8.8	20.7 ± 7.0	538	27.6 ± 7.3	13.2 ± 6.3
Asian or Pacific Islander	1,077	83.0 ± 5.2	56.4 ± 6.3	32.8 ± 6.5	1,048	34.1 ± 6.0	14.5 ± 4.3
Asian	886	86.4 ± 5.7	58.6 ± 7.1	34.8 ± 7.5	860	34.5 ± 6.6	16.8 ± 5.2
Native Hawaiian and other	239	72.4 ± 11.1	45.3 ± 12.1	23.9 ± 10.8	234	31.0 ± 11.8	6.5 ± 3.9
Black or African American	2,606	59.7 ± 2.9	27.9 ± 2.5	12.9 ± 1.9	2,569	22.7 ± 2.4	8.2 ± 1.5
White	1,3425	77.7 ± 1.2	45.1 ± 1.5	23.6 ± 1.3	13,194	35.3 ± 1.4	14.4 ± 1.0
Hispanic or Latino	2,895	80.6 ± 2.4	46.0 ± 3.1	24.7 ± 2.8	2,855	33.4 ± 3.0	13.4 ± 2.2
Not Hispanic or Latino (NH)	13,734	72.8 ± 1.3	41.9 ± 1.4	21.5 ± 1.2	13,481	32.9 ± 1.3	13.2 ± 0.9
NH Black or African American	2,309	58.1 ± 3.1	27.5 ± 2.7	12.5 ± 1.9	2,276	21.9 ± 2.5	8.0 ± 1.5
NH White	10,937	76.2 ± 1.4	44.7 ± 1.5	23.3 ± 1.3	10,738	35.8 ± 1.5	14.8 ± 1.0

Table 1-4. Any and Exclusive Breastfeeding Rates by Sociodemographic Factors, Among Children Born in 2007 (percent ± half 95% confidence interval) (continued)

Sociodemographic Factors	n	Ever Breastfeeding	Breastfeeding* at 6 Months	Breastfeeding* at 12 Months	n	Exclusive Breastfeeding[†] Through 3 Months	Exclusive Breastfeeding[†] Through 6 Months
Birth order							
Firstborn	8,834	74.5 ± 1.6	44.1 ± 1.8	23.7 ± 1.6	8,679	33.4 ± 1.7	13.8 ± 1.2
Not firstborn	7,795	75.6 ± 1.6	41.8 ± 1.9	20.8 ± 1.7	7,657	32.6 ± 1.8	12.6 ± 1.2
Receiving WIC							
Yes	6,814	67.5 ± 1.8	33.7 ± 2.0	17.5 ± 1.7	6,725	25.5 ± 1.8	9.2 ± 1.2
No, but eligible	939	77.5 ± 4.7	48.2 ± 5.7	30.7 ± 5.4	916	39.9 ± 5.6	19.2 ± 4.8
Ineligible	8,143	84.6 ± 1.4	54.2 ± 1.9	27.6 ± 1.6	8,007	41.9 ± 1.8	17.7 ± 1.3
Maternal age, yr							
<20	360	59.7 ± 7.9	22.2 ± 7.5	10.7 ± 5.7	356	18.1 ± 6.4	7.9 ± 4.7
20–29	5,449	69.7 ± 2.1	33.4 ± 2.1	16.1 ± 1.7	5,370	28.8 ± 2.1	10.2 ± 1.3
≥30	10,820	79.3 ± 1.4	50.5 ± 1.7	27.1 ± 1.6	10,610	36.6 ± 1.6	15.5 ± 1.2
Maternal education							
Not a high school graduate	1,808	67.0 ± 3.4	37.0 ± 3.8	21.9 ± 3.5	1,784	23.7 ± 3.3	9.2 ± 2.3
High school graduate	3,056	66.1 ± 2.5	31.4 ± 2.5	15.1 ± 2.0	3,017	25.8 ± 2.5	8.9 ± 1.5
Some college	4,290	76.5 ± 2.1	41.0 ± 2.5	20.5 ± 2.2	4,224	34.1 ± 2.5	14.4 ± 2.1
College graduate	7,475	88.3 ± 1.1	59.9 ± 1.8	31.1 ± 1.7	7,311	45.9 ± 1.9	19.6 ± 1.4

Table 1-4. Any and Exclusive Breastfeeding Rates by Sociodemographic Factors, Among Children Born in 2007 (percent ± half 95% confidence interval) (continued)

Sociodemographic Factors	n	Ever Breastfeeding	Breastfeeding* at 6 Months	Breastfeeding* at 12 Months	n	Exclusive Breastfeeding[†] Through 3 Months	Exclusive Breastfeeding[†] Through 6 Months
Maternal marital status							
Married	12,444	81.7 ± 1.3	51.6 ± 1.6	27.5 ± 1.5	12,200	39.0 ± 1.5	16.7 ± 1.2
Unmarried[‡]	4,185	61.3 ± 2.4	25.5 ± 2.3	11.9 ± 1.8	4,136	20.9 ± 2.2	6.4 ± 1.2
Residence							
MSA, central city	7,163	75.5 ± 1.8	43.9 ± 2.1	24.4 ± 2.0	7,051	32.8 ± 2.0	13.3 ± 1.3
MSA, non-central city	6,004	77.9 ± 1.7	45.3 ± 2.1	22.3 ± 1.8	5,880	34.9 ± 2.0	13.9 ± 1.5
Non-MSA	3,462	66.4 ± 2.9	35.0 ± 2.6	17.4 ± 2.0	3,405	28.8 ± 2.4	11.8 ± 1.7
Poverty income ratio,[§] %							
<100%	3,196	67.0 ± 2.7	34.7 ± 3.0	19.0 ± 2.7	3,153	25.0 ± 2.7	8.6 ± 1.7
100%–184%	2,520	71.2 ± 2.8	36.9 ± 3.0	18.9 ± 2.4	2,487	31.7 ± 3.0	12.7 ± 2.1
185%–349%	3,745	77.7 ± 2.4	45.0 ± 2.7	23.9 ± 2.2	3,670	36.0 ± 2.5	14.6 ± 1.7
≥350%	5,755	84.4 ± 1.7	54.0 ± 2.2	26.7 ± 2.0	5,675	41.1 ± 2.1	17.6 ± 1.6

*Breastfeeding with or without the addition of complementary liquids or solids.
[†] Exclusive breastfeeding is defined as ONLY human milk—NO solids, no water, and no other liquids.
[‡] Unmarried includes never married, widowed, separated, or divorced.
[§] Poverty income ratio is the ratio of self-reported family income to the federal poverty threshold value depending on the number of people in the household.
WIC = Special Supplemental Nutrition Program for Women, Infants, and Children; MSA = Metropolitan Statistical Area defined by the Census Bureau.
Adapted from Centers for Disease Control and Prevention, Department of Health and Human Services. 2009 National Immunization Survey (NIS) breastfeeding tables are slightly
http://www.cdc.gov/breastfeeding/data/NIS_data/index.htm. Sample sizes appearing in the National Immunization Survey. Available at:
smaller than the numbers published in other NIS publications because of the fact that in the Division of Nutrition, Physical Activity, and Obesity breastfeeding analyses,
the sample was limited to records with valid responses to the breastfeeding questions.

The US Surgeon General in 2011 issued a *Call to Action to Support Breastfeeding* to address obstacles and strategies to overcome in the United States.

Obstacles identified include:

- Lack of experience or understanding among family members of how best to support mothers and babies
- Not enough opportunities to communicate with other breastfeeding mothers
- Lack of up-to-date instruction and information from health care professionals
- Hospital practices that make it hard to get started with successful breastfeeding
- Lack of accommodation to breastfeed or express milk at the workplace

Opportunities for health care professionals to help include:

- More hospitals can incorporate the recommendations of the United Nations Children's Fund/World Health Organization's (UNICEF/WHO's) Baby-Friendly Hospital Initiative.
- Provide breastfeeding education for health care practitioners who care for women and children.
- Ensure access to lactation specialists, such as those credentialed as International Board Certified Lactation Consultants (IBCLC) or are Fellows of the Academy of Breastfeeding Medicine (FABM).

Moreover, it is important to address the cultural and linguistic diversity of our nation. Traditional practices and beliefs can and do influence the way breastfeeding is practiced and how families respond to promotional and educational efforts, as well as to medical advice about breastfeeding. Health care professionals will be most successful in supporting breastfeeding if they learn and understand the basis of these traditional practices.

Breastfeeding Education

Education is necessary for mothers to meet their breastfeeding goals and may be targeted for a variety of audiences, including health care professionals, parents, and the general public. Several studies have documented the need to improve education and skills necessary to support breastfeeding. Furthermore, generations of low breastfeeding rates have led to a population lacking confidence in support and management of breastfeeding. Recognition of this deficiency has led to the development of new curricula, including breastfeeding education in schools from kindergarten to medical school. In addition, core competencies for health care professionals have been delineated by the US Breastfeeding Committee (USBC; Box 1-5) and endorsed by the AAP.

Box 1-5. US Breastfeeding Committee Core Competencies

At a minimum, every health professional should understand the role of lactation, human milk, and breastfeeding in:
- The optimal feeding of infants and young children
- Enhancing health and reducing:
  - Long-term morbidities in infants and young children
  - Morbidities in women

All health professionals should be able to facilitate the breastfeeding care process by:
- Preparing families for realistic expectations
- Communicating pertinent information to the lactation care team
- Following up with the family, when appropriate, in a culturally competent manner after breastfeeding care and services have been provided

US Breastfeeding Committee proposes to accomplish this by recommending that health professional organizations:
- Understand and act on the importance of protecting, promoting, and supporting breastfeeding as a public health priority
- Educate their practitioners to:
  - Appreciate the limitations of their breastfeeding care expertise
  - Know when and how to make a referral to a lactation care professional
- Regularly examine the care practices of their practitioners and establish core competencies related to breastfeeding care and services

Adapted from United States Breastfeeding Committee. *Core Competencies in Breastfeeding Care and Services for All Health Professionals.* Rev. ed. Washington, DC: US Breastfeeding Committee; 2010.

Specific Audiences

Physicians

Deficiencies in residency preparation for primary care residency programs were identified in the mid-1990s. To address these deficiencies, the AAP in collaboration with American Congress of Obstetricians and Gynecologists (ACOG) and American Academy of Family Physicians (AAFP) developed a multispecialty curriculum for residents and published findings from the pilot implementation of the program Breastfeeding Residency Curriculum. Not only did systematic education and training of residents improve their knowledge, confidence, and practice patterns, but implementation of the curriculum resulted in higher rates of breastfeeding. The most dramatic effect was seen in increased exclusive breastfeeding rates at 6 months. The inclusion of breastfeeding questions on board examinations also has been a standard for more than a decade, and more activities are available for physicians to achieve Maintenance of Certification by completing online activities to enhance the quality of breastfeeding care provided. Physicians are also being educated as a result of increased activity among hospitals and health systems that are seeking designation as a Baby-Friendly facility. One mandatory component of the designation process is that physicians must be educated and trained to acquire the same level of knowledge and clinical skills as their nursing colleagues. As a result, record numbers of physicians associated with these facilities are being educated and trained to provide basic breastfeeding support and management.

Midwives, Advanced Practice Nurses, and Perinatal Nurses

All nurses and midwives have become increasingly effective members of the perinatal health team, practicing either within an obstetric group or hospital, or independently. Many have been educated and trained in lactation and breastfeeding and can provide excellent support for the breastfeeding mother. Some have additional training and are certified lactation specialists. Their specialized skills may be used as part of an obstetric team, and they can provide the additional breastfeeding help many mothers need.

Parents

Because it is no longer assumed that parents and families are prepared with basic knowledge about breastfeeding and there are many myths, it is incumbent on all parts of the health system to provide prenatal and continuing education about the benefits and management of breastfeeding. The education should be culturally sensitive and conducted, when possible, in relation to the understandings and misunderstandings that individuals bring with them. Motivational interviewing is a useful strategy to gather information and guide families through the decision pathways that enable optimal feeding behaviors. Every health care contact, prenatal and postnatal, is an opportunity to educate parents about breastfeeding.

Although there are many considerations for potential influences in a mother's decision to breastfeed, one important person, the father, should not be overlooked. Breastfeeding education programs, particularly in the prenatal period, are most effective when they include the father to provide critical encouragement and emotional support. The knowledgeable father can often provide direct assistance in the breastfeeding process by helping with positioning, evaluating latch and milk transfer, and taking responsibility for baby and household duties, freeing the mother to give more attention to breastfeeding. Although fathers may fear their exclusion from baby care when the mother is breastfeeding, physicians can encourage the father to be an active partner in the nurturing of the baby.

The mother-infant dyad may be best supported by others in the community. Grandmothers, friends, and even strangers may act on behalf of a breastfeeding mother to provide encouragement, self-efficacy, and even answers to simple questions that may not be addressed in the clinical setting. Peer-to-peer support is facilitated by the establishment of community-based support groups. These standing support groups have been shown to enhance breastfeeding exclusivity and duration.

Legislators, Business Leaders, and the Public

Government officials, legislators, judges, and public administrators are uniquely positioned in their role overseeing health and general welfare of the population to support breastfeeding through laws and their enforcement, funding of programs, and education. Over the past few years, many state and local health departments have made funds available for special projects that increase breastfeeding. Two main initiatives funded through the American Recovery and Reinvestment Act and the CDC have involved maternity care practices in hospitals and workplace support programs. In addition, the Affordable Care Act requires workplace accommodations for breastfeeding women. Human resources departments are just now becoming educated about how to comply with this legislation and support their employees' efforts to continue breastfeeding after returning to work. Implementation of such programs decreases employees' absenteeism, enhances employee satisfaction and productivity, as well as saves industry money. Because most US women work, and return is, on average, within 3 months of delivery, support for breastfeeding after return to work is necessary to meet Healthy People 2020 goals for breastfeeding (see Chapter 10). The Maternal and Child Health Bureau, together with the Office on Women's Health, produced the Business Case for Breastfeeding along with a toolkit to help businesses achieve compliance with the Affordable Care Act.

Medical Offices and Staff

Physicians function both as individual providers of breastfeeding care and as managers in the operations of their medical practices or clinics. In their role as manager, they have a unique opportunity to develop an office setting that supports breastfeeding patients, eliminates the marketing of human milk substitutes, and provides employee support for breastfeeding (see Chapter 17). The ability to provide complete support, however, is limited by the constraints of the clinical setting, including time.

Physicians may influence members of a mother's support system, give lectures to educate other physicians and child care providers, add breastfeeding to the curriculum of residents and medical students, help create and adopt policies or regulations supportive of breastfeeding in the hospital or health department, testify on behalf of fair reimbursement for breastfeeding management to third-party payers or employers, advocate for inclusion of breastfeeding in credentialing, and help implement recommendations set forth by The Joint Commission (TJC), the Institute of Medicine, and other national organizations and agencies. In addition, pediatricians can identify their role in implementing the 2011 *Surgeon General's Call to Action to Support Breastfeeding* by mapping their own influences among 20 identified strategies (Table 1-6).

Hospitals

The environment that a mother delivers in is strongly associated with her breastfeeding outcomes, including the rate of supplementation and overall likelihood of any breastfeeding. Hospitals that follow the Ten Steps to Successful Breastfeeding (see Chapter 6, Box 6-3) and uphold the International Code of Marketing of Breastmilk Substitutes may become designated as a Baby-Friendly hospital, and this designation is associated with increased rates of overall and exclusive breastfeeding among healthy newborns, as well as increased breastfeeding and use of human milk in preterm infants. Hospitals should establish policies and practices to support breastfeeding that are based on evidence and should eliminate policies and practices that are known to disrupt or interrupt breastfeeding.

Supportive hospitals involve key administrators, managers, nursing staff, physicians, allied health, and all ancillary support staff that may interact with the mother and her infant during this critical time in establishing breastfeeding (see Chapter 6). Hospitals should convene a multidisciplinary task force, involving leaders, community partners, and families who have experienced deliveries there, to meet on a regular basis and establish a culture of breastfeeding support and ongoing quality improvement, like skin-to-skin contact and no supplementation without medical indication. Hospitals can establish support groups linked to the hospital and to which patients can then be referred.

Managed Care Organizations

Breastfeeding is associated with improved health outcomes and can reduce health care costs of children during the first year of life. Thus, some health insurance companies including managed care organizations have adopted extensive programs to promote and support breastfeeding among their enrollees. Recently, Kaiser Permanente announced the goal that all of their

Table 1-6. Recommended Strategies for Health Care Professionals in response to
The Surgeon General's Call to Action to Support Breastfeeding

Strategies	Settings and Potential Actors	Examples
Improve the breastfeeding content in health professional education (undergraduate and graduate)	Faculty in medical schools and other health professional schools	Implement the AAP Residency Curriculum; integrate breastfeeding and human lactation into basic courses such as anatomy, physiology, nutrition, and health promotion/disease prevention
Establish and incorporate minimum competencies in breastfeeding for health care professionals	Health Care Organizations such as AAP, ACOG, AAFP, as well as credentialing boards such as ABP	AAP endorsement of the USBC Core Competencies; ABP and other credentialing boards add content to certifying examinations, add structures assessments for medical students and residents to ensure skills
Increase opportunities for continuing education and MOC that focuses on breastfeeding	Health professional organizations, academic medical centers, and board certifying entities	AAP NCE educational opportunities, ABM annual meeting and Summit, university-based courses and online learning opportunities, MOC offered by ABP
Define standards for clinical practice that ensures continuity of care, especially for the first 4 weeks of life	Physicians providing maternal and pediatric care, and community support groups working with federal partners and quality improvement entities to adopt standards	Support initiatives such as pay for performance and accountable care that defines optimal and evidence-based breastfeeding care to reduce unnecessary expenditures on health care while supporting continued exclusive breastfeeding
Study the comparative effectiveness of different models of care integrating skilled support for breastfeeding by maternal and pediatric care providers	Physicians, Health and Human Services, and Quality Improvement entities such as AHRQ	Study the cost and effectiveness of learning collaboratives in making breastfeeding support more comprehensive and efficient

AAP = American Academy of Pediatrics; ACOG = American Congress of Obstetricians and Gynecologists; AAFP = American Academy of Family Physicians; USBC = US Breastfeeding Committee; ABM = Academy of Breastfeeding Medicine; MOC, Maintenance of Certification; AHRQ = Agency for Healthcare Research and Quality; NCE = National Conference and Exhibit; ABP = American Board of Pediatrics.

Adapted from Appendix 1 of the US Department of Health and Human Services. *The Surgeon General's Call to Action to Support Breastfeeding*. Washington, DC: US Department of Health and Human Services, Office of the Surgeon General; January 20, 2011.

delivery hospitals should be designated as Baby-Friendly institutions. Physicians who participate with managed care organizations have incentives to enhance their support of breastfeeding and develop strong programs for health and economic reasons (see Chapter 2).

Federal and State Governments

The WIC program in 2010 served 9 million mothers and young children, 1.5 million pregnant and breastfeeding mothers, and 2.17 million infants. The program has significant effects on protection, promotion, and support of breastfeeding offered to women and families in the United States. In October 2009, a major revision in the program allowed for the first time in the history of the program for participants who are exclusively breastfeeding to receive 100% of their nutrient needs as food with an enhanced package recommended by the Institute of Medicine to support the exclusively breastfed infant (compared with the traditional supplement of infant formula—not 100% of the needed nutrition), in effect, enhancing the food allowances given to the mother. In addition to food for the mother, the WIC program, although variable by state, offers breastfeeding support in providing lactation consultations, peer support, warm lines, and equipment such as breast pumps. Compared with the historical operations of WIC where mothers access free infant formula, these new provisions have resulted in substantial increases in the rates of breastfeeding among WIC clients. Nevertheless, there continue to be disparities between mothers who receive WIC benefits and those who do not, and these disparities transcend the predicted racial and economic disparities that also result in lower rates of breastfeeding. In 2010, among the 2.2 million infants who participated in the WIC program, merely 27% were breastfed, with 10% exclusively (fully) breastfed. The Healthy, Hunger-Free Kids Act of 2010 was enacted to prevent states from restricting use of WIC funds despite budgets constraints, effectively preserving the functions of the WIC program through 2015. Thus, breastfeeding support may be enhanced by the continued coordination of WIC personnel, such as lactation specialists and peer counselors, with the health system and hospitals.

The Surgeon General of the United States, US Department of Health and Human Services, Office on Women's Health, Health Resources and Services Administration, Maternal and Child Health Bureau, US Food and Drug Administration, and CDC have all contributed to the education and support of breastfeeding by the publication of multiple reports, documents, and programs, such as the 2011 *Surgeon General's Call to Action to Support Breastfeeding,* the CDC's Vital Signs August 2011, *Hospital Support for*

Breastfeeding: Preventing Obesity Begins in Hospitals, and research related to the longitudinal Infant Feeding Study, the Maternal and Child Health Bureau publication of the *Business Case for Breastfeeding* toolkit for worksite lactation support, Health Resources and Services Administration's education and grants programs that led to education and training about breastfeeding including the *AAP Breastfeeding Residency Curriculum,* and the Office on Women's Health's *Breastfeeding Helpline,* Web pages, and magazines for new moms in multiple languages, *Your Guide to Breastfeeding.* Given the number of free publications aimed at educating health care professionals and consumers produced by the federal government, there is essentially no need to use industry-sponsored materials any longer. Furthermore, ongoing federally sponsored published materials permit enhancements to our existing knowledge about how best to support breastfeeding, manage complications of breastfeeding, and increase breastfeeding among populations least likely to try. In its 2012 publication, *Accelerating Progress in Obesity Prevention: Solving the Weight of the Nation,* the Institute of Medicine identified employers and health care professionals as key change agents for obesity prevention. The recommendation is for health care professionals to encourage healthy weight gain during pregnancy and breastfeeding, and promote breastfeeding-friendly environments, including, but not limited to, adopting policies consistent with the Baby-Friendly Hospital Initiative.

Nongovernmental Organizations

The USBC is an advisory organization to the US government, established in 2000 and composed of representative organizations in the United States. Along with the initial National Agenda and recently with its 5-year Strategic Plan, 2009–2013, the USBC's mission is to improve the nation's health by working collaboratively to protect, promote, and support breastfeeding, and do so by collaboration, leadership, and advocacy. In addition, the *Core Competencies in Breastfeeding Care and Services for All Health Professionals* were developed to delineate the core minimum standards for all health care professionals in their ability to provide breastfeeding-related care (Box 1-5).

The Joint Commissions (TJC) is an independent not-for-profit organization established in 1951 to evaluate and accredit more than 19,000 health care organizations and programs in the United States. In 2003, the Centers for Medicare & Medicaid Services and TJC established a set of Core Measure Sets, one of which is the Perinatal Care Core Measure Set. It includes five measures, including Exclusive Breastmilk Feeding. TJC has defined the numerator and denominator for delivery hospitals to collect data with the concept that tracking these data will permit greater rates of initiation of exclusive human milk feeding. The USBC followed with the publication of a toolkit to educate health care professionals on ways to implement and collect these data (http://www.usbreastfeeding.org/HealthCare/HospitalMaternityCenterPractices/ToolkitImplementingTJCCoreMeasure/tabid/184/Default.aspx). Implementation of processes necessary to collect accurate data on exclusive human milk feeding in all US hospitals will require considerable education and resources, yet provides tremendous opportunity in terms of eliminating unnecessary supplementation. As a companion to the development of TJC Core Measures, the *Speak Up: What You Need to Know About Breastfeeding* campaign and brochure was created to enhance consumer awareness and support for hospital practices that support breastfeeding, including the Ten Steps to Successful Breastfeeding. The brochure is ideal for distribution in prenatal settings to augment education about the benefits and management of breastfeeding.

The World Health Organization and UNICEF have been among the most effective organizations worldwide in supporting breastfeeding through education, direct services, and development of special programs, such as the Baby-Friendly Hospital Initiative of UNICEF.

Professional physician organizations providing and/or advocating breastfeeding support and education include the AAP, ACOG, AAFP, and Academy of Breastfeeding Medicine (ABM), an international physician organization dedicated to professional breastfeeding education and translation of research into practice. The ABM recognizes physicians who distinguish themselves in lactation as Fellows (FABM). In addition, research in the field has been advanced and advocated by the multidisciplinary International Society for Research in Human Milk and Lactation. There are also multiple non–physician-based organizations that coordinate in a multidisciplinary fashion to advocate and educate about breastfeeding. These include the Academy of Nutrition and Dietetics (AND, formerly ADA), American Public Health Association (APHA), and multiple nursing organizations such as the National Association of Pediatric Nurse Practitioners (NAPNAP), Association of Women's Health, Obstetric and Neonatal Nurses (AWHONN), and American College of Nursing (ACN), and National Database of Nursing Quality Indicators (NDNQI) that participate in education and setting standards of care.

Wellstart International has been providing physician education in breastfeeding and lactation worldwide and has developed a physician curriculum that now serves as the basis for the knowledge component of the AAP Breastfeeding Residency Curriculum. Wellstart has created multiple levels of curricula to train health care professionals at all levels of care, from the minimum standard to the consultative level of tertiary breastfeeding care. Breastfeeding experts may be recognized by the IBCLC credential, and are represented by the International Lactation Consultant Association (ILCA), as well as the newer ILCA affiliate, the US Lactation Consultant Association (USLCA). The AAP has a history of collaboration with ILCA, as well as La Leche League International, a peer support organization, to provide education for both health care professionals and consumers about breastfeeding.

Ethics

As with all medical care, ethical issues must be considered in the field of breastfeeding promotion and management. These include informed choice, mothers who choose not to breastfeed, medical care responsibilities, custody rights in parental separation and divorce, workplace rights, breastfeeding in public places, duration of breastfeeding, and formula marketing. For many of these ethical concerns, there are no simple answers, only questions.

Informed Choice

It is incumbent upon the physician and all health care professionals to inform the pregnant woman and new mother of the risks of formula feeding in health outcomes for herself and her child. With this knowledge, the mother can then make a choice appropriate to her own circumstances (see Chapter 2).

Medical Home

The management of breastfeeding is often a shared responsibility with participation by the obstetric and pediatric care providers and lactation specialists. To provide this coordination, it is important for both the mother and the infant to have an identified medical home. The medical home is defined as an approach to providing health care services that are accessible, continuous, comprehensive, family centered, coordinated, compassionate, and culturally effective. Health care professionals and parents act as partners in a medical home to identify and access the medical and nonmedical services needed. Through this structure, communications among all involved are conveyed effectively.

Workplace Rights

The right of the mother who is returning to work to maintain her breastfeeding has been the subject of much recent discussion and legislative efforts. Only a few states have enacted laws that give mothers the right to pump their breasts while on the employment site. Child care policies at work also have been addressed (see Chapter 10).

Breastfeeding in Public Places

The right of the mother to breastfeed in a public location in which she is legally entitled to be has been ensured by legislation in the majority of the states and at US federal sites. These laws either eliminate indecent exposure restrictions from the breastfeeding situation or provide a specific right of the mother to breastfeed in public.

"Extended" Breastfeeding

The question of whether there is an upper limit to the duration of breastfeeding has been asked. Data on the scientific foundation for an age above which it is inappropriate or harmful to the child to continue breastfeeding do not exist. Nor are there reported risks to this method of social/nutritional interactions. Questions may arise as to the ethics of allowing a mother to put her child to the breast for as long as they both wish (see Chapter 8). Although these may be raised, cultural norms exist and should be supported.

Formula Marketing

Marketing practices that have been shown to adversely affect the choice of breastfeeding or continuation of breastfeeding should be recognized by physicians and other health care workers. No subject in the ethical realm of breastfeeding has received as much attention as the issues related to the marketing of human milk substitutes. The International Code of Marketing of Breast-milk Substitutes (http://www.who.int/nutrition/publications/infantfeeding/9241541601/en/) and a subsequent WHO resolution provide detailed guidelines on formula marketing to ensure that it does not diminish breastfeeding initiation or continuation. Although virtually all countries in the world (including the United States) have endorsed the Code of Marketing, many (including the United States) have not enacted legislation to give the force of law to these guidelines. Despite this absence of legal authority, the principles of the Code provide a sound ethical basis for examination of marketing practices by manufacturers and distributors of infant formulas.

Physicians should work toward eliminating policies and practices that discourage breastfeeding in the hospital and office (see Chapters 6 and 15).

Custody Rights

Some of the most difficult and intense controversies occur in the course of marital separation and divorce proceedings when a breastfeeding child is involved. Separate visitation with the father is the issue that leads to confrontation over breastfeeding, particularly when the child is older than 1 year. The health and welfare of the child should be given highest priority, including the maintenance of breastfeeding. Determining whether the breastfeeding is a legitimate need or is being used inappropriately to deny visitation rights is extremely difficult, with experts supporting both sides.

Recommended Practices

Box 1-7 summarizes obstacles identified in the Surgeon General's report. Barriers including lack of knowledge, inconsistent social norms, poor family and social support, embarrassment, lactation problems, employment, and health services may all be offset by improving the knowledge, attitudes, and skills among physicians who are in ideal positions to support breastfeeding (see Table 1-6). Box 1-8 summarizes the recommended practices for breastfeeding identified in the 2012 AAP policy statement, Box 1-9 presents the pediatrician's role in supporting breastfeeding, and Box 1-10 summarizes the obstetrician's role.

Box 1-7. Obstacles to Breastfeeding in the United States

- Insufficient prenatal education
- Disruptive hospital policies and practices
- Inappropriate interruption of breastfeeding
- Early hospital discharge among some populations
- Lack of timely routine follow-up care and postpartum home health visits, including the fragmentation between hospital care and pediatric follow-up care
- Maternal employment
- Lack of family and broad-based societal support
- Media portrayal of bottle-feeding as normative
- Commercial promotion of infant formula
- Misinformation and lack of health care professional concern and involvement

Box 1-8. Recommended Breastfeeding Practices

1. **Exclusive breastfeeding for about 6 months**
   - Breastfeeding preferred; alternatively expressed mother's milk, or donor milk
   - To continue for at least the first year and beyond for as long as mutually desired by mother and child
   - Complementary foods rich in iron and other micronutrients should be introduced at about 6 months of age
2. **Peripartum policies and practices that optimize breastfeeding initiation and maintenance should be compatible with the American Academy of Pediatrics and Academy of Breastfeeding Medicine Model Hospital Policy and include:**
   - Direct skin-to-skin contact with mothers immediately after delivery until the first feeding is accomplished and encouraged throughout the postpartum period
   - Delay in routine procedures (weighing, measuring, bathing, blood tests, vaccines, and eye prophylaxis) until after the first feeding is completed
   - Delay in administration of intramuscular vitamin K until after the first feeding is completed but within 6 hours of birth
   - Ensure 8 to 12 feedings at the breast every 24 hours
   - Ensure formal evaluation and documentation of breastfeeding by trained caregivers (including position, latch, milk transfer, examination) at least for each nursing shift
   - Give no supplements (water, glucose water, commercial infant formula, or other fluids) to breastfeeding newborn infants unless medically indicated using standard evidence-based guidelines for the management of hyperbilirubinemia and hypoglycemia.
   - Avoid routine pacifier use in the postpartum period
   - Begin daily oral vitamin D drops (400 IU) at hospital discharge

3. **All breastfeeding newborn infants should be seen by a pediatrician at 3 to 5 days of age, which is within 48 to 72 h after discharge from the hospital**
   - Evaluate hydration (elimination patterns)
   - Evaluate body weight gain (body weight loss no more than 7% from birth and no further weight loss by day 5: assess feeding and consider more frequent follow-up)
   - Discuss maternal/infant issues
   - Observe feeding

4. **Mother and infant should sleep in proximity to each other to facilitate breastfeeding**
5. **Pacifier should be offered, while placing infant in back-to-sleep position, no earlier than 3 to 4 weeks of age and after breastfeeding has been established**

Adapted from American Academy of Pediatrics policy on breastfeeding and the use of human milk. *Pediatrics*. 2012;129:e827–e841.

Box 1-9. Role of the Pediatrician

1. Promote breastfeeding as the norm for infant feeding.
2. Become knowledgeable in the principles and management of lactation and breastfeeding.
3. Develop skills necessary for assessing the adequacy of breastfeeding.
4. Support training and education for medical students, residents, and postgraduate physicians in breastfeeding and lactation.
5. Promote hospital policies that are compatible with the American Academy of Pediatrics and Academy of Breastfeeding Medicine Model Hospital Policy and the World Health Organization/United Nations Children's Fund (WHO/UNICEF)
6. Ten Steps to Successful Breastfeeding.
7. Collaborate with the obstetric community to develop optimal breastfeeding support programs.
8. Coordinate with community-based health care professionals and certified breastfeeding counselors to ensure uniform and comprehensive breastfeeding support.

Box 1-10. Role of the Obstetrician

Antepartum
1. **Ask early and often about breastfeeding.**
   - Each annual gynecologic examination
   - First prenatal visit
   - Subsequent visits
   - Predelivery pediatrician visit

2. **Examine the breasts.**
   - Inverted nipples
   - Prior surgery
   - Asymmetry
   - Tubular breasts

3. **Offer resources for prenatal education.**

Intrapartum
4. **Delay routine postpartum procedures.**
   - Limit unnecessary interventions.
   - Place baby skin-to-skin.
   - Initiate breastfeeding in first hour.
   - Delay vitamin K and routine eye prophylaxis.
   - Avoid traumatic interventions (suctioning).

5. **Encourage the Ten Steps (see Box 6-3).**

Postpartum
6. **Offer resources.**
   - Lactation specialists

In the Office
7. **Remove formula advertising from the office.**

8. **Know medical management of common issues.**
   - Perceived insufficient supply
   - Engorgement
   - Mastitis/Candidal infection
   - Breast pain

9. **Know what products/medications are safe for breastfeeding women.**
   - Contraception
   - LactMed

10. **Educate yourself.**
    - American Congress of Obstetricians and Gynecologists resources
    - American Academy of Pediatrics resources including learning modules
    - Gold Book
    - Academy of Breastfeeding Medicine journal, *Breastfeeding Medicine*

Selected References

1. American Academy of Pediatrics Section on Breastfeeding. Breastfeeding and the use of human milk. *Pediatrics*. 2012;129:e827–e841

2. Avery AB, Magnus JH. Expectant fathers' and mothers' perceptions of breastfeeding and formula feeding: a focus group study in three US cities. *J Hum Lact*. 2011;27:147–154

3. Bernard JY, De Agostini M, Forhan A, et al. Breastfeeding duration and cognitive development at 2 and 3 years of age in the EDEN mother-child cohort. *J Pediatr*. 2013;163(1):36–42

4. Centers for Disease Control and Prevention. Breastfeeding among US children born 2000–2010, CDC National Immunization Survey. http://www.cdc.gov/breastfeeding/data/NIS_data/index.htm. Accessed August 30, 2013

5. Centers for Disease Control and Prevention. Breastfeeding report card: United States/2013. http://www.cdc.gov/breastfeeding/data/reportcard.htm. Accessed August 30, 2013

6. Centers for Disease Control and Prevention. Racial and ethnic differences in breastfeeding initiation and duration, by state—National Immunization Survey, United States, 2004–2008. *MMWR Morb Mortal Wkly Rep*. 2010;59:327–338

7. Chantry CJ, Howard CR. Clinical protocols for management of breastfeeding. *Pediatr Clin North Am*. 2013;60:75–113

8. Cohen R, Mrtek MB, Mrtek RG. Comparison of maternal absenteeism and infant illness rates among breast-feeding and formula-feeding women in two corporations. *Am J Health Promot*. 1995;10:148–153

9. Department of Health and Human Services. *The Surgeon General's Call to Action to Support Breastfeeding*. Washington, DC: Department of Health and Human Services, Office of the Surgeon General; 2011

10. Feldman-Winter L. Evidence-based interventions to support breastfeeding. *Pediatr Clin North Am*. 2013;60:169–187

11. Feldman-Winter L, Barone L, Milcarek B, et al. Residency curriculum improves breastfeeding care. *Pediatrics*. 2010;126:289–297

12. Freed G, Clark SJ, Sorenson J, Lohr JA, Cefalo R, Curtis P. National assessment of physicians' breast-feeding knowledge, attitudes, training, and experience. *JAMA*. 1995;273:472–476

13. Handa D, Schanler RJ. Role of the pediatrician in breastfeeding management. *Pediatr Clin North Am*. 2013;60:1–10

14. Howard C, Howard F, Lawrence R, Andresen E, DeBlieck E, Weitzman M. Office prenatal formula advertising and its effect on breast-feeding patterns. *Obstet Gynecol*. 2000;95:296–303

15. Institute of Medicine. *Accelerating Progress in Obesity Prevention: Solving the Weight of the Nation*. Washington, DC: Institute of Medicine of the National Academies; 2012

16. Labbok MH. Breastfeeding: population-based perspectives. *Pediatr Clin North Am*. 2013;60:11–30

17. National Conference of State Legislatures. Breastfeeding laws. Washington, DC: National Conference of State Legislatures; 2011

18. US Department of Health and Human Services Office of Disease Prevention and Health Promotion. Healthy People 2010. http://www.healthypeople.gov. Accessed August 30, 2013

19. US Department of Health and Human Services Office of Disease Prevention and Health Promotion. Healthy People 2020. http://www.healthypeople.gov. Accessed August 30, 2013

20. Perez-Escamilla R, Pollitt E, Lonnerdal B, Dewey KG. Infant feeding policies in maternity wards and their effect on breastfeeding success: an analytical overview. *Am J Public Health.* 1994;84:89–97

21. Shealy KR, Li R, Benton-Davis S, Grummer-Strawn LM. Support for breastfeeding in the workplace. In: *The CDC Guide to Breastfeeding Interventions.* Atlanta, GA: Centers for Disease Control and Prevention; 2005:7–12

22. Taveras EM, Capra AM, Braveman PA, Jensvold NG, Escobar GJ, Lieu TA. Clinician support and psychosocial risk factors associated with breastfeeding discontinuation. *Pediatrics.* 2003;112:108–15

23. US Breastfeeding Committee. *Core Competencies in Breastfeeding Care and Services for All Health Professionals.* Rev ed. Washington, DC: US Breastfeeding Committee; 2010

24. US Breastfeeding Committee. *Workplace Accommodations to Support and Protect Breastfeeding.* Washington, DC: US Breastfeeding Committee; 2010

25. US Department of Health and Human Services. *Executive Summary: The Surgeon General's Call to Action to Support Breastfeeding.* Washington, DC: US Department of Health and Human Services, Office of the Surgeon General; 2011

26. Washington Business Group on Health. *Business, Babies and the Bottom Line: Corporate Innovations and Best Practices in Maternal and Child Health.* Washington, DC: Washington Business Group on Health; 1996

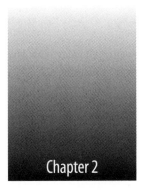

Chapter 2

Rationale for Breastfeeding: Benefits to Infants, Mothers, and Society

A woman's decision to breastfeed has far-reaching benefits, not only for her infant and her own health, but also for the economic and environmental benefits to society. Given the well-documented short-term and long-term medical and neurodevelopmental advantages, breastfeeding should be considered a public health priority and not just a lifestyle choice. This chapter outlines the preventive benefits for acute and chronic illness for both infant and mother, and the economic effects of breastfeeding.

Benefits of Breastfeeding for the Infant

Extensive data confirm that many acute and chronic pediatric disorders, such as otitis media, acute diarrheal disease, lower respiratory illnesses, sudden infant death syndrome (SIDS), inflammatory bowel disease, childhood leukemia, diabetes mellitus, obesity, asthma, and atopic dermatitis, occur less frequently among children who were breastfed as infants (see Box 2-1). To date, the most comprehensive publication that reviews and analyzes published scientific literature comparing breastfeeding and formula feeding regarding health outcomes is the report prepared by the Evidence-Based Practice Centers of the Agency for Healthcare Research and Quality (AHRQ) of the US Department of Health and Human Services entitled

Box 2-1.
Human Milk Feeding Protects Against Many Diseases in Childhood

Acute disorders
- Diarrhea and gastrointestinal infections
- Respiratory infections and hospitalizations
- Otitis media, acute and chronic
- Urinary tract infection
- Septicemia and bacterial meningitis
- Necrotizing enterocolitis
- Sudden infant death syndrome
- Postneonatal infant mortality

Chronic disorders
- Insulin-dependent diabetes mellitus (type 1)
- Non–insulin-dependent diabetes mellitus (type 2)
- Obesity and overweight
- Allergy and asthma
- Inflammatory bowel disease (celiac and Crohn diseases)
- Childhood leukemia (acute lymphocytic leukemia and acute myelogenous leukemia)

Source: American Academy of Pediatrics Section on Breastfeeding. Breastfeeding and the use of human milk. *Pediatrics*. 2012; 129(3):e827–41.

"Breastfeeding and Maternal and Infant Health Outcomes in Developed Countries." A dose-response for breastfeeding and these acute and chronic outcomes can be measured (see Table 2-2).

Acute Illness

Breastfeeding provides a number of physical and biochemical factors that prevent infectious agents to enhance the infant's host defenses (see Chapter 3, Table 3-2). Not only is the illness rate lower in breastfed infants, but the duration and severity of illness are shortened as well. Breastfed infants experience the same infections but generally are asymptomatic or have milder symptoms than formula-fed infants. These effects are observed in both developing and industrialized countries. In addition, breastfeeding limits infants' exposure to environmental pathogens (microorganisms, chemicals) that may be introduced through contaminated formula, foods, fluids, or feeding devices. Breastfed infants also have significantly higher responses to bacille Calmette-Guérin(BCG), Haemophilus influenzae type b, polio, tetanus, and diphtheria toxoid immunizations.

Table 2-2.
Dose-Response for Beneficial Effects of Breastfeeding

Condition	% Lower Risk*	Comment	OR	95% CI
Otitis media	50	EBF ≥ 6 versus 3 mo	0.50	0.36–0.70
Recurrent otitis media	49	EBF ≥ 6 versus 4–6 mo	0.51	0.28–0.94
Upper respiratory tract infection	70	EBF > 6 versus < 6 mo	0.30	0.18–0.74
Lower respiratory tract infection	77	EBF 4–6 versus ≥ 6 mo	0.23	0.07–0.79
Asthma	40	EBF ≥ 3 mo, positive atopic family hx	0.60	0.43–0.82
Asthma	27	EBF ≥ 3 mo, negative atopic family hx	0.73	0.60–0.92
RSV bronchiolitis	74	EBF > 4 mo	0.26	0.07–0.90
Necrotizing enterocolitis	77	Exclusive human milk diet	0.23	0.51–0.94
Atopic dermatitis	27	EBF > 3 mo, negative family hx	0.84	0.59–1.19
Atopic dermatitis	42	EBF > 3 mo, positive family hx	0.58	0.41–0.92
Gastroenteritis	64	Any	0.36	0.32–0.40
Inflammatory bowel disease	31	Any	0.69	0.51–0.94
Obesity	24	Any	0.76	0.67–0.86
Celiac disease	52	>2 mo gluten exposure when BF	0.48	0.40–0.89
Type 1 diabetes	30	EBF > 3 mo	0.71	0.54–0.93
Type 2 diabetes	40	Any	0.61	0.44–0.85
Leukemia (ALL)	20	>6 mo	0.80	0.71–0.91
Leukemia (AML)	15	>6 mo	0.85	0.73–0.98
Sudden infant death syndrome	73	EBF	0.27	0.24–0.31

*% lower risk refers to lower risk while breastfeeding compared with feeding commercial infant formula or referent group specified.

ALL = acute lymphocytic leukemia; AML = acute myelogenous leukemia; CI = confidence interval; EBF = exclusive breastfeeding; hx = history; OR = odds ratio; RSV = respiratory syncytial virus.

Source: American Academy of Pediatrics Section on Breastfeeding. Breastfeeding and the use of human milk. *Pediatrics.* 2012; 129(3):e827–41.

Gastrointestinal Infection

The severity of gastrointestinal infection is attenuated if not prevented in breastfed infants, with specific effects against enteric pathogens such as rotavirus, Giardia, Shigella, Campylobacter, and enterotoxigenic Escherichia coli. Taking into account the role of potential confounders, infants who were breastfeeding had a 64% reduction in the risk for nonspecific gastroenteritis compared with infants who were not breastfeeding.

Respiratory Illnesses

Wheezing and lower respiratory tract disease, among other respiratory illnesses, are reduced in frequency and duration in breastfed infants. The AHRQ reported a 72% reduction in the risk for hospitalization because of lower respiratory tract diseases in infants younger than 1 year who were exclusively breastfed for 4 months or longer. The results remained consistent after adjustment for potential confounders. Before the immunization for these diseases, breastfeeding prevented a major portion of illness from H influenzae type b and Streptococcus pneumoniae.

Otitis Media

Large prospective studies of otitis media have shown a protective effect of breastfeeding. Comparing ever breastfeeding with exclusive formula feeding, AHRQ estimated the risk reduction of acute otitis media to be 23%. Exclusive breastfeeding for 3 to 6 months, compared with exclusive formula feeding, was associated with a 50% reduction in the incidence of otitis media. These associations remain significant after controlling for a number of confounders, including socioeconomic status, sibling factors, and maternal smoking.

Sudden Infant Death Syndrome

Breastfeeding is protective against SIDS, and this effect is stronger when breastfeeding is exclusive. At all ages studied, control infants were breastfed more than SIDS victims, and the protective effect of partial or exclusive breastfeeding is significant even after adjustment for confounding factors, and independent of sleep position. When studies reporting adjusted Odd's Ratios were included in a meta-analysis, the OR for reduction of SIDS with breast-feeding was 0.55 (95% CI: 0.44–0.69). The recommendation to breastfeed infants should be included with other SIDS risk-reduction messages to both reduce the risk of SIDS and promote breastfeeding for its many other infant and maternal health benefits.

Chronic Diseases of Childhood

Diabetes

Nearly a 30% reduction in the incidence of type 1 diabetes mellitus has been reported for infants who exclusively breastfed for at least 3 months, thus avoiding exposure to cow milk protein. The putative mechanism in the development of type 1 diabetes mellitus is postulated to be the infant's exposure to cow milk β-lactoglobulin, which stimulates an immune-mediated process cross-reacting with pancreatic β cells. Breastfeeding offers several potential mechanisms for protection against type 1 diabetes, including protection against infections, effects on maturation of gut-associated lymphoid tissue, and modulation of immune response to insulin. Elevated concentrations of specific IgG antibodies to bovine serum albumin that cross-react with β-cell–specific surface protein have been identified in children with insulin-dependent diabetes mellitus.

In addition, there is a reduction of 39% in the incidence of type 2 diabetes mellitus in breastfed infants, possibly reflecting the long-term positive effects of breastfeeding on weight control and feeding self-regulation.

Obesity

Because rates of obesity are significantly lower in breastfed infants, national campaigns to prevent obesity begin with breastfeeding support. Although complex factors may confound studies of obesity, there is a modest reduction in adolescent and adult obesity rates if any breastfeeding occurred in infancy compared with no breastfeeding. Findings from systematic reviews and meta-analyses suggest a significant reduction even when accounting for the role of potential confounders. One study reported the reduction in the risk for overweight/obesity in breastfeeders compared with nonbreastfeeders was 24% (95% confidence interval [CI] 14%–33%); another study reported 7% (95% CI 1%–12%). A third study using meta-regression found that the duration of breastfeeding is inversely related to the risk for overweight; each month of breastfeeding was associated with a 4% reduction in risk for overweight/obesity.

The protective effect of breastfeeding against overweight and obesity appears to be greater for exclusively breastfed infants, compared with those fed formula or combined breastfeeding and formula fed. Mothers who use combined breastfeeding and formula feeding, or exclusive formula feeding, may be less attuned to feeding and satiety cues in their infants. Other postulated mechanisms for this association relate to how nursing infants self-regulate milk intake volume irrespective of maneuvers that increase available milk volume, and the early programming of self-regulation, in turn, affects adult weight gain. This concept is supported by the observations that infants who are fed by bottle, formula, or expressed breast milk will have increased bottle emptying, poorer self-regulation, and excessive weight gain in later infancy (older than 6 months) compared with infants who only nurse from the breast. In addition, among formula-fed infants, introduction of solid foods before 4 months has been associated with a six-fold increase in the odds of obesity at age 3 years. However, among breastfed infants, the timing of solid food introduction was not associated with an increased risk for obesity. In conclusion, there is an association between breastfeeding and a lower risk for being overweight or obese in adolescence and adult life.

Asthma and Allergy

Exclusive breastfeeding is recommended to reduce the incidence of atopic dermatitis, early-onset wheezing (before 4 years), and cow's milk allergy in the first 2 years. The benefit may be larger (up to 40%) in infants with positive family history of atopic disease. Conflicting data remain regarding protection against allergy afforded by breastfeeding, possibly because in some studies, maternal diet did not exclude the potentially offending antigens, particularly bovine milk proteins. Most recommendations strongly endorse exclusive breastfeeding for at least 4 months and up to 6 months for the primary prevention for allergic disease.

Inflammatory Bowel Disease

Breastfeeding is associated with a 31% reduction in the risk for childhood inflammatory bowel disease. The protective effect may result from the interaction of the immunomodulating effect of human milk and the underlying genetic susceptibility of the infant, or from altered intestinal colonization in formula-fed infants. There is a reduction of 52% in the risk for development of celiac disease in infants who were breastfed at the time of gluten exposure.

Childhood Leukemia

Breastfeeding for at least 6 months' duration was associated with a 19% reduction in the risk for childhood acute lymphocytic leukemia and a 15% reduction in the risk for acute myelogenous leukemia.

Preterm Infants

Necrotizing Enterocolitis

Randomized clinical trials summarized in meta-analyses, support the conclusion that feeding preterm infants human milk is associated with a significant reduction (58%) in the incidence of necrotizing enterocolitis. Preterm infants fed an exclusive human milk diet compared with those fed human milk supplemented with bovine milk-based formula products have a 77% reduction in necrotizing enterocolitis. Human milk feeding protects the preterm infant from nosocomial infection and necrotizing enterocolitis probably as a result of numerous factors in human milk, such as secretory IgA, acetylhydrolase, epidermal growth factor, and cytokines. In addition, the benefits of feeding human milk to preterm infants have been observed not only in the neonatal intensive care unit (NICU) but also in fewer hospital readmissions for illness in the first year after NICU discharge.

Neurobehavior

Maternal-infant bonding is enhanced during breastfeeding. Improved long-term cognitive development in preterm infants has been correlated with being fed human milk, including pasteurized, banked donor human milk during hospitalization. A meta-analysis of studies, where a multitude of confounding factors (including maternal education and intelligence) were considered, concluded that breastfeeding conferred significant benefit to cognitive function well beyond the period of actual breastfeeding. More recently, extremely low-birth-weight preterm infants receiving the greatest proportion of human milk while in the NICU had significantly higher scores for mental, motor, and behavioral ratings at later follow-up at ages 18 and 30 months. Moreover, these data showed significant improvements for babies fed more human milk after adjustment for important confounding factors, such as maternal age, education, marital status, race, and infant morbidities.

Other Benefits

Breastfeeding has been reported to provide analgesia to infants during painful procedures. Lower rates of retinopathy of prematurity (ROP) have been associated with human milk feedings in preterm infants. Visual acuity, particularly in preterm infants, seems to be enhanced by breastfeeding compared with formula feeding. The long-chain polyunsaturated fatty acids (LCPUFAs) have been implicated as factors associated with better visual acuity in breastfed infants. Long-term studies of preterm infants also suggest that human milk feeding may be associated with lower rates of metabolic syndrome, and in adolescents, it is associated with lower blood pressures and low-density lipoprotein concentrations.

Benefits of Breastfeeding for the Mother

Immediate Health Benefits

Postpartum of Hemorrhage

Women who breastfeed have uterine contractions similar to those stimulated by the administration of oxytocin. Breastfeeding mothers have decreased postpartum blood loss and more rapid involution of the uterus. Increased uterine activity from oxytocin release during milk letdown reduces maternal blood loss, supporting the World Health Organization recommendation to decrease postpartum hemorrhage by nipple stimulation and/or breastfeeding in areas where oxytocin-like medications are not readily available.

Bonding and Stress Reduction

Psychological advantages to breastfeeding are obvious because it creates a quiet time for the nursing mother and fosters bonding. Human data show decreased levels of steroid hormones in lactating women. The blunted response of stress hormones is thought to be an adaptive mechanism for negotiating the stressful time of the puerperium. In addition to decreasing the stress response, oxytocin also may foster maternal-infant bonding and play a role in blunting the perception of pain via the dopaminergic pathway.

Postpartum Depression

Postpartum depression is associated with a history of short breastfeeding or not breastfeeding. Prospective cohort studies have noted an increase in postpartum depression in mothers who do not breastfeed or who wean early because of painful nursing. It is not clear whether difficulties with breastfeeding predispose a fragile mother to depression, or whether depressed mothers lack interest in breastfeeding. Some researchers have hypothesized that there may be a shared neuroendocrine mechanism contributing to both failed lactation and perinatal mood disorders.

Weight Loss

Postpartum weight loss may be facilitated in breastfeeding women. However, studies of the overall effect of breastfeeding on the return of mothers to their prepregnancy weight are inconclusive, given the large numbers of confounding factors on weight loss (eg, diet, activity, baseline body mass index, and ethnicity).

Long-term Health Benefits

Amenorrhea and Birth Spacing

Exclusive breastfeeding delays the resumption of normal ovarian cycles and the return of fertility in most mothers. As such, the contraceptive effects of breastfeeding contribute globally to increased child spacing (see Chapter 13). Amenorrhea is most likely to occur in women exclusively breastfeeding, particularly in the first 6 months postpartum. This allows for repletion of maternal iron stores and correction of anemia. Epidemiologic data from around the world indicate that prolonged breastfeeding into the second year, but not exclusively beyond 6 months, prolongs the interpregnancy interval to 1 year, resulting in the birth of the next infant 20 to 24 months after the previous infant. This longer interval may be a factor in reducing infant mortality.

Cardiovascular Disease

An association between cumulative duration of breastfeeding and the incidence of adult cardiovascular disease was reported by the Women's Health Initiative in a longitudinal study of more than 139,000 postmenopausal US women. Women with a cumulative breastfeeding history of 12 to 23 months had a significant reduction in metabolic syndrome (hypertension, hyperlipidemia, cardiovascular disease, and diabetes).

Cancer

Breastfeeding has been associated with a decrease in the risk for both breast and ovarian cancers. Cumulative duration of breastfeeding of longer than 12 months is associated with a 28% reduction in breast cancer (predominantly premenopausal) and ovarian cancer. In global epidemiologic studies, each year of breastfeeding has been calculated to result in a 4.3% reduction in breast cancer. The relative risk for premenopausal breast cancer was significantly reduced in women who, when younger than 20 years, breastfed their infants for at least 6 months. A reduced risk for breast cancer also was observed in women who, when older than 20 years, breastfed from 3 to 6 months compared with women who did not breastfeed. The anovulation associated with lactation also may protect against ovarian cancer, which has been shown to increase with greater frequency of ovulation.

Maternal Type 2 Diabetes

In parous women in the United States without a history of gestational diabetes, each additional year of breastfeeding has been associated with a reduced risk (4%–12%) for development of type 2 diabetes. In women with a history of gestational diabetes, breastfeeding has no significant effect on the already increased risk for diabetes.

Effect on Bone Density

Losses in bone density (approximately 5%) are seen during lactation, with remineralization occurring during weaning. Increased calcium supplementation beyond the normal intake does not prevent bone mineral loss. Calcium needs during this time may be compensated for by decreased urinary excretion. Epidemiologic studies suggest that breastfeeding does not have an effect on long-term changes in bone mineral density and does not increase the risk for postmenopausal osteoporosis. Currently, the association between lifetime breastfeeding duration and the risk for fractures caused by osteoporosis is inconclusive.

Economic Impact of Breastfeeding

The economic advantages of breastfeeding can be calculated at the personal, community, and national levels. The obvious personal advantage is in the savings accrued by not purchasing infant formula, a figure conservatively estimated to range from $750 to $1,200 per year. Studies conducted by managed care organizations indicate that breastfeeding for 3 months significantly reduces the direct costs of medical care (for medicines and doctor visits) compared with no breastfeeding.

From the population perspective of overall costs of illness in 2001, the impact (on three diseases) of increasing the breastfeeding rate to the Healthy People 2010 targets (75% initiating, 50% at 6 months) was estimated to be a savings of $3.6 billion. A more recent detailed pediatric cost analysis based on the 2007 AHRQ report concluded that if 90% of US mothers breastfeed exclusively for 6 months, there would be a cost savings of $13 billion per year. Moreover, these estimated savings did not include those related to a reduction in parental absenteeism from work or adult deaths from diseases acquired in childhood, such as asthma, type 1 diabetes mellitus, or obesity-related conditions.

In addition, the expected savings for infants in the US Special Supplemental Nutrition Program for Women, Infants, and Children who were breastfed exclusively for 6 months were estimated to be more than $950 million annually in 1997 compared with not breastfeeding for 6 months. These savings would come from a combined reduction in household expenditure for formula, as well as reductions in health care expenditures.

The Maternal and Child Health Bureau of the US Department of Health and Human Services, with support from the Office of Women's Health, created "The Business Case for Breastfeeding," a program that provides details of economic benefits to employers and toolkits for the creation of mother-friendly worksites. A mother-friendly worksite provides proven benefits to employers, including a reduction in company health care costs, lower employee absenteeism, reduction in employee turnover, and increased employee morale and productivity. The return on investment has been calculated that for every $1 invested in creating and maintaining a mother-friendly worksite and lactation support program (including a designated pump site, privacy, availability of refrigeration and a hand-washing facility, and appropriate maternal break time), there is a $2 to $3 return on investment.

In summary, breastfeeding results in reduced burden of both acute and chronic infant illnesses, reduced burden of maternal illness, reduced annual health care costs, reduced public health and Women, Infants, and Children costs for formula, reduced employer costs and parental employee absenteeism (with associated loss of family income), reduced environmental burden for disposal of formula cans and bottles, and reduced energy demands for production and transport of artificial feeding products.

Selected References

1. Ball TM, Wright AL. Health care cost of formula-feeding in the first year of life. *Pediatrics.* 1999;103:870–876
2. Bartick M, Reinhold A. The burden of suboptimal breastfeeding in the United States: a pediatric cost analysis. *Pediatrics.* 2010;125:e1048–e1056
3. Centers for Disease Control and Prevention. *National Diabetes Fact Sheet, 2011.* Atlanta, GA: Centers for Disease Control and Prevention; 2011
4. Chua S, Arulkumaran S, Lim I, Selamat N, Ratnam SS. Influence of breastfeeding and nipple stimulation on postpartum uterine activity. *Br J Obstet Gynaecol.* 1994;101:804–805
5. Cumming RG, Klineberg RJ. Breastfeeding and other reproductive factors and the risk of hip fractures in elderly women [published erratum appears in *Int J Epidemiol.* 1993;22:962]. *Int J Epidemiol.* 1993;22:684–691
6. Dewey KG, Lönnerdal B. Infant self-regulation of breast milk intake. *Acta Paediatr Scand.* 1986;75:893–898
7. Dieterich CM, Felice JP, O'Sullivan E, Rasmussen KM. Breastfeeding and health outcomes for the mother-infant dyad. *Pediatr Clin North Am.* 2013;60:31–48
8. Fleischer DM, Spergel JM, Assa'ad AH, Pngracic JA. Primary prevention of allergic disease through nutritional interventions. *J Allergy Clin Immunol.* 2013;1:29–36
9. Harder T, Bergmann R, Kallischnigg G, Plagemann A. Duration of breastfeeding and risk of overweight: a meta-analysis. *Am J Epidemiol.* 2005;162:397–408
10. Hatsu IE, McDougald DM, Anderson AK. Effect of infant feeding on maternal body composition. *Int Breastfeed J.* 2008;3:18

11. Hauck FR, Thompson JMD, Tanabe KO, Moon RY, Vennemann MM. Breastfeeding and reduced risk of sudden infant death syndrome: a meta-analysis. *Pediatrics.* 2011;128:1–8

12. Heinig MJ. Host defense benefits of breastfeeding for the infant. Effect of breastfeeding duration and exclusivity. *Pediatr Clin North Am.* 2001;48:105–123

13. Holmes AV, Auinger P, Howard CR. Combination feeding of breast milk and formula: evidence for shorter breastfeeding duration from the National Health and Nutrition Examination Survey. *J Pediatr.* 2011;159:186–191

14. Huh SY, Rifas-Shiman SL, Taveras EM, Oken E, Gillman MW. Timing of solid food introduction and risk of obesity in preschool-aged children. *Pediatrics.* 2011;127:e544–e551

15. Ip S, Chung M, Raman G, Trikalinos TA, Lau J. A summary of the Agency for Healthcare Research and Quality's evidence report on breastfeeding in developed countries. *Breastfeed Med.* 2009;4(S1):S17–S30

16. Ivarsson A, Hernell O, Stenlund H, Persson LA. Breast-feeding protects against celiac disease. *Am J Clin Nutr.* 2002;75:914–921

17. Kennedy KI, Visness CM. Contraceptive efficacy of lactational amenorrhoea. *Lancet.* 1992;339:227–230

18. Kurian AK, Cardarelli KM. Racial and ethnic differences in cardiovascular disease risk factors: a systematic review. *Ethn Dis.* 2007;17:143–152

19. Labbok MH. Effects of breastfeeding on the mother. *Pediatr Clin North Am.* 2001;48:143–158

20. Melton LJ 3rd, Bryant SC, Wahner HW, et al. Influence of breastfeeding and other reproductive factors on bone mass later in life. *Osteoporos Int.* 1993;3:76–83

21. Montgomery DL, Splett PL. Economic benefit of breast-feeding infants enrolled in WIC. *J Am Diet Assoc.* 1997;97:379–385

22. Owen CG, Martin RM, Whincup PH, Smith GD, Cook DG. Effect of infant feeding on the risk of obesity across the life course: a quantitative review of published evidence. *Pediatrics.* 2005;115:1367–1377

23. Rogan WJ, Gladen BC. Breast-feeding and cognitive development. *Early Hum Dev.* 1993;31:181–193

24. Rosenbauer J, Herzig P, Giani G. Early infant feeding and risk of type 1 diabetes mellitus—a nationwide population-based case-control study in pre-school children. *Diabetes Metab Res Rev.* 2008;24:211–222

25. Rosenblatt KA, Thomas DB. Lactation and the risk of epithelial ovarian cancer. The WHO Collaborative Study of Neoplasia and Steroid Contraceptives. *Int J Epidemiol.* 1993;22:192–197

26. Schanler RJ. The use of human milk for premature infants. *Pediatr Clin North Am.* 2001;48:207–219

27. Schwarz EB, Ray RM, Stuebe AM, et al. Duration of lactation and risk factors for maternal cardiovascular disease. *Obstet Gynecol.* 2009;113:974–982

28. Steube AL, Grewen K, Pedersen CA, Propper C, Meltzer-Brody S. Failed lactation and perinatal depression: common problems with shared neuroendocrine mechanisms? *J Women Health.* 2012;21:1–9

29. Steube AL, Rich-Edwards JF, Willett WC, Manson JE, Michels KB. Duration of lactation and incidence of type 2 diabetes. *JAMA.* 2005;294:2601–2610

30. Stuebe AM, Schwarz EB, Grewen K, et al. Duration of lactation and incidence of maternal hypertension: a longitudinal cohort study. *Am J Epidemiol.* 2011;174:1147–1158

31. Sullivan S, Schanler RJ, Kim JH, et al. An exclusively human milk-based diet is associated with a lower rate of necrotizing enterocolitis than a diet of human milk and bovine milk-based products. *J Pediatr.* 2010;156:562–567, e1

32. Task Force on Sudden Infant Death Syndrome, Moon RY. SIDS and other sleep-related infant deaths: expansion of recommendations for a safe infant sleeping environment. *Pediatrics.* 2011;128(5):1030–1039

33. Task Force on Sudden Infant Death Syndrome, Moon RY. Technical report: SIDS and other sleep-related infant deaths: expansion of recommendations for a safe infant sleeping environment. *Pediatrics.* 2011;128(5):e1341–1367

34. United Kingdom Cancer Study Investigators. Breastfeeding and childhood cancer. *Br J Cancer.* 2001;85:1685–1694

35. Watkins S, Meltzer-Brody S, Zolnoun D, Stuebe A. Early breastfeeding experiences and postpartum depression. *Obstet Gynecol.* 2011;118:214–221

36. Weimer J. *The Economic Benefits of Breast Feeding: A Review and Analysis.* Washington, DC: Food and Rural Economics Division, Economic Research Service, US Department of Agriculture; 2001. Food Assistance and Nutrition Research Report No. 13

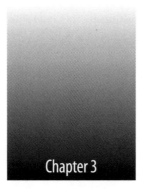

Chapter 3

Composition of Human Milk

There is no other stage in life where a single food serves as the sole source of adequate nutrition as human milk does for us in early infancy. Human milk is a dynamic, complex fluid that contains nutrients and bioactive factors needed for infant health and development. This chapter outlines the unique nutritional and other non-nutritional protective components found in human milk.

Nutritional Components

Human milk has a changing nutrient composition that may vary through lactation, over the course of a day, within a feeding, and from woman to woman. The variable composition of human milk provides nutrients specifically adapted to the changing needs of the infant, and also provides an array of flavors and tastes to stimulate sensory integration. It is important to understand that human milk has unique specificity for human babies. Many components in human milk serve dual roles; a single component may enhance nutrition and host defense, or nutrition and neurodevelopment.

Colostrum is the milk produced in the first few days, a relatively denser milk characterized by high concentrations of protein and antibodies. The transition to mature milk begins around days 3 to 5 postpartum with the onset of lactogenesis II, and mature milk appears by about day 10 postpartum. Table 3-1 lists representative values for the constituents of mature human milk.

Table 3-1.
Representative Values for Constituents of Human Milk

Constituent (per liter)	Mature Milk (after 2 weeks' lactation)
Energy (kcal)	650–700
Macronutrients	
Lactose (g)	67–70
Oligosaccharides (g)	12–14
Total nitrogen (g)	1.9
Nonprotein nitrogen (% total nitrogen)	23
Protein nitrogen (% total nitrogen)	77
Total protein (g)	9
Total lipids (g)	35
Triglyceride (% total lipids)	97–98
Cholesterol (% total lipids)	0.4–0.5
Phospholipids (% total lipids)	0.6–0.8
Water-Soluble Vitamins	
Ascorbic acid (mg)	100
Thiamin (µg)	200
Riboflavin (µg)	400–600
Niacin (mg)	1.8–6.0
Vitamin B_6 (mg)	0.09–0.31
Folate (µg)	80–140
Vitamin B_{12} (µg)	0.5–1.0
Pantothenic acid (mg)	2–2.5
Biotin (µg)	5–9
Fat-Soluble Vitamins	
Retinol (mg)	0.3–0.6
Carotenoids (mg)	0.2–0.6
Vitamin K (µg)	2–3
Vitamin D (µg)	0.33
Vitamin E (mg)	3–8
Calcium (mg)	200–250
Magnesium (mg)	30–35
Phosphorus (mg)	120–140
Sodium (mg)	120–250
Potassium (mg)	400–550
Chloride (mg)	400–450

Trace Elements	
Iron (mg)	0.3–0.9
Zinc (mg)	1–3
Copper (mg)	0.2–0.4
Manganese (µg)	3
Selenium (µg)	7–33
Iodine (µg)	150
Fluoride (µg)	4–15

Adapted from Picciano MF. Representative values for constituents of human milk. *Pediatr Clin North Am.* 2001;48:263–264, with permission from Elsevier.

Nitrogen

Nitrogen is provided by protein (80%) and by nonprotein nitrogen-containing compounds (20%). In the first few weeks postpartum, the total nitrogen content of milk from mothers who have preterm infants (preterm milk) is greater than the milk of women who have term infants (term milk). The content of protein nitrogen declines over 2 to 4 weeks postpartum and then remains relatively constant until weaning. The content of nonprotein nitrogen, such as free amino acids, nucleotides, carnitine, creatinine, and urea, remains relatively constant throughout lactation and accounts for a larger fraction of total nitrogen (20%) than in bovine milk (5%).

Whey and Casein

The protein quality of human milk differs greatly from that in bovine milk. Human milk is 70% whey and 30% casein, whereas bovine or cow milk is 18% whey and 82% casein. The caseins are proteins with low solubility in acid media. Whey proteins are soluble and remain in solution after acidification. Generally, the whey fraction is more easily digested and associated with more rapid gastric emptying.

The plasma amino acid pattern in breastfed infants serves as the model on which enteral and parenteral amino acid solutions are based. The whey protein fraction provides lower concentrations of phenylalanine, tyrosine, and methionine, again specific for human infants.

The protein constituents of human milk serve many diverse functions, ranging from nutrients (amino acids) to protective factors in host defense (immunoglobulins, lysozyme, and lactoferrin) to enzymatically active factors (amylase and bile salt–stimulated lipase) and other biologically active factors (insulin and epidermal growth factor [EGF]). Different proteins comprise the whey fraction of human milk when compared with those of bovine milk. The major human whey protein is α-lactalbumin, notably distinct from the major whey protein in bovine milk, β-lactoglobulin. Human milk lactoferrin, lysozyme, and secretory immunoglobulin A (sIgA) are specific whey proteins, present only in human milk, and are involved in host defense. Because these host defense proteins resist proteolytic digestion, they serve as a first line of defense by lining the gastrointestinal tract.

Carbohydrates

The major carbohydrate in human milk is lactose, a disaccharide that increases in content as lactogenesis progresses from colostrum to mature milk. The lactose content of mature milk remains relatively constant. A small proportion of the lactose is not absorbed. This unabsorbed lactose promotes a softer stool consistency, reduced pathogenic bacterial fecal flora, and improved absorption of minerals. Oligosaccharides are carbohydrate polymers that comprise approximately 5% to 10% of total carbohydrates in human milk. There are more than 100 different oligosaccharides in human milk. In addition to their role in nutrition, oligosaccharides exert an important role in host defense of the infant as "prebiotic" agents, stimulating beneficial intestinal colonization of bacteria and reducing colonization with pathogens.

Lipids

Lipids compromise the major energy-yielding fraction of human milk, approximately 50% of the calories in the milk.

Components of the Lipid System

The lipid system in human milk is composed of an organized milk fat globule, a bile salt-stimulated lipase, and an abundance of essential fatty acids (linoleic [C18:2 ω6] and linolenic [C18:3 ω3] acids). The fatty acids exist in the form of triglycerides.

Fat Absorption

The resulting products of lipase action on the triglyceride molecule in the proximal small intestine are free fatty acids and 2-monoglycerides. Palmitic acid is the predominant fatty acid esterified in the 2-position of the triglyceride molecule. As such, after hydrolysis it remains bound to the 2-position of the glycerol molecule which prevents it from interacting with minerals to form soaps. Thus, this structural relationship enhances net fat and mineral absorption. Fat and mineral absorption from human milk are superior to bovine milk in part because of this interaction.

Fatty Acids

The pattern of fatty acids in human milk is unique in its composition of long-chain polyunsaturated fatty acids. Arachidonic acid (C20:4 ω6) and docosahexaenoic acid (C22:6 ω3), derivatives of the essential fatty acids linoleic and linolenic acids, respectively, are found only in human and not bovine milk. Acids in young infants is important not only for energy for growth, but also for the function of retinal and neural tissues. Arachidonic acid and docosahexaenoic acid are constituents of retinal and brain phospholipid membranes, and have been associated with improved visual function and neurodevelopmental outcome.

Variability of Fat Content

Of all the components of human milk, the total fat content is the most variable. Milk fat content increases slightly throughout lactation, changes over the course of one day, increases during a feed (as foremilk progresses to hindmilk), and varies from mother to mother. During a feeding, the lipid content of milk increases 2- to 3-fold from beginning (foremilk) to end (hindmilk). Milk from overweight and obese mothers has been found to have higher fat content. On standing in a container, the fat in human milk may separate from the other components because it is not homogenized. This nonhomogeneity in human milk has implications for the collection and storage of milk (see Chapter 11).

Too Much Foremilk?

If a mother limits breastfeeding time and doesn't drain one breast before nursing on the second breast, her infant may feed more frequently but will consume a lower calorie milk. Infant weight gain may be adversely affected, the infant's hunger may not be satiated, and because of the higher proportion of lactose (and less fat) in the diet, the stools may be large and frothy. In that scenario, the infant wishes to feed sooner and the frequency of nursing increases. This stimulates more milk production but the infant appears hungry despite good milk volume and transfer. Lengthening the nursing period to ensure adequate draining of the breast often solves the problem. Similarly, incomplete breast draining during mechanical milk expression might not provide sufficient fat from the hindmilk.

Minerals and Trace Elements

Although relatively constant through lactation, the human milk content of calcium and phosphorus is significantly lower than in bovine milk and infant formula. The macrominerals in human milk are more bioavailable (easily absorbable) than those in infant formula because they are bound to digestible proteins, are less bound to fatty acid, and are present in complexed and ionized states, which are more readily absorbed. Despite lower mineral intake, the bone mineral content of breastfed infants is considered the norm on which bone mineralization in formula-fed infants is based.

The concentration of iron is low in human milk, whereas those of zinc are initially several fold higher and sharply decline through lactation. For the first several months of life, infants are primarily dependent on their iron endowment at birth to meet physiologic iron needs. By approximately 6 months, the stores are typically expended, and the demands for iron to support erythropoiesis dictate that other sources will be necessary to avoid deficiency. The physiologic decline in milk zinc concentrations also results in dependence on complementary foods to meet requirements after about 6 months of age.

Vitamins

In general, the vitamin content in human milk is affected by maternal vitamin intake and nutritional status.

Vitamin K

Deficiencies of vitamin K with resulting abnormalities in blood coagulation and hemorrhagic disease can occur in the young infant without supplementation. The content of vitamin K in human milk is low. Therefore, to ensure adequate vitamin K, all infants should receive a single intramuscular dose (0.5–1.0 mg) of vitamin K at birth. However, a single dose of oral vitamin K is inadequate to prevent hemorrhagic disease of the newborn (see Chapter 8).

Vitamin D

There are limited natural dietary sources of vitamin D for infants since its content in human milk is low. Adequate sunshine exposure for the cutaneous synthesis of vitamin D is also not easily determined for a given individual. In addition, oral supplementation of vitamin D to lactating mothers may not provide adequate vitamin D intake for her breastfed infant unless she is given very large doses. As a result, the recommendations to ensure vitamin D sufficiency have been revised to include all infants, including those who are exclusively breastfeeding. All infants should receive daily oral doses (400 IU) of vitamin D starting at hospital discharge or soon after birth (see Chapter 8).

Non-nutritional Components in Human Milk

Bioactive Proteins

Specific factors such as lactoferrin, lysozyme, and sIgA reside in the whey fraction of human milk (see Table 3-2). Lactoferrin is an acute-phase protein that exhibits antimicrobial activity when not conjugated to iron (apolactoferrin). By binding excess iron, it prevents bacterial iron uptake and fosters nonpathogenic bacterial growth. Lactoferrin also functions with other host defense proteins to kill bacteria and viruses. A growth-promoting effect on intestinal epithelium also has been attributed to lactoferrin. Lysozyme has antibacterial effects through cleaving amino acids in bacterial cell walls.

Secretory IgA (sIgA) is the most common immunoglobulin in human milk. SIgA is synthesized by maternal intestinal lymphoid tissue in response to challenge by specific antigens and rapidly transfers into milk. It acts to neutralize foreign antigens. The concentration of sIgA is greatest in colostrum and declines in the first 4 weeks postpartum. The lowest content is observed at 6 months, and thereafter the values increase slightly to levels that remain relatively constant through 2 years of lactation. IgM, IgG, IgD, and IgE also are present in human milk.

Cytokines are multifunctional proteins that are produced by immune cells and affect the function and development of the immune system. Proinflammatory cytokines include the interleukins (ILs). IL-6 and IL-8 are proinflammatory, stimulating B cell activation and recruitment of neutrophils. Anti-inflammatory cytokines include IL-10 and transforming growth factor-β.

Certain free amino acids may exert dual roles in infants. Taurine is trophic for intestinal growth, and glutamine is a fuel for the enterocyte and also affects the gut immune system.

Bioactive Lipids and Carbohydrates

The products of lipid hydrolysis, free fatty acids and monoglycerides, exhibit antimicrobial activity against a variety of pathogens by preventing their attachment and subsequent infection (see Table 3-2). Oligosaccharides and glycoproteins serve as microbial ligands to mimic bacterial epithelial receptors in the respiratory and gastrointestinal tracts and, in doing so, prevent attachment of pathogenic agents to the epithelial lining of mucosal surfaces. The predominant bacterium found in the gastrointestinal tract of breastfed infants is *Lactobacillus bifidus*. A nitrogen-containing carbohydrate factor in human milk (bifidus factor), not found in other mammalian milks, supports the

Table 3-2. Selected Bioactive Factors in Human Milk

Secretory immunoglobulin A (sIgA)	Specific antigen-targeted anti-infective action
Lactoferrin	Immunomodulation, iron chelation, antiadhesive, trophic for intestinal growth
Lysozyme	Bacterial lysis, immunomodulation
κ-Casein	Antiadhesive for bacterial flora, promotes growth
Oligosaccharides	Prebiotic, stimulate beneficial colonization and block attachment of bacterial pathogens
Cytokines	Modulate intestinal epithelial barrier function
Interleukins (IL-6, IL-8)	Proinflammatory
Interferon (IFN)	Proinflammatory
Tumor necrosis factor (TNF)	Stimulates inflammatory immune activation
Growth factors	
Epidermal growth factor (EGF)	Gut luminal surveillance, repair of intestine
Transforming growth factor (TGF)	Promotes epithelial cell growth, suppresses lymphocyte function
Nerve growth factor (NGF)	Growth of neuronal, hepatic, and intestinal cells and tissues
Insulin-like growth factor (IGF)	
Granulocyte colony-stimulation factor (G-CSF)	
Vascular endothelial growth factor (VEGF)	Promotes angiogenesis and tissue repair
Enzymes	
Bile salt-stimulating lipase (BSSL)	Produces free fatty acids, antibacterial activity
Platelet-activating factor-acetylhydrolase	Blocks action of platelet-activating factor
Glutathione peroxidase	Prevents lipid peroxidation, anti-inflammatory
Nucleotides	Enhance T cell maturation, antibody responses, bacterial flora
Vitamins A, E, and C	Antioxidants (scavenge oxygen radicals)
Amino acids	
Glutamine	Intestinal cell fuel, immune response

Table 3-2. Selected Bioactive Factors in Human Milk

Secretory immunoglobulin A (sIgA)	Specific antigen-targeted anti-infective action
Hormones	Anti-infective properties, immunomodulation
Leptin	Regulation of food intake and energy metabolism
Adiponectin	Reduction of proinflammatory cytokines, improves insulin sensitivity, increases fatty acid metabolism
Erythropoietin (EPO)	Stimulates production of red blood cells

Adapted from Hamosh M. Bioactive factors in human milk. *Pediatr Clin North Am.* 2001;48:69–86, with permission from Elsevier.

growth of the nonpathogenic *Lactobacillus,* which results in an inhibition of the growth of pathogenic bacteria.

Cellular Elements

Human milk contains living cells, including macrophages, lymphocytes, neutrophils, and epithelial cells. Colostrum contains the most cells, predominantly neutrophils. As milk matures, the number of cells decreases and the type of cells changes to mononuclear cells such as macrophages (90%) and lymphocytes (10%). The neutrophils in colostrum promote bacterial killing, phagocytosis, and chemotaxis. Some investigators view the neutrophil as a protector of the mammary gland in defense of inflammation with less of a role in the infant. The macrophage in human milk functions in phagocytosis, secretion of lysozyme, bacterial killing, and interactions with lymphocytes to aid in host defense.

Nucleotides

The immediate precursors for RNA and DNA synthesis, dietary nucleotides have been reported to affect immune function, iron absorption, intestinal flora, lipoprotein metabolism, and cellular growth of intestinal and hepatic tissues.

Hormones and Growth Factors

Many hormones (eg, cortisol, somatomedin-C, insulin-like growth factors, insulin, thyroid hormone), growth factors (eg, EGF, nerve growth factor), and gastrointestinal mediators (eg, neurotensin, motilin) that may affect gastrointestinal function or body composition, or both, are present in human milk (see Table 3-2). The EGF, for example, is a polypeptide that stimulates

DNA synthesis, protein synthesis, and cellular proliferation and maturation of intestinal cells. EGF resists proteolytic digestion, and one of its functions is intestinal lumen surveillance, repairing any disruptions in intestinal integrity. Nerve growth factor may play a role in the innervation of the intestinal tract by promoting neuronal growth and maturation.

Leptin and adiponectin are hormones produced in the breast and found in human milk. They may play important roles in the regulation of food intake and energy metabolism, and insulin sensitivity and fatty acid metabolism, respectively. Leptin and adiponectin levels in human milk vary with maternal adiposity, ethnicity, and duration of lactation. The impact of maternal phenotype on these and other bioactive compounds in human milk and their effects on infant growth are areas of intensive research.

Enteromammary and Bronchomammary Immune System

The enteromammary and bronchomammary immune system of the mother produces sIgA antibody when exposed to foreign antigens either via her gastrointestinal or respiratory tracts. The plasma cells traverse the lymphatic system and are secreted at mucosal surfaces, including the mammary gland. Ingestion of human milk, therefore, provides the infant with passive sIgA antibodies against a variety of antigens. This response is quite rapid; within 3 to 4 days after maternal exposure to a foreign antigen, antibodies appear in the milk. The intimate contact of the breastfeeding mother and infant allows for such a system to operate. Skin-to-skin protocols for hospitalized preterm infants facilitate this biological intimacy.

Changes in some of the immunomodulatory constituents of human milk have been measured in response to infection in the nursing infant. During active infection in nursing infants, both macrophages and tumor necrosis factor-α levels were increased in mother's milk, suggesting a dynamic interaction between an infant's health status and the mother's immunologic defenses in her milk.

Selected References

1. Ballard O, Morrow AL. Human milk composition: nutrients and bioactive factors. *Pediatr Clin North Am.* 2012;60:49–74

2. Carver JD, Walker WA. The role of nucleotides in human nutrition. *Nutr Biochem.* 1995;6:58–72

3. Goldman AS, Frawley S. Bioactive components of milk. *J Mammary Gland Biol Neoplasia.* 1996;1:241–242

4. Hamosh M. Bioactive factors in human milk. *Pediatr Clin North Am.* 2001;48:69–86

5. Lawrence R. Host resistance factors and immunologic significance of human milk. In: Lawrence RL, Lawrence R, eds. *Breastfeeding: A Guide for the Medical Profession.* 5th ed. St Louis, MO: Mosby; 1999:159–195

6. Martin LJ, Woo JG, Gerahty SR, et al. Adiponectin is present in human milk and is associated with maternal factors. *Am J Clin Nutr.* 2006;83:1106–1111

7. Miralles O, Sanchez J, Palou A, Pico C. A physiological role of breast milk leptin in body weight control in developing infants. *Obesity.* 2006;14:1371–1377

8. Newburg DS, Woo JG, Morrow AL. Characteristics and potential functions of human milk adiponectin. *J Pediatr.* 2012;156:S41–S46

9. Picciano MF. Representative values for constituents of human milk. *Pediatr Clin North Am.* 2001;48:263–264

10. Riskin A, Almog M, Peri R, Halasz K, Srugo I, Kessel A. Changes in immunomodulatory constituents of human milk in response to active infection in the nursing infant. *Pediatr Res.* 2012;71:220–225

11. Wagner CL, Greer FR. Prevention of rickets and Vitamin D deficiency in infants, children, and adolescents. *Pediatrics.* 2008;122:1142–1152

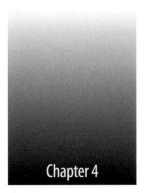

Chapter 4

Anatomy and Physiology of Lactation

The defining characteristic of mammals is the provision of milk, a fluid whose composition exactly mirrors the needs of the young of the species. In the human breast, milk is produced and stored in differentiated alveolar units, often called lobules. These lobules contain small ducts, which coalesce into main ducts that drain sectors of the gland and open directly on the nipple. The amount of milk produced is regulated by prolactin and local factors. Removal of the milk from the breast is accomplished by a process called milk ejection brought about by a neuroendocrine reflex. Afferent stimuli lead to the secretion of oxytocin from the posterior pituitary into the bloodstream, where it is carried to the myoepithelial cells that surround the ducts and alveoli. Contraction of these cells leads to milk ejection.

Anatomy of the Breast

The breast contains a tubuloalveolar parenchyma embedded in a connective and adipose tissue stroma. In the mature breast of the nonpregnant, nonlactating woman, 6 to 10 branching ducts form a treelike pattern that extends from the nipple to the edges of a specialized fat pad on the anterior wall of the thorax. Lobules of varying complexity extend from these ducts. These lobules form the acinar structures that will become the milk-secreting organ. The milk-secreting unit is composed of a single layer of epithelial cells with surrounding supporting structures that include myoepithelial cells, contractile cells responsible for milk ejection, and a connective tissue stroma containing a large number of adipocytes and a copious blood supply.

Stages in Breast Development

The breast, or mammary gland, like most reproductive organs, is not fully developed until sexual maturity. Development of the mammary gland can be divided into five major stages: embryogenesis, pubertal development, development in pregnancy, lactation, and involution.

Embryogenesis

This stage begins in the 18- to 19-week fetus when a bulb-shaped mammary bud can be discerned extending from the epidermis into the dense subepidermal mesenchyme. At the same time, a loose condensation of mesenchyme extends subdermally to form the fat pad precursor. The ducts elongate to form a mammary sprout, invade the fat pad precursor, branch, and canalize to form the rudimentary mammary ductal system that is present at birth in the connective tissue just below the nipple. Limited milk secretion may take place at birth under the influence of changes in maternal hormones. After birth, the gland remains as a set of small branching ducts that grow in parallel with the child. The breast then remains inactive until puberty.

Pubertal Breast Development

Mammogenesis During Puberty

Thelarche, which indicates the beginning of puberty, is the period during which breast development occurs. The initial stages are increase in size and pigmentation of the areola and development of a mass of tissue underneath the areola (breast bud). Thelarche typically begins at a mean age of 9.6 years but may begin as early as 8 years of age, with ethnic and environmental factors accounting for the variation. Normal breast development takes an average of 3 to 3½ years. Thelarche typically occurs approximately 2½ to 3 years before the onset of menstruation (menarche).

At puberty, estrogen and a pituitary factor that is probably growth hormone stimulate the growth of the mammary ducts into the preexisting mammary fat pad. In early puberty, bare ducts course through the fat. With the onset of the menses and ovulatory cycles, the progesterone secreted by the ovary during the luteal phase brings about some lobuloalveolar development. The alveolar clusters are dynamic structures that increase in size and complexity during each luteal phase but tend to regress with the onset of the menses and the loss of hormonal support. However, there is a gradual accretion of epithelial tissue with each successive cycle.

The Mature Mammary Gland

Each of the 6 to 10 lobes of a mature mammary gland has a single opening (galactophore) in the nipple. Each mammary acinus consists of epithelial-lined ductules that form a round alveolus. Myoepithelial cells surround the cuboidal cells of the alveolus and contract under the influence of oxytocin during milk ejection. Multiple alveoli are clustered into lobules, which are then connected via lactiferous ducts to form a distinct mammary lobe. Each lobe is anatomically separate from other lobes. This is important to remember when examining the breast for abnormal nipple discharge. Ultrasound studies have shown that the number of mammary ducts is lower than thought previously, with a mean of nine ducts in each breast, and that they do not dilate into small sinuses, but rather open directly at the galactophore at the nipple (Figure 4-1). The areola contains numerous small sebaceous glands, Montgomery tubercles, which usually are not visible before pregnancy and

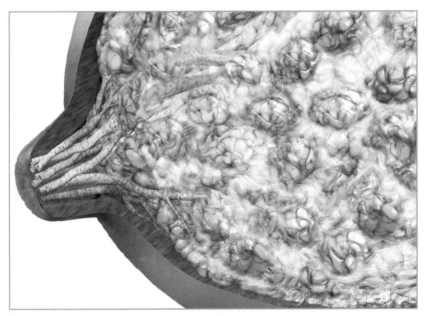

Figure 4-1. The ratio of glandular tissue to fat tissue increases to 2:1 in the lactating breast, compared with a 1:1 ratio in nonlactating women. Much of the glandular tissue is concentrated near the nipple. The milk is transported through the milk ducts to the nipple. The ducts near the nipple do not act as reservoirs for milk. Source: ©2006 Medela AG.

lactation. Their function is to secrete a cleansing and lubricating fluid that is bacteriostatic.

Breast Development in Pregnancy

Lactogenesis I

The breast undergoes marked changes during pregnancy. Physically, the breasts experience a doubling of weight, an increase in blood flow, lobular and alveolar growth, and increased secretory activity. Pregnancy hormones bring about full alveolar development. In addition to increasing levels of progesterone, a lactogenic hormone, either prolactin or human placental lactogen, is thought to be essential for the final stages of mammary growth and differentiation. By midpregnancy, the gland has developed extensive lobular clusters and, indeed, small amounts of secretion product are formed and lactose can be detected in the blood and urine. This maturation process is sometimes referred to as lactogenesis stage 1. Some women will notice a slight leakage of colostrum in the second half of the pregnancy, which is normal. Furthermore, patients will begin to notice superficial veins as their breasts enlarge, as well as enlargement and darkening in pigmentation of the areola; the Montgomery tubercles will begin to protrude from the areola. The gland continues to develop until parturition, with the secretory process being held in check by the high circulating concentrations of progesterone.

Lactogenesis Stage 2

This stage, signaled by the change from small quantities of colostrum to copious amounts of human milk, occurs after delivery, and is due to a dramatic decrease in progesterone, removal of milk from the breast, and maintenance of prolactin levels. A major volume increase around 40 hours postpartum often is referred to as the "coming in" of the milk. For most women, this change in the volume of the breasts is noticeable between the second and fifth postpartum day, with the process occurring later in primiparous women than in multiparous women. Although milk volume is low during the first 2 days postpartum, the amount of colostrum is usually sufficient to meet the needs of the term infant.

Lactation is initiated regardless of whether the newborn breastfeeds, so even nonbreastfeeding mothers experience breast fullness and leaking of milk. The process is marked by an increase in blood flow to the breasts, an increase in milk volume, and a change in composition so that the milk appears somewhat creamy in color and consistency, compared with the thick, yellow colostrum. Some women experience engorgement, or extreme fullness of the breasts, during this stage, especially if the newborn is not feeding frequently. During this stage and after, continued milk production becomes dependent on regular milk removal.

Delayed Lactogenesis Stage 2

Commonly defined as the maternal perception of lactogenesis occurring after 72 hours postpartum, the prevalence of delayed lactogenesis 2 is greater in the United States than in less developed countries. For example, the prevalence of delayed lactogenesis stage 2 was 44% among first-time mothers in California, but was 17% in first-time mothers in Peru. In the California study, significant independent risk factors were maternal body mass index in the overweight or obese range, maternal age older than 30 years, infant birth weight more than 3,600 g, and lack of effective breastfeeding in the first 24 hours. The later lactogenesis stage 2 seen in the United States may be related to a delayed time for first breastfeeding or to differences in maternal diet. Mothers of preterm infants who express milk within the first hour have earlier lactogenesis stage 2. One study in rats fed a high-fat diet found a reduction in the number of intact alveolar units needed for lactogenesis to occur normally. Factors associated with maternal glucose tolerance also are important; 56% of the variation in time to lactogenesis stage 2 has been explained by maternal insulin and adiponectin concentrations. Insulin availability to the mammary alveoli is thought to be a limiting factor in the upregulation of lactose synthesis, which is the key determinant of lactogenesis stage 2, whereas the hormone adiponectin increases sensitivity to insulin. The number of glands on the areola (Montgomery tubercles) also has been associated with the speed to lactogenesis stage 2. A possible mechanism is that more secreting glands on the areola cause the newborn to suck more effectively, leading to more stimulation and earlier onset of lactation. Whatever the cause, a recent study has found that delayed lactogenesis stage 2 is an independent risk factor for the cessation of any and exclusive breastfeeding in the first month. At first postpartum visits, health professionals should ask mothers if their milk "came in" within 3 days, and thereby identify mothers at risk for breast-feeding cessation.

Lactation

The process of milk secretion, lactation, continues as long as milk is removed from the gland on a regular basis. Prolactin is required to maintain milk secretion and oxytocin to produce letdown, to allow the infant to extract milk from the gland.

Involution

The process of involution takes place at weaning (ie, when regular extraction of milk from the gland ceases or in many, but not all species, when prolactin is withdrawn). Like the initiation of lactation, this stage involves an orderly sequence of events to bring the mammary gland back nearly to the prepregnant state.

Physiology of Lactation

Regulation of Milk Synthesis, Secretion, and Ejection

Milk is synthesized continuously and secreted into the alveolar lumen, where it is stored until milk removal from the breast is initiated. This means that two levels of regulation must exist: regulation of the rate of synthesis and secretion and regulation of milk ejection. Although both processes ultimately depend on sucking by the infant or other stimulation of the nipple, the mechanisms involved, central and local, are very different. Prolactin is necessary for milk secretion, and its secretion is directly linked to suckling stimulation at the breast, the intensity of suckling being related to the height of the prolactin peak. However, as described later, the level of plasma prolactin is not directly related to the amount of milk produced, which is a function of poorly understood local factors that depend on milk removal from the breast. Oxytocin participates in a neuroendocrine reflex that results in stimulation of the myoepithelial cells that surround the alveoli and ducts (Figures 4-2 and 4-3). When these cells contract, milk is forced out of the alveoli to the nipple (the letdown reflex). Only then does it become available to the suckling

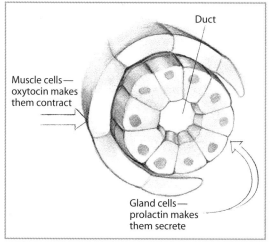

Duct

Muscle cells—
oxytocin makes
them contract

Gland cells—
prolactin makes
them secrete

Figure 4-2. Breastfeeding stimulates the increase of hormones oxytocin and prolactin.

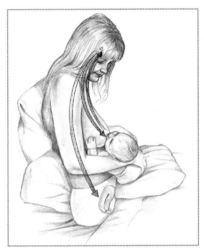

Figure 4-3. An infant's mouth on the mother's nipple signals the brain to release oxytocin, which causes the milk ducts to contract and expel milk, and the uterus to contract.

infant. If the letdown reflex is inhibited, milk cannot be removed from the breast, and local mechanisms bring about an inhibition of milk secretion. With partial removal of milk on a consistent basis, these local factors adjust milk secretion to a new steady-state level. If milk removal ceases altogether, involution sets in and the gland loses its competency to secrete milk.

Milk Production

Infant demand regulates milk production in lactating women. When the milk has a lower caloric density, increased suckling by the infant is thought to result in increased emptying of the breast, in turn bringing about an increase in milk secretion. Mothers of twins, and occasionally even triplets, are able to produce volumes of milk sufficient for complete nutrition of their multiple infants. However, if infants are supplemented with foods other than human milk, milk secretion is proportionately reduced. Therefore, it is important that the baby suckle at the breast 8 to 12 times per day or when the baby displays cues for feeding.

Prolactin Secretion

Secretion of prolactin occurs episodically with peaks of up to 75 minutes in duration that occur 7 to 20 times a day. During pregnancy, serum prolactin levels increase steadily from about 10 ng/mL in the prepregnant state to about 200 ng/mL at term. After parturition, the basal prolactin levels decrease, returning to prepregnancy values at 2 to 3 weeks in the woman who is not breastfeeding. In the lactating woman, suckling usually leads to a rapid increase in prolactin secretion. If the activity of the nerves to the nipple is inhibited, the prolactin increase is abolished.

Although prolactin levels are consistently above basal values for the duration of lactation, they are not proportional to milk volume secretion. Thus, although prolactin is necessary for milk secretion in women, plasma prolactin concentrations do not directly regulate milk synthesis and secretion.

Local Regulation of Milk Production

Two local mechanisms have been implicated in the regulation of milk volume production. An inhibitor of milk secretion, the protein called Feedback Inhibitor of Lactation builds up as milk accumulates in the lumen of the mammary gland. Thus, the actual volume of milk secreted may be reduced if the breast is not drained adequately. Distention or stretch of the alveoli also may regulate milk synthesis and secretion.

Oxytocin Stimulation of Milk Ejection

Milk removal from the breast is accomplished by the contraction of myoepithelial cells, whose processes form a basket-like network around the alveoli where milk is stored, in concert with sucking by the infant. When the infant is suckled, afferent impulses from sensory stimulation of nerve terminals in the areolae travel to the central nervous system, where they promote the release of oxytocin from the posterior pituitary. Oxytocin release often is associated with such stimuli as the sight or sound, or even the thought, of the infant, indicating a significant psychological component in this neuroendocrine reflex. Oxytocin is transported systemically to the mammary gland, where it interacts with specific receptors on myoepithelial cells, initiating their contraction and expelling milk from the alveoli into the ducts. The process by which milk is forcibly moved out of the alveoli is called milk ejection reflex or letdown and is essential to milk removal from the lactating breast. Clinically, there is a great deal of individual variation in women's perception of letdown. In the first few days after delivery, uterine contractions, or "after pains," associated with suckling indicate oxytocin release, which probably aids in uterine involution. Some women experience leaking of milk, some feel sensations in the breast, and some have none of these physical sensations in the presence of letdown. If present, the sensations are confirmatory; if absent, no specific conclusions can be drawn without further investigation into the feeding process.

Effect of Suckling

During correct suckling, the nipple and much of the areola are drawn well into the mouth. Milk removal from the breast occurs because of a combination of positive pressure occurring from the mother's milk ejection reflex and negative pressure (vacuum) created by the infant's tongue. This negative pressure results from a downward motion of the infant's tongue during the first half of the suck cycle. Tongue compression during the second half of the suck cycle is thought to clear the milk from the oral cavity (Figure 4-4).

Effect of Emotional State and Drugs

Psychological stress, pain, or fatigue can decrease milk output because of inhibition of oxytocin release. Oxytocin release begins with the onset of suckling in relaxed, undisturbed mothers, but may occur before suckling if the infant cries or becomes restless. Alcohol and opioids inhibit oxytocin release.

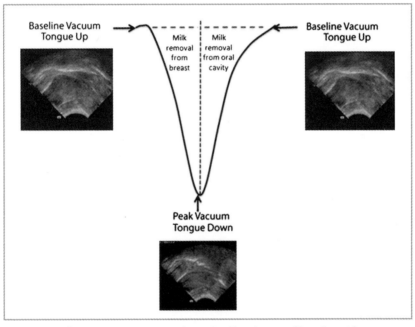

Figure 4-4. Infant's tongue position as determined by ultrasound imaging with respect to the suck cycle. At baseline, the mid-tongue is in contact with the palate and baseline vacuum is applied. When the tongue is drawn down during the first half of the suck cycle, vacuum increases and milk flows into the intraoral cavity. During the second half of the suck cycle, the vacuum decreases when the tongue moves upward and milk is cleared from the oral cavity. Reprinted from Geddes DT, Sakalidis VS, Hepworth AR, et al. Tongue movement and intraoral vacuum of term infants during breastfeeding and feeding from an experimental teat that released milk under vacuum only. *Early Hum Dev.* 2012;88:443–449. Copyright 2011, with permission from Elsevier.

Selected References

1. Arthur PG, Kent JC, Potter JM, Hartmann PE. Lactose in blood in nonpregnant, pregnant, and lactating women. *J Pediatr Gastroenterol Nutr.* 1991;13:254–259

2. Brownell E, Howard CR, Lawrence RA, Dozier AM. Delayed onset lactogenesis II predicts the cessation of any or exclusive breastfeeding. *J Pediatr.* 2012;161:608–614

3. Chiodera P, Salvarani C, Bacchi-Modena A, et al. Relationship between plasma profiles of oxytocin and adrenocorticotropic hormone during suckling or breast stimulation in women. *Horm Res.* 1991;35:119–123

4. Crowley WR, Armstrong WE. Neurochemical regulation of oxytocin secretion in lactation. *Endocr Rev.* 1992;13:33–65

5. Doucet S, Soussignan R, Sagot P, Schaal B. An overlooked aspect of the human breast: areolar glands in relation with breastfeeding pattern, neonatal weight gain, and the dynamics of lactation. *Early Hum Dev.* 2012;88:119–128

6. Geddes DT, Kent JC, Mitoulas LR, Hartman PE. Tongue movement and intra-oral vacuum in breastfeeding infants. *Early Hum Dev.* 2008;84:471–477

7. Geddes DT, Sakalidis VS, Hepworth AR, et al. Tongue movement and intra-oral vacuum of term infants during breastfeeding and feeding from an experimental teat that released milk under vacuum only. *Early Hum Dev.* 2012;88:443–449

8. Giraldi A, Enevoldsen AS, Wagner G. Oxytocin and the initiation of parturition. A review. *Dan Med Bull.* 1990;37:377–383

9. Hernandez LL, Grayson BE, Yadav E, Seeley RJ, Horseman ND. High fat diet alters lactation outcomes: possible involvement of inflammatory and serotonergic pathways. *PLoS One.* 2012;7:e32598

10. Kleinberg DL. Early mammary development: growth hormone and IGF-1. *J Mammary Gland Biol Neoplasia.* 1997;2:49–57

11. Neville MC. Anatomy and physiology of lactation. *Pediatr Clin North Am.* 2001;48:13–34

12. Neville MC. Volume and caloric density of human milk. In: Jensen RG, ed. *Handbook of Milk Composition.* San Diego, CA: Academic Press; 1995:101–113

13. Neville MC, Morton J, Umemura S. Lactogenesis. The transition from pregnancy to lactation. *Pediatr Clin North Am.* 2001;48:35–52

14. Peaker M, Wilde CJ. Feedback control of milk secretion from milk. *J Mammary Gland Biol Neoplasia.* 1996;1:307–315

15. Ramsay DT, Kent JC, Hartmann RL, Hartmann PE. Anatomy of the lactating human breast redefined with ultrasound imaging. *J Anat.* 2005;206:525–534

16. Ueda T, Yokoyama Y, Irahara M, Aono T. Influence of psychological stress on suckling-induced pulsatile oxytocin release. *Obstet Gynecol.* 1994;84:259–262

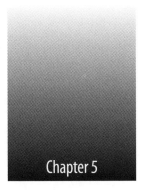

Chapter 5

Breastfeeding: Management Before and After Conception

The annual office encounter and other preconception visits for teens and women of childbearing age offer practitioners opportunities to discuss the benefits of breastfeeding and the importance of a strong support system. With recurring visits to a breastfeeding-friendly medical office, the notion of breastfeeding can become normalized, and many natural occasions for patients to ask questions and seek resources may arise, maximizing the chances for successful breastfeeding. To further optimize breastfeeding, the practitioner can also assess the patient's personal and family history, perform a breast examination to identify any problems, or suggest lifestyle or medication changes. Furthermore, cancer detection is easier before pregnancy or lactation, so this opportunity should not be missed.

Initial Visit

Once a patient presents for prenatal care, the initial and subsequent prenatal visits are excellent opportunities for the obstetric care professional to introduce and encourage breastfeeding. Most women make their feeding choice early; in fact, one study reported that 78% of women made their feeding decision before the pregnancy or during the first trimester. Early intervention by the obstetric care professional positively affects initiation and continuation of breastfeeding. The initial input from the obstetric care professional may give the mother confidence to pursue her goal of breastfeeding. Ideally, the patient and practitioner will discuss breastfeeding and decide on a plan well before the patient presents in labor. If the advantages and benefits of breastfeeding are reinforced at multiple visits, patients may be more likely to succeed. Where specific circumstances of the pregnancy or the mother's health raise concerns regarding successful breastfeeding, referral to a lactation specialist can often avert difficulties or allay fears. For example, if a prenatal diagnosis of cleft palate is suspected, plans can begin for pump acquisition, the learning of optimal techniques for the pumping mother, and the referral of a prosthesis that may create a seal for the suckling infant. Likewise, a mother with gestational diabetes can learn how to express small amounts of colostrum soon after delivery anticipating the possibility of neonatal hypoglycemia.

History

Whether a woman presents for a preconception or prenatal visit, a database should be compiled that would form the basis for her future care and aid in detecting any concerns that may arise with respect to future breastfeeding. In addition to an obstetric history, a complete medical history, including tabulation of chronic conditions, medications, diet and dietary supplements, smoking, alcohol use, and substance use/abuse, should be included. These data can be revisited at the first obstetric visit. Box 5-1 lists factors that can be identified before delivery, or even pregnancy, that potentially may affect the success of lactation.

Medical History

Medical Conditions
Any medical condition that may affect breastfeeding should be discussed, including a history of human immunodeficiency virus infection or herpetic breast lesions.

Medications
Certain medications that are known to be problematic during lactation can be identified and alternative medications may be suggested (see Chapter 12). The use of complementary and alternative medicine can be assessed.

Prior Breast Surgery
All forms of prior breast surgery, breast disease, or trauma should be explored, especially that which involved the areolar area, because periareolar incisions

Box 5-1.
Risk Factors for Lactation Problems That Can Be Identified Before Delivery

History/Social Factors
- Early intention to breastfeed and bottle-feed
- History of previous breastfeeding problems or breastfed infant with slow weight gain
- History of hormone-related infertility; intended use of hormonal contraceptives
- Significant medical problems (eg, untreated hypothyroidism, diabetes, cystic fibrosis)
- Maternal age (eg, adolescent mother)
- Psychosocial problems, especially depression

Anatomic/Physiologic Factors
- Flat or inverted nipples
- Variation in breast appearance (marked asymmetry, hypoplastic, tubular)
- Previous breast surgery that severed milk ducts or nipple afferent nerves
- Previous breast surgery to correct abnormal appearance or developmental variants
- Previous breast abscess

See Box 7-1 for additional factors identified after delivery. Source: Neifert MR. Prevention of breastfeeding tragedies. *Pediatr Clin North Am.* 2001;48:273–297.

are most likely to interrupt the ducts and innervation. Breast reduction surgery may be more disruptive to adequate milk supply than other breast surgeries (see Chapter 16).

Nutritional Assessment

Adequate dietary intake should be assessed. When indicated, motivational interviewing can be used to improve dietary habits. Even before conception, patients should begin taking a prenatal multivitamin (including folic acid, iron, and vitamin D). To reduce maternal anxiety, practitioners should reinforce that usual diets do not affect milk composition.

Social History

Substance use/abuse and other potentially harmful habits should be discussed. Discontinuation before conception is recommended, and appropriate support services should be provided. In addition, appropriate support for breastfeeding can be assessed.

Prior Breastfeeding History

The documentation of prior breastfeeding history allows for an excellent opportunity to broach the topic of future breastfeeding and can help the patient address barriers to breastfeeding she may have experienced, as well as concerns the patient and her family and friends have expressed regarding breastfeeding.

Physical Examination

A breast examination should be performed at an annual or preconception visit. If a recent breast examination is not documented, at the first prenatal visit, one should be performed gently, yet thoroughly, because breasts are generally more tender in early pregnancy. The examination offers an ideal opportunity to reassure the patient that she is physically capable of providing nutrition to her infant. It may be appropriate to describe the stage of breast development in the medical record (Figure 5-1).

Ideal Timing

When a patient is not pregnant, the ideal time for a breast examination is in the early follicular phase, after completion of the menses and before the mid-cycle increases in edema, mastalgia, and cutaneous tactile sensitivity.

Structural Evaluation of the Breast

Structural evaluation should include identification of scars or lesions, as well as the maturational stage and symmetry of the breasts. Inverted nipples and tubular or hypoplastic breasts can also be identified.

Breast Symmetry

Patients with hypoplastic or inadequately developed breasts should be evaluated further for prior hormonal deficiencies in the developmental process. Many patients will present with slight breast asymmetry, which is normal. Significant asymmetry between breasts warrants further consideration, especially if the asymmetry is a recent occurrence.

Inverted Nipples

Nipple size and shape generally do not affect the ability to breastfeed (Figure 5-2). Patients may complain of inverted (turned in) nipples (Figure 5-3) and question the effect on future breastfeeding. A woman who has flat (Figure 5-4) or inverted nipples is able to breastfeed if her nipples can become erect. The use of breast shells for inverted nipples, however, has not been shown to be effective in the limited research done to date. Similarly, stretching or rolling the nipples during pregnancy has not been found to be beneficial. Indeed, nipple rolling may result in oxytocin release, which might induce uterine contractions.

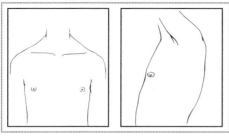

Figure 5-1A. Breast stage 1. There is no development. Only the papilla is elevated.

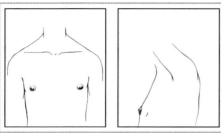

Figure 5-1B. Breast stage 2. The "breast bud" stage. The areola widens, darkens slightly, and elevates from the rest of the breast as a small mound. A bud of breast tissue is palpable below the nipple.

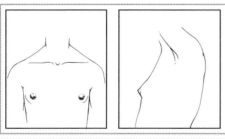

Figure 5-1C. Breast stage 3. The breast and areola further enlarge and present a rounded contour. There is no separation of contour between the nipple and areola. Note that lack of separation of contour between the areola and the rest of the breast also is a feature of stage 5. These stages may be distinguished from one another by the greater diameter of breast tissue in stage 5. At stage 3, the breast tissue creates a small cone as opposed to the wider cone in stage 5.

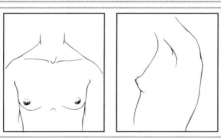

Figure 5-1D. Breast stage 4. The breast continues to expand. The papilla and areola project to form a secondary mound above the rest of the breast tissue. Approximate median age is 12 years.

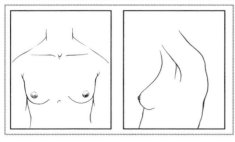

Figure 5-1E. Breast stage 5. The mature adult stage. The secondary mound made by the nipple and areola present in stage 4 disappears. Only the papilla projects. Even in a small-breasted individual, the diameter of the breast tissue (as opposed to the height) has extended to cover most of the area between the sternum and lateral chest wall.

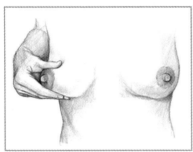

Figure 5-2. A normally protruding, or everted nipple, becomes erect when you press the areola between two fingers.

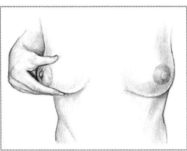

Figure 5-3. Inverted nipples retract toward the breast when pressure is applied to the areola.

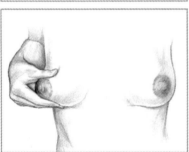

Figure 5-4. Flat nipples neither retract nor protrude.

Breast Size

Patients with small breasts should be reassured that their breastfeeding potential is not affected by breast size.

Suspicious Lumps

Any suspicious lumps should be managed appropriately, with surgical consultation as appropriate (see Chapter 9).

Education

The history and physical examination of a patient allow ample opportunity to initiate discussion and encouragement for breastfeeding. Anatomic considerations, practical concerns, and fears can be addressed. It is important to provide complete information on human milk, breastfeeding, and other infant feeding in relation to the health of women and their infants, and to offer resources and support for breastfeeding. Attending a breastfeeding education class will increase breastfeeding success. The clinician's recommendations and reassurance to the patient are essential and should not be underestimated. The timing of implementing various breastfeeding-related interventions is summarized in Table 5-2.

Educating the Individual

Patient Education Resources

The importance of early and continuing discussion about the decision to breastfeed cannot be overemphasized. Individual and group discussions between health care professionals and mothers-to-be have been shown to be effective. Contact information from pediatric health care professionals, nurses, and lactation specialists, as well as breastfeeding support groups, can augment the education efforts of the woman's health care professional. Finally, Internet-based resources allow the patient to explore the many benefits of breastfeeding (see the Appendix).

Planning and Expectations

Proper planning during antepartum care can help ensure successful breastfeeding. More than 60% of all new mothers will be returning to school or work, and these women often do not breastfeed. Patients should be assured that successful breastfeeding is possible even if the mother will be apart from the child at times. Early discussions of practical issues and plans, including breast pumps and milk storage, can help mothers continue breastfeeding when separated from their infants (see Chapter 10). It is helpful to suggest that the patient discuss breastfeeding and pumping locations and timing with her school administrator or employer before delivery.

Family and Friends

The previous experiences that family and friends have had with breastfeeding may be helpful in predicting the type of support the mother will receive. Negative experiences and attitudes can be discussed to allay the patient's fears and suggest solutions to any problems encountered. The partner and other significant family members should be included in breastfeeding discussions, if feasible and culturally appropriate. The partner can be the mother's most important support person (see Chapter 1).

Visit to Pediatric Care Professional

A third trimester visit to a pediatric care professional should be encouraged in order to discuss plans for infant nutrition and address any concerns about the

...ide for Prenatal Breastfeeding Support During Obstetric Visits

Obstetric Visit	Discussion	Examination
Initial visit	• Breastfeeding plans: reinforce and/or explore reasoning, education, correction of myths. • Note prior breast surgical history. • Note breast growth during pregnancy. • Note prior breastfeeding experience. • Review impact of medical conditions and applicable drugs on pregnancy and lactation.	• Palpate for masses or adenopathy. • Evaluate for inverted nipples and prior surgical scars.
14–20 weeks	• Discuss breast growth (if not previously noted). • Discuss feeding plans.	
24–28 weeks	• Recommend birthing classes. • Reinforce breastfeeding decision.	• Repeat breast examination with patient-voiced breast complaints at ANY subsequent visit.
32 weeks	• Readdress prior breast surgeries if applicable.	• Consider routine examination around this time.
34–36 weeks	• Discuss potential obstacles placed by hospital practices and strategies to overcome (eg, separation of mother and infant). • Encourage breastfeeding during first hour after delivery, rooming-in, avoiding supplementation unless medical indication, avoiding bottle nipples, pacifiers, etc. • Discuss return to work, breast pumps, child care choices, etc. • Review pertinent medical conditions and medications, and potential changes after delivery and during breastfeeding. • Reexplore prior breastfeeding experiences if relevant. • Discuss pediatric care professional visit.	
36+ weeks	• Review patient knowledge and pertinent questions. • Discuss pediatric care professional visit. • Discuss plans for additional childbearing/family planning.	

pregnancy. The patient should select a pediatric care professional who meets her needs, especially one who is a knowledgeable supporter of breastfeeding (Box 5-3).

Educating the Public

Mass Media

There is an opportunity for mass media to impact many potential current and future mothers and their supporting families. More focus should be provided by the media in portraying breastfeeding as the standard or normative form of infant nutrition. It is important that accurate information, in content and in portrayal, be provided. Subtle marketing strategies may undermine breastfeeding; health care professionals should recognize the risk these

Box 5-3. Prenatal Visit

Gathering Information/Anticipatory Guidance

- Discuss the family's thoughts and feelings about breastfeeding.
- Acknowledge the family's concerns.
- Provide accurate information on the topics that concern the family.
- State your support for exclusive breastfeeding.
- Review the benefits of exclusive breastfeeding.
- Review important aspects of breastfeeding management.
- As per The Joint Commission Speak Up initiatives, the mother should be informed about the World Health Organization/United Nations Children's Fund Ten Steps to Successful Breastfeeding and that she can request that her birth center provide her this opportunity.
- Explain importance of skin-to-skin and of first breastfeed within the first 30 minutes to 1 hour of life.
- Obtain information about previous breastfeeding experiences.
- Review medical history about breast-related conditions, including surgery or injury.
- Discuss importance of prenatal breast examination to assess breast changes in pregnancy. Pediatrician may perform the examination or refer to mother's physician.
- Discuss the importance of exclusive human milk feedings until about 6 months of age.
- Discuss available breastfeeding classes in the community.
- Have appropriate videos and books for parents to purchase or borrow.
- Ask about maternal medications.

Closing the Visit

- "Do you have any other questions about breastfeeding?"
- Encourage parents to call with other questions.
- Reinforce the importance of optimal maternity care practices and empower families to request care consistent with the Ten Steps to Successful Breastfeeding.
- Use positive, encouraging statements about breastfeeding.
- Discuss options of who can give professional breastfeeding support.

Adapted from Checklists for Breastfeeding Health Supervision. Elk Grove Village, IL: American Academy of Pediatrics; 2013.

strategies represent, help their patients understand these risks, and work to minimize their influence. Public art projects and nurse-ins have contributed to conversations about a baby's right to eat in public.

Legislative Initiatives

Many legislative initiative have improved the climate for mothers who wish to breastfeed in public spaces or need to express human milk at work. Legislation exists in much of the United States to protect various concerns related to breastfeeding. State laws fall into three categories: (1) protecting the right to breastfeed, (2) breastfeeding in the workplace, and (3) exempting breastfeeding mothers from jury duty. Most states have laws that protect a mother breastfeeding in public. The 2010 Affordable Healthcare Act mandates support by employers for breastfeeding employees. The Business Case for Breastfeeding helps employers create breastfeeding support programs. In some states, companies that provide specific features that promote and support breastfeeding for their employees are designated as breastfeeding-friendly worksites (see Chapter 10). Businesses meeting certain criteria can then advertise this benefit to their employees. Currently, legislation is under way to require minimum standards for breast pumps and potential tax-free status for breastfeeding devices.

Selected References

1. American Academy of Pediatrics. *New Mother's Guide to Breastfeeding.* Meek JY, ed. 2nd ed. New York, NY: Bantam Books; 2011
2. American Academy of Pediatrics Committee on Psychosocial Aspects of Child and Family Health. The prenatal visit. *Pediatrics.* 2001;107:1456–1458
3. American Academy of Pediatrics Section on Breastfeeding. *Ten Steps to Support Parents' Choice to Breastfeed Their Baby* [brochure]. Elk Grove Village, IL: American Academy of Pediatrics; 2003
4. American Academy of Pediatrics Work Group on Breastfeeding. *Checklists for Breastfeeding Health Supervision.* Elk Grove Village, IL: American Academy of Pediatrics; 2013
5. American College of Obstetricians and Gynecologists. *Breastfeeding Your Baby* [pamphlet]. Washington, DC: American College of Obstetricians and Gynecologists; 2011
6. American College of Obstetricians and Gynecologists. *Planning Your Pregnancy and Birth.* 3rd ed. Washington, DC: American College of Obstetricians and Gynecologists; 2000
7. Fritz, MA, Speroff L. *Clinical Gynecologic Endocrinology and Infertility.* 8th ed. Baltimore, MD: Lippincott Williams & Wilkins; 2010
8. Lawrence RA, Lawrence RM. *Breastfeeding: A Guide for the Medical Profession.* 6th ed. Philadelphia, PA: Elsevier Mosby; 2005
9. Snyder R, Zahn C. Breast disease during pregnancy and lactation. In: Gilstrap LC 3rd, Cunningham FG, VanDorsten JP, editors. *Operative Obstetrics.* 2nd ed. New York, NY: McGraw-Hill; 2002
10. Wolfberg AJ, Michels KB, Shields W, O'Campo P, Bronner Y, Bienstock J. Dads as breastfeeding advocates: results from a randomized controlled trial of an educational intervention. *Am J Obstet Gynecol.* 2004;191:708–712

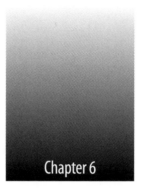

Chapter 6

Peripartum Care:
The Transition to Lactation

The labor and delivery period represents a vulnerable time for the success of breastfeeding. Many women who state before delivery that they wish to exclusively breastfeed are discharged from the hospital either not exclusively breastfeeding or not breastfeeding at all. The obstetric and perinatal care professional should have the knowledge and resources to support a woman who chooses to breastfeed. Immediate management issues are discussed in this chapter, whereas issues dealing with the entire hospital stay are described in Chapter 7.

Labor and Delivery Care

Hospital policies and practices, including those in the obstetric suite, can make a critical difference in the successful establishment of breastfeeding (Table 6-1).

Early Initiation of Breastfeeding

Within the first hour after birth, early initiation of breastfeeding should be practiced unless the medical condition of the mother or infant indicates otherwise. Infants who are placed on their mother's abdomen after birth and who attach to the breast within 1 hour of birth have better breastfeeding outcomes than infants who do not self-attach early. Indeed, early nursing in the delivery room is associated with a marked increase in the percentage of mothers who continue breastfeeding at 2 to 4 months postpartum compared with later

Table 6-1. Hospital Practices That Influence Breastfeeding

Strongly Encouraging	Encouraging	Discouraging	Strongly Discouraging
Physical Contact			
• Baby put to breast immediately in delivery room • Baby not taken from mother after delivery • Mother helped by staff to suckle baby in recovery room • Rooming-in; staff help with baby care in room, not only in nursery	• Staff sensitivity to cultural norms and expectations of mother	• Scheduled feedings regardless of mother's breastfeeding wishes	• Mother-infant separation at birth • Mother-infant housed on separate floors in postpartum period • Mother separated from newborn because of bilirubin problem • No rooming-in policy
Verbal Communication			
• Staff initiates discussion of mother's intention to breastfeed prepartum and intrapartum • Staff encourages and reinforces breastfeeding immediately on labor and delivery • Staff discusses use of breast pump and realities of separation from infant	• Appropriate language skills of staff, teaching how to handle breast engorgement and nipple problem • Staff's own skills and comfort regarding art of breastfeeding and time to teach mother on one-to-one basis	• Staff instructs woman to "get a good night's rest and miss the feed" • Strict times allotted for breastfeeding regardless of mother/baby's feeding "cycle"	• Mother told to "take it easy," "get your rest," giving impression that breastfeeding is effortful/tiring • Mother told she doesn't "do it right," staff interrupts her efforts, corrects her regarding positions, etc.

Strongly Encouraging	Encouraging	Discouraging	Strongly Discouraging
Nonverbal Communication			
• Staff (physicians as well as nurses) give reinforcement for breastfeeding (respect, smiles, affirmation) • Nurse (or any attendant) making mother feel comfortable and helping to arrange baby at breast for nursing • Mother sees others breastfeeding in hospital	• Pictures of mothers breastfeeding • Literature on breastfeeding in understandable terms • Closed circuit TV show in hospital on breastfeeding	• Pictures of mothers bottle-feeding • Staff interrupts breastfeeding session for laboratory tests, etc. • Mother does not see others breastfeeding	• Mother given infant formula kit and infant food literature • Mother sees official-looking nurses authoritatively caring for newborns by bottle-feeding (leads to mother's own insecurities regarding own capability of care)
Experiential			
• If breastfeeding is not immediately successful, staff continues to be supportive • Previous success with breastfeeding experience in hospital			• Previous failure with breastfeeding experience in hospital

Source: US Department of Health and Human Services. Report of the Surgeon General's Workshop on Breastfeeding & Human Lactation. Rockville, MD: US Department of Health and Human Services, Public Health Service, Health Resources and Services Administration; 1984. DHHS publication HRS-D-MC 84-2.

initiation. Successful lactation management includes encouraging nursing in the delivery room and avoiding maternal-infant separation in the first hours.

Initial Breastfeeding

Although the mother may have read about proper positioning and latch-on, the real-life situation is different. Many newborns placed on the mother's chest or abdomen during their usually alert and active first hour after delivery will spontaneously find the nipple/areola and latch on to it, but others may require assistance. Although infant identification bands may be essential immediately after delivery, eye prophylaxis, vitamin K, weighing, and other routine procedures may be postponed until opportunity for the first breastfeed has been successful. Ideally, the initial feed should not be interrupted, and as long as medically safe, the mother and infant should remain together. Skin-to-skin contact in the delivery room will maintain the newborn's body temperature in a normal range.

Breastfeeding Technique

General

Breastfeeding is natural, but it is also a learned skill. Teaching the mother the basics of correct breastfeeding technique reduces the chance of physical discomfort during feedings, improves infant attachment to the breast, and enhances milk transfer to the infant. Bedside teaching should be reinforced with written materials or videos, or both, that may be reviewed in the hospital or at home.

Care must be used to prevent mother and babies from bed-sharing directly after feeding. Avoid use of soft surfaces. Ideally, the newborn should be placed on a proximate but separate sleep surface, on their back, after feeding.

Positioning

A nursing mother can use many different positions, but regardless of position, she should be comfortable. Pillows and footstools may provide assistance. The baby should be positioned so that the head, shoulders, and hips are in alignment and the infant faces the mother's body. The football (or clutch) and side-lying positions may be more comfortable after cesarean delivery. No matter which position is used, it is important to avoid pushing on the back of the infant's head because doing so may cause the infant to arch away from the breast.

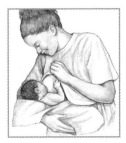

Figure 6-1. The cradle hold.

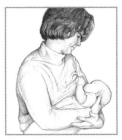

Figure 6-2. The cross-cradle hold.

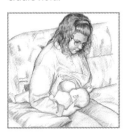

Figure 6-3. The clutch or football hold is an easy position to maintain and is particularly helpful after a cesarean delivery because it keeps the infant's weight off the incision.

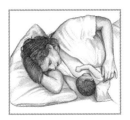

Figure 6-4. Side-lying position.

Cradle Hold

With the cradle hold, the mother's same-sided arm supports the infant at the breast on which the infant is nursing (Figure 6-1). The infant's head is cradled near the mother's elbow while the arm supports the infant along the back, facing the mother, chest-to-chest. Care must be taken in this position to prevent too lateral a position of the infant with regard to the breast. Lining the infant's nose up with the nipple allows for direct attachment and prevents neck flexion to reach the nipple.

Cross-Cradle or Transitional Hold

This hold uses the opposite arm to support the infant with the back of the head (below the occiput) and neck held in the mother's hand (Figure 6-2). This leaves the hand closest to the breast to support and position the breast as needed. This position is ideal for the early breastfeeding infant because it provides excellent support and the ability to present the breast in a molded fashion with the free hand. It is also easier to assess a wide gap of the mouth and appropriate lip flange.

Football (or Clutch) Hold

The infant is positioned at the mother's side (Figure 6-3). The infant's feet and body are tucked under her arm, and the infant's head is held in her hand facing the breast. It can be difficult in this position to determine whether the infant's mouth is open wide enough and whether lower lip is flanged.

Side-Lying Position

In the side-lying position, the mother lies on her side facing the infant, who is also lying on his or her side (Figure 6-4). The infant faces the mother with the mouth at the level of the nipple. Special care should be taken that the infant is not surrounded by loose clothing or bedding, and careful precautions should be made if the mother is drowsy to prevent entrapment or suffocation.

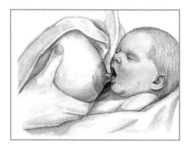

Figure 6-5A. The C-hold.

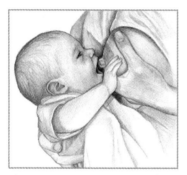

Figure 6-5B. Ensure the infant's mouth is wide open.

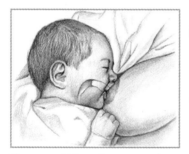

Figure 6-5C. This infant is properly latched on, with lips covering the areola and the nipple well inside the mouth.

Latch-on

To ensure proper latch-on, the infant should be held so that the mouth is opposite the mother's nipple and the neck is slightly extended, with the head, shoulders, and hips in alignment. While the infant is learning to breastfeed, proper latch-on is facilitated if the breast is supported with 4 fingers underneath and the thumb on top (C-hold; Figure 6-5), or U-hold with fingers wrapped under breast and thumb on outside, at 3 o'clock and 9 o'clock positions, respectively. Another way to present the nipple and areola is the scissors or V-hold, but only if the mother's fingers can open wide enough to keep the areola exposed to ensure adequate latch-on. An effective latch is crucial to breastfeeding success because it prevents sore nipples, ensures sufficient milk transfer, and adequately stimulates the breast to ensure plentiful continued milk production.

Rooting Reflex

The mother may elicit the rooting reflex by stroking the newborn's lip with her nipple. The mother should wait patiently until the infant opens his or her mouth wide, and then quickly draw the baby to her breast, aiming the nipple toward the hard palate to facilitate the lower jaw taking in an adequate amount of the breast.

Areola Grasp

The infant should grasp the entire nipple and as much of the areola as comfortably possible (about 1–2 inches from the base of the nipple) and draw it into the mouth, perhaps as far as the circumareolar line. If the infant is well positioned, the nose and chin will touch the breast, and the lips will be flanged outward around the breast tissue. The infant's tongue should be cupped beneath the nipple/areola complex and may be visible if the infant's lower lip is pulled down slightly. The partner, spouse, or other family members can be helpful in looking for these signs of good positioning and latch-on. When the infant is latched correctly, the mother will feel a gentle undulating motion but no pain with each suck.

Sucking and Swallowing and Milk Transfer

Once the infant is latched to the breast, suckling begins with rapid bursts and intermittent pauses. In the immediate newborn period, sucking occurs but swallowing may not be audible. After about 24 hours, sucking will elicit the milk letdown response and soft audible swallows may be heard. Initially, this may take a few minutes. As milk flow is established, the rhythm of suckling, swallowing, and pauses becomes slower and more rhythmic, approximately one suckle/swallow per second. Audible swallowing indicates milk transfer to the infant. Ultrasound imaging of the submental region of the infant during feeding suggests that milk flow from the nipple into the mouth coincides with the lowering of the infant's tongue and the peak vacuum pressure developed by the infant. This suggests that a vacuum effect is likely to serve a major role in milk removal from the breast.

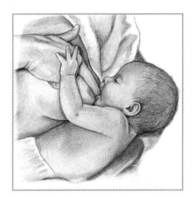

Figure 6-6. Releasing the latch.

Releasing the Latch

At the end of nursing, the infant will often come off the breast spontaneously. If that does not occur, the mother can release the suction by retracting the infant's cheek to break the seal or inserting her finger gently into the corner of the infant's mouth (Figure 6-6). This will minimize trauma to the nipple. The nipple should be observed; it should be elongated but otherwise have no creases or signs of trauma.

Signs of Incorrect Latch

Many signs may indicate incorrect latch, including indentation of the infant's cheeks during suckling, clicking noises, lips curled inward, frequent movement of the infant's head, lack of swallowing, and maternal complaint of pain. Swallowing may be difficult to hear when the newborn is taking small sips of colostrum, but as milk volume increases, swallowing should be heard easily. Later signs of incorrect latch-on include trauma to the nipples, pain, poor infant weight gain, and low milk supply.

Problem Solving

Pain Management During and After Labor and Delivery

To support the mother's desire to breastfeed, pain management should be balanced to ensure pain relief for the mother while avoiding excessive amounts of medication, particularly narcotics, that can have adverse effects on the infant's ability to nurse effectively.

Intrapartum Narcotics

The narcotic choice and dosing interval should be managed with the goal of minimizing adverse effects on the infant's ability to nurse effectively (Table 6-2). Many products for pain control are available; however, meperidine is the most problematic and therefore is not routinely used in obstetrical anesthesia. Meperidine is metabolized by mother and infant via N-demethylation to form normeperidine, an active metabolite. Normeperidine is lipophilic, has a long half-life in the newborn and may accumulate with regular breastfeeding. If possible, meperidine should be avoided intrapartum and postpartum in breastfeeding mothers. Morphine also is metabolized by mother and infant via N-demethylation but forms inactive morphine-3-glucuronide and active morphine-6-glucuronide in a 9:1 ratio. Therefore, it has primarily inactive metabolites. Morphine is hydrophilic, so there is less transfer into human milk. Nalbuphine is a synthetic narcotic with agonist-antagonist properties. It is excreted in the milk in clinically insignificant amounts and has a short half-life. Butorphanol has similar properties to nalbuphine.

Epidural Anesthesia

Although the effect of epidural or intrathecal narcotics on sucking behavior, lactation success, or both has not been adequately studied, there is ample evidence that regional administration of narcotics results in lower maternal levels than with parenteral administration and does not inhibit the breastfeeding process. Epidural anesthesia provides excellent and safe pain relief during labor.

Trained Labor Support Personnel

Labor support personnel, or a companion, other than family, such as a doula or other trained health professional providing one-to-one support, is an effective method to support some women's desire to decrease the need for labor analgesia. Although not necessarily formally trained breastfeeding experts, doulas have been shown to enhance the success of breastfeeding by providing experience, consistent advice, encouragement, and reassurance.

Table 6-2. Postpartum Pain Management

Drug	Onset IV	Onset IM	Neonatal Half-life
Meperidine	5 min	30–45 min	13–22 h (63 h for active metabolites)
Morphine	5 min	30–40 min	7 h
Nalbuphine	2–3 min	15 min	4 h
Butorphanol	1–2 min	10–30 min	Unknown (similar to nalbuphine in adults)

IM = intramuscular; IV = intravenous.

Postpartum Pain Relief

Pain relief in the postpartum period is usually well managed by non-narcotic medications such as nonsteroidal anti-inflammatory drugs or acetaminophen. When stronger medication is needed, oral narcotics are safely used and have minimal transfer to the breastfeeding infant. When possible, aspirin-containing products should be avoided.

- Acetaminophen is excreted into human milk in extremely low concentrations and is not highly protein bound. It is considered compatible with breastfeeding.
- Nonsteroidal anti-inflammatory drugs generally have short half-lives and primarily inert metabolites. They are excreted into human milk in low or undetectable amounts and are considered compatible with breastfeeding.
- Oral narcotics (fentanyl, codeine, propoxyphene, methadone, morphine) are excreted in milk, but at low concentrations with short half-lives. They are compatible with breastfeeding.
- Meperidine given orally or as intramuscular injection may accumulate with regular use and should be avoided in breastfeeding mothers.
- Aspirin is metabolized into salicylate. Although transport into milk is limited, neonates eliminate salicylate very slowly. Therefore, caution must be exercised with more than occasional use.

Postsurgical Pain Relief

The same medications mentioned previously may also be used to manage postsurgical pain. Severe pain may be managed by intrathecal narcotic, continuous epidural, use of a patient-controlled analgesia pump, or parenteral narcotics. Pain relief that requires parenteral administration of medication is best achieved with narcotics other than meperidine.

Cesarean Delivery

The incidence rate of breastfeeding may be 10% to 20% lower after cesarean compared with vaginal delivery. After cesarean deliveries, clinicians concerned about maternal rest and recovery also may be less likely to help the mother put the infant to the breast immediately or to encourage frequent feeding in the first 24 hours. While important, rest and recovery should not preclude breastfeeding. Women undergoing planned cesarean delivery are more likely to breastfeed than those for whom the cesarean was not anticipated. Sometimes the unanticipated cesarean follows a long and difficult labor. In addition, some mothers view unplanned cesarean delivery as a distressing turn of events, a loss of control, or even a failure, factors that contribute to stress that may inhibit milk letdown.

With active interventions to support breastfeeding in these high-risk situations, the initiation and duration of breastfeeding can be preserved. With assistance, the infant can be placed at the breast while avoiding the incision area. A side-by-side lying down position may be helpful initially. Later, an upright position in a supportive chair with other positioning adaptations allows breastfeeding in the sitting or semi-reclining position. After cesarean delivery, the mother usually needs more help from the nursing staff and family members in lifting and positioning the infant. Compared with general anesthesia, regional anesthesia for cesarean delivery is preferable for maternal health and also has been associated with improved breastfeeding rates.

Exhaustion

Long and difficult labor and the exhaustion that comes with it may affect breastfeeding outcome and make it more difficult for the new mother to initiate breastfeeding and learn proper technique. Adequate support by educated personnel after delivery will help to overcome these obstacles to establishing successful breastfeeding. In addition, when the new mother leaves the hospital, the many tasks facing her may be overwhelming. The new mother will be able to focus her energies on bonding with and breastfeeding her infant, as well as resting and recuperating from delivery, if she requests visitors and family members to help by changing diapers, cooking, and assisting with other children and household tasks. Postpartum depression is not uncommon, and new parents should be informed regarding the need for rest and how to identify more severe symptoms that would warrant contacting their physician. Screening tools are available to assist the caregiver in determining the need for intervention in mothers who may be at risk for depression. Validated tools include the Edinburgh Postpartum Depression Scale screening (see Chapter 9).

Hospitals Can Affect Breastfeeding Success

In 1984, the Report of the Surgeon General's Workshop on Breastfeeding and Human Lactation commented on hospital practices that influence breastfeeding. This was the first national effort to promote breastfeeding as normative and vitally necessary from a public health perspective. In 2012, the Surgeon General reiterated the national interest and importance of breastfeeding (see Chapter 1), calling to action many community partners to remove barriers to successful lactation.

Although a majority of women intend to breastfeed before delivery, many begin artificial milk feedings or are offered supplementation before discharge without medical indication. The Academy of Breastfeeding Medicine has a detailed peer-reviewed protocol on indications for supplementation. Before any supplementary feedings are begun, it is important that a formal evaluation of each mother-baby dyad, including a direct observation of breastfeeding, is completed. Special consideration is given to those infants who are late preterm deliveries as these infants likely will require supplementation.

Hospitals or birth centers can facilitate breastfeeding success by implementing criteria set forth in the Ten Steps to Successful Breastfeeding. Hospitals have used a variety of strategies to encourage breastfeeding (Box 6-3). Some traditional hospital practices such as taking the newborn away from the mother for routine procedures, supplementation of the breastfeeding infant without a medical indication, requiring pediatric clearance prior to the first feeding, and limiting maternal access to the infant can work against the physiology of lactation. Policies drive hospital systems. A written breastfeeding policy (Step 1) is an important tool for establishing routines that endorse breastfeeding. The following elements should be included in written hospital breastfeeding policy.

Staff Training

At all levels, staff training (Step 2) is critical to the successful support and promotion of breastfeeding. Without adequate staff education, families receive conflicting advice. Evidence-based lactation policies implemented by trained staff that offer accurate, consistent advice can make the difference between success and failure for breastfeeding women. Updating the breastfeeding knowledge of perinatal staff is essential, given that most indicate their professional preparation did not result in adequate breastfeeding education. All staff should receive formal training in current breastfeeding management.

Steps to Successful Breastfeeding

Step 1—	Have a written breastfeeding policy that is routinely communicated to all health care staff.
Step 2—	Train all health care staff in skills necessary to implement this policy.
Step 3—	Inform all pregnant women about the benefits and management of breastfeeding.
Step 4—	Help mothers initiate breastfeeding within 1 hour of birth.
Step 5—	Show mothers how to breastfeed and how to maintain lactation even if they should be separated from their infants.
Step 6—	Give breastfeeding newborns no food or drink other than human milk, unless medically indicated.
Step 7—	Practice rooming-in—allow mothers and infants to remain together 24 hours a day.
Step 8—	Encourage breastfeeding on demand.
Step 9—	Give no artificial teats or pacifiers to breastfeeding infants.
Step 10—	Foster the establishment of breastfeeding support groups and refer mothers to them on discharge from the hospital or clinic.

The 1994 report of the Healthy Mothers, Healthy Babies National Coalition Expert Work Group recommends that the UNICEF-WHO Baby-Friendly Hospital Initiative be adapted for use in the United States as the US Breastfeeding Health Initiative, using these adapted 10 steps.
Source: Randolph L, Cooper L, Fonseca-Becker F, York M, McIntosh M. Baby-Friendly Hospital Initiative feasibility study: Final report. Alexandria, VA: Healthy Mothers, Healthy Babies National Coalition Expert Work Group; 1994.

As described before, the latch-on is one of the most important factors in breastfeeding. The latch describes the way the infant takes the breast and transfers milk from the breast into the mouth. In some situations, it may be helpful to use objective tools such as a LATCH score to communicate effectively among hospital caregivers.

Infant Practices

Several strategies with regard to newborn feeding can enhance breastfeeding success, particularly when they are part of standard hospital practice.

Breastfeeding on Demand

Infant cues should be used as signs of hunger (hand-to-mouth activity, smacking lips, rooting, eye movement in light sleep, movement of extremities) to determine when an infant should be fed, rather than adherence to a rigid feeding schedule (Step 8). Putting infants to breast frequently, and whenever they demonstrate these cues, stimulates milk production and allows the full milk supply to develop as soon as possible, usually in 2 to 5 days. Breastfeeding should continue at each breast without a time limit until the infant falls asleep or unlatches. Complete draining of the breast is essential for establishing a full milk supply.

Rooming-in

The practice of rooming-in, where mother and infant are in close proximity so that the mother can recognize and respond to the feeding cues, allows a better chance for successful initiation and establishment of breastfeeding (Step 7).

Supplementation

No Supplements

There is no need for supplements (water, glucose water, formula) for breastfeeding newborns unless a medical indication exists. Giving such supplements is likely to interfere with the process of successful initiation of breastfeeding by the mother and newborn (Step 6).

Patient Incentives

The practice of routine distribution of discharge formula packs to new mothers is discouraged. Merely providing samples of formula and commercial literature has been shown to decrease successful breastfeeding outcomes (Step 6). Parents should not be marketed to prenatally or in the postpartum period by offers of free formula, gifts, and discounts. Families routinely receive mailings because of information sharing from the physician's office to formula companies or tracking of family product purchases at retail stores.

Separation of Mothers and Infants

To support mothers in their desire to breastfeed, they should be taught how to express milk by hand or pump (see Chapter 11) in case there is a need for separation from the infant (Step 5). If the infant is admitted to the neonatal intensive care unit, the need for this teaching will be immediate, but it should, in any case, take place before discharge and be reinforced in early visits together with other breastfeeding skills. When mothers and infants need to be separated, expression of milk is important, not only for infant feeding, but also to initiate and maintain the woman's milk supply during the separation (see Chapter 10).

Pacifiers

The most common reason women stop breastfeeding in the hospital setting is because of perceived inadequacy of their milk supply. Offering anticipatory guidance about normal milk production and normal weight loss for the newborn in the first few days can reassure the mother. The time a newborn spends sucking on a pacifier is time not spent suckling on the mother's breast, and the lack of stimulation can delay the arrival of the full milk supply. The use of pacifiers in the early breastfeeding period has been shown to be associated with shorter breastfeeding duration and should be avoided until breastfeeding is well established; it should be avoided under routine circumstances (Step 9). However, newborns who are ill or who are undergoing painful procedures may be calmed with non-nutritive sucking. Similarly small amounts of sucrose have been shown to help newborns coping with painful procedures, usually given by a syringe to prevent nipple confusion. The AAP recommends pacifiers be used after breastfeeding is well established, usually by 3 to 4 weeks.

Support Following Discharge

Discharge planning includes referrals and contact information for ongoing assistance with breastfeeding (Step 10). The AAP recommends that all newborns be seen by a knowledgeable health care professional by 3 to 5 days of age. It has been shown that early follow-up contributes to breastfeeding duration and may prevent complications such as failure to thrive and severe hyperbilirubinemia (see Chapter 7).

Selected References

1. The Academy of Breastfeeding Medicine Protocol Committee. ABM clinical protocol #3: Hospital guidelines for the use of supplementary feedings in the healthy term breastfed neonate, Revised 2009. *Breastfeed Med.* 2009;4:175–182

2. Berens PD. Prenatal, intrapartum, and postpartum support of the lactating mother. *Pediatr Clin North Am.* 2001;48:365–375

3. Dewey KG, Nommsen-Rivers LA, Heinig MJ, Cohen RJ. Risk factors for suboptimal infant breastfeeding behavior, delayed onset of lactation, and excess neonatal weight loss. *Pediatrics.* 2003;112:607–619

4. Ferber SG, Makhoul IR. The effect of skin-to-skin contact (kangaroo care) shortly after birth on the neurobehavioral responses of the term newborn: a randomized, controlled trial. *Pediatrics.* 2004;113:858–865

5. Geddes DT, Kent JC, Mitoulas LR, Hartmann PE. Tongue movement and intra-oral vacuum in breastfeeding infants. *Early Hum Dev.* 2008;84:471–477

6. Hauck FR, Thompson JM, Tanabe KO, Moon RY, Vennemann MM. Breastfeeding and reduced risk of sudden infant death syndrome: A meta-analysis. *Pediatrics.* 2011;128:103–110

7. Howard CR, Howard FM, Lanphear B, et al. Randomized clinical trial of pacifier use and bottle-feeding or cupfeeding and their effect on breastfeeding. *Pediatrics.* 2003;111:511–518

8. Jacqz-Aigrain E, Serreau R, Boissinot C, et al. Excretion of ketoprofen and nalbuphine in human milk during treatment of maternal pain after delivery. *Ther Drug Monit.* 2007;29:815–818

9. Jensen D, Wallace S, Kelsay P. LATCH: A breastfeeding charting system and documentation tool. *J Obstet Gynecol Neonatal Nurs.* 1994;23:27–32

10. Kramer MS, Barr RG, Dagenais S, et al. Pacifier use, early weaning, and cry/fuss behavior. *JAMA.* 2001;286:322–326

11. Kramer MS, Chalmers B, Hodnett ED, et al. Promotion of Breastfeeding Intervention Trial (PROBIT): a randomized trial in the Republic of Belarus. *JAMA.* 2001;285:413–420

12. Langer A, Campero L, Garcia C, Reynoso S. Effects of psychosocial support during labour and childbirth on breastfeeding, medical interventions, and mothers' well-being in a Mexican public hospital: a randomized clinical trial. *Br J Obstet Gynaecol.* 1998;105:1056–1063

13. Powers NG, Naylor AJ, Wester RA. Hospital policies: crucial to breastfeeding success. *Semin Perinatol.* 1994;18:517–524

14. Spigset O. Analgesics and breast-feeding: safety considerations. *Pediatric Drugs.* 2000;2:223–238

15. Task Force on Sudden Infant Death Syndrome, Moon R. SIDS and other sleep related infant deaths, expansion of recommendations for a safe infant sleeping environment. *Pediatrics.* 2011;128:1030–1039

16. Teissedre F, Chabrol H. A study of the Edinburg Postnatal Depression Scale (EPDS) on 859 mothers: detection of mothers at risk for postpartum depression. *Encephale.* 2004;30:376–381

17. US Department of Health and Human Services. *Report of the Surgeon General's Workshop on Breastfeeding & Human Lactation.* Rockville, MD: US Department of Health and Human Services, Public Health Service, Health Resources and Services Administration; 1984. DHHS publication HRS-D-MC 84-2

18. World Health Organization Division of Child Health and Development. *Evidence for the Ten Steps to Successful Breastfeeding.* Geneva, Switzerland: World Health Organization; 1998

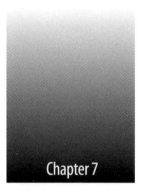

Chapter 7

Breastfeeding in the Hospital: The Postpartum Period

Adequate communication between obstetric and pediatric care professionals in the immediate postdelivery period will greatly facilitate helping the breast-feeding woman. It is equally important that all health care personnel involved in caring for mothers and infants possess basic breastfeeding knowledge so that they can provide accurate and consistent information. This chapter discusses issues relating to infants and mothers after delivery and before hospital discharge. Before discharge, anticipatory guidance regarding the breastfeeding process should be provided to the patient, her partner, and other supporting family members. Follow-up visits should be arranged. The patient should be given information on how to easily access further breast-feeding support if it is needed.

Breastfeeding Risk Factor History

General

Although most mothers can produce an adequate quantity of milk and most infants can nurse effectively and consume an adequate volume, specific maternal and infant factors can place an infant at risk for breastfeeding problems (Boxes 7-1 and 7-2). It is assumed that risk factors for breastfeeding problems are assessed as part of routine prenatal care, although some mothers may present with limited or no prenatal care. Findings of the prenatal maternal breast examination that may adversely affect adequacy of milk production (eg, inverted nipples, severely asymmetrical or tubular breasts, and prior breast surgeries) should be discussed with the patient as well as potential strategies to optimize successful breastfeeding. This information also should be discussed with the patient in a supportive and realistic fashion. In particular, lack of breast growth during pregnancy is a red flag and this information should be communicated from the obstetric to the pediatric care professional, as well as any other pertinent information about maternal perinatal conditions and delivery events.

Maternal History

Appropriate maternal history includes amount and timing of prenatal care and education, medical complications, obstetric complications, medical

Box 7-1. Maternal Risk Factors for Lactation Problems

History/Social Factors
- Early intention to breastfeed and bottle-feed
- History of previous breastfeeding problems or breastfed infant with slow weight gain
- History of hormone-related infertility
- Significant medical problems (eg, untreated hypothyroidism, diabetes, cystic fibrosis)
- Maternal age (eg, adolescent mother or advanced age)
- Psychosocial problems, especially depression
- Perinatal complications (eg, hemorrhage, hypertension, infection)
- Intended use of combined oral contraceptives before breastfeeding is well established

Anatomic/Physiologic Factors
- Lack of noticeable breast enlargement during pregnancy
- Flat or inverted nipples
- Variation in breast appearance (marked asymmetry, hypoplastic, tubular)
- Previous breast surgery that severed milk ducts or nipple afferent nerves
- Previous breast surgery to correct abnormal appearance or developmental variants
- Previous breast abscess
- Extremely or persistently sore nipples
- Failure of lactogenesis stage 2 (milk did not noticeably come in)

Environmental Factors
- Mother and infant separation or mother needing to pump

Adapted with permission from Neifert MR. Prevention of breastfeeding tragedies. *Pediatr Clin North Am.* 2001;48:273–297.

Box 7-2. Infant Risk Factors for Lactation Problems

Medical/Anatomic/Physiologic Factors
- Low birth weight or preterm (<37 weeks)
- Multiples
- Difficulty latching on to one or both breasts
- Ineffective or unsustained suckling
- Oral anatomic abnormalities (cleft lip/palate, micrognathia, macroglossia)
- Medical problems (jaundice, hypoglycemia, respiratory distress, infection)
- Neurologic problems (genetic syndromes, hypotonia, or hypertonia)
- Persistently sleepy infant
- Excessive infant weight loss

Environmental Factors
- Formula supplementation
- Effective breastfeeding not established by hospital discharge
- Early discharge from hospital
- Early pacifier use

Adapted with permission from Neifert MR. Prevention of breastfeeding tragedies. *Pediatr Clin North Am.* 2001;48:273–297.

history (especially breast surgeries, infertility, endocrine problems, and past breastfeeding difficulties), family history (atopy, breastfeeding problems), and psychosocial history (substance abuse, mental illness, sexual abuse, family support of breastfeeding).

Infant History

Appropriate history includes medical complications, postnatal feeding and elimination patterns, and infant temperament and sleep patterns.

Feeding Patterns

New mothers should be encouraged to nurse at each breast starting with the breast offered last at the prior feeding. This will help her achieve an optimal milk supply (Table 7-3). However, it is perfectly normal for a newborn to fall asleep after the first breast and refuse the second. It is preferable to allow infants to drain the first breast well before switching them to the other breast. The mother should not interrupt a feeding just to switch to the second side. Typically, the infant will spontaneously release the first breast after sufficient draining. Timing each side is not necessary or desirable. Limiting the time at the breast has no effect on nipple soreness, but correct latch and positioning are crucial.

Table 7-3. Milk Supply for Breastfed Neonates: The First Week

First 24 hours	Some milk may be expressed
Day 2	Milk should come in (lactogenesis stage 2)
Day 3	Milk should come in (lactogenesis stage 2)
Day 4	Milk should come in (lactogenesis stage 2)
Day 5	Milk should be present; breasts may be firm or leaking
Day 6+	Breasts should feel softer after nursing

Adapted with permission from Neifert MR. Clinical aspects of lactation. *Clin Perinatol.* 1999;26:281–306.

Hunger Cues

Many new parents expect their infants to cry when they are hungry, and the parents need to be informed that crying is a late sign of hunger and can result in an infant who is difficult to calm and latch to the breast. Anticipatory guidance and rooming-in 24 hours a day allow the parents to notice early infant hunger cues such as increased alertness, flexion of the extremities, mouth and tongue movements, cooing sounds, rooting, bringing the fist toward the mouth, or sucking on fingers or the hand. Signs of satiety also need to be taught, such as non-nutritive sucking with longer pauses between sucking bursts, infant taking himself or herself off the breast, disappearance of hunger cues, relaxed posture, and sleep.

Feeding Frequency

In addition to information regarding latch-on and positioning of the infant (see Chapter 6), the mother should be instructed on expected breastfeeding routines, which can vary widely (Table 7-4). Typically, newborns will nurse 8 to 12 times or more in 24 hours for at least 10 to 15 minutes per breast. The interval between feedings is figured from the beginning of one nursing to the beginning of the next. Frequent breastfeeding in the first few days minimizes postnatal weight loss, decreases bilirubin levels, and helps establish a good milk supply. Although every 2 to 3 hours is the average, there is a great deal of variation from infant to infant and during a 24-hour period. Human milk empties from the stomach faster than formula. Without anticipatory guidance, new mothers often compare their infants to bottle-fed infants and misinterpret the normal frequency of breastfeeding to mean they have insufficient milk. As infants get older, they nurse more efficiently, and the frequency and duration of feedings decrease.

Table 7-4. Breastfed Newborn Intake/Output Norms

Day	Age (h)	Milk Volume per Feeding (mL)	Milk Volume That Mother Sees	Characteristic of the Day	No. of Feeds	No. of Voids*	No. of Stools*,†	Color of Stools	Weight Loss Norms‡	Excess Weight Loss‡	Supplement Volume (mL)
1	0–24	0–5	Drops	"Anything goes"	>6	≥1	≥1	Meconium	Birth weight	—	5–10
2	24–48	5–10	1 tsp	"Feeding frenzy"	≥8§	2–3	1–2	Meconium	≤3%	>5%	10–20
3	48–72	10–20	1 tbsp	"Starting to get milk"	≥8§	4–6	≥3	Transitional	≤6%	>8%	20–30
4	72–96	20–30	1 oz	"Dealing with milk volume"	≥8	4–6	≥4	Transitional	≤8% (may gain)	>10%	30–40
5	>96	>30	>1 oz	"Growing"	≥8	6–8	≥4	Yellow	Newborn should gain	>10%	40–50*

Newborn has 24 hours to void and 48 hours to stool after birth.
*There may be a lull in stooling after meconium is cleared while newborn waits for milk to come in.
‡Weight loss norms and excess weight loss numbers are ballpark figures and may be different for more robust or more vulnerable newborns.
§Newborns may feed VERY frequently before the milk comes in, even hourly for the first few nights.
Adapted from Stellwagen L, Schanler RJ. Breastfeeding the newborn. *AAP Textbook of Pediatric Care*. Elk Grove Village, IL: American Academy of Pediatrics; 2013.

Nursing Styles

Infants have been classified by their feeding behaviors. The key to appropriate counseling is recognizing the difference in infants and responding to them (Table 7-5).

Infant Behaviors

Sleepy Infant

After the usual 1 to 2 hours of quiet alertness immediately after birth (the ideal time to initiate breastfeeding), many infants fall into deep sleep, with only brief, partial arousals for several hours. This is a normal pattern and does not indicate a need for supplementation. Sometimes unwrapping, gentle massage, holding upright, motion, changing a diaper, talking, or holding the infant skin-to-skin against the mother's chest may arouse the sleepy infant. Infants have short wakeful periods throughout the first couple of days that can be missed. Rooming-in, where the infant sleeps in close proximity to the mother, allows the mother to recognize subtle hunger cues. The newborn whose mother received a large quantity of narcotics or sedatives may have longer periods of sleep and may need to be awakened after 4 hours to feed.

Fussy/Unsettled Infants

An infants who appears fussy or unsettled may be fretful after a feed, especially before lactogenesis stage 2 is complete. An extra minute or 2 at the breast, a diaper change, or a cuddle will usually satisfy the infant. If the

Table 7-5. Infant Breastfeeding Styles

Attention to infant cues for feeding and the acceptance of a range of styles is helpful in optimizing breastfeeding.	
Type	**Description**
Barracuda (or "Excited, effective")	Grabs the nipple and sucks energetically for 10–20 minutes
Excited ineffective	Very eager and active at the breast, frustrated and crying when no milk results
Procrastinator ("Slow to start")	Waits until the milk appears before sucking, does well once started
Gourmet ("Slow feeder")	Licks and tastes little drops of milk before latch-on; attempts to hurry are met with vigorous infant protest
Rester ("Protracted feeder")	Prefers to breastfeed for a few minutes, then rest a few minutes, resulting in a longer than usual nursing time

infant is consistently fussy after every feeding, even after the milk supply is established, the breastfeeding mother and infant should be carefully assessed with regard to milk supply, milk transfer, and infant weight gain. Breastfeeding should commence when the infant is in the quiet alert state. If the infant is at an active alert or crying state, the infant may need to be consoled before he or she can be successfully breastfed.

Crying

Interpreted through the years as a sign of vigor, "good lungs," and general health, crying results in increased work, energy expenditure, and swallowing of air, which may precipitate vomiting. In addition, crying depletes metabolic reserves, which may precipitate hypoglycemia, and disrupts early breastfeeding behavior. Crying is a very late sign of hunger. Infants who cry for a long time may become exhausted and go to sleep without nursing or before they have finished the entire feeding. Frequent feeding will diminish crying episodes. Efforts should be made to minimize crying.

Assessment of the Infant

Physical Examination

The physical examination of the infant should include a general examination, vital signs, growth percentiles and percentage weight change from birth, and a detailed oral-motor examination including assessment of mandible size, frenulum, rooting, and sucking. Presence of congenital anomalies and overall tone should be noted.

Breastfeeding Observation

It is helpful for the physician, or the staff under a physician's guidance, to observe a feeding and evaluate positioning, latch, milk letdown, and milk transfer, as well as maternal responses to the feeding (eg, painful, pleasurable, anxious, relaxed) also should be noted. The hospital staff should observe and document these breastfeeding observations at least twice daily (Box 7-6).

Latch

The infant's mouth should be wide open with lips flanged outward ("fish lips") encompassing the nipple and a significant part of the areola. Some of the factors that are important in assessing latch include the ability of the infant to latch, quality of the latch, presence of audible swallowing, characteristics of the anatomy and physiology of the nipple, maternal sensation, and whether the caregiver provides assistance with feeding.

Box 7-6. Overview: In-hospital Newborn Breastfeeding Health Supervision

Breastfeeding Assessment
- Review maternal prenatal record, intrapartum record, and newborn recovery and transition records.
- Discuss timing and events of first feeding.
- Has mother previously breastfed?
- How is mother doing, and how is she feeling about breastfeeding?
- Does newborn need to be awakened to feed?
- Does newborn easily latch on to breast and nurse eagerly?
- How many times has the newborn been to the breast within the first 24 to 48 hours?
- Is newborn receiving any supplements?
- What is the number of wet diapers in last 24 hours?
- What is the number of stools in last 24 hours?
- What is the color of the stools?
- Are mother's breasts comfortable (no tenderness or pain)?
- Is mother taking any medications?
- How do family members feel about breastfeeding?

Examination of the Newborn and Mother
- Obtain birth weight and gestational age.
- Evaluate neurobehavioral condition of the newborn.
- Calculate newborn's weight gain or loss since birth.
- Observe breastfeeding.
- Examine mother's breasts or refer for examination, if needed.
- Perform newborn examination with attention to oral-motor examination.
- Assess state of hydration.
- Observe for jaundice.

Anticipatory Guidance
- Encourage breastfeeding on demand, approximately 8 to 12 times per 24 hours.
- During the first 24 to 48 hours, newborn may show little interest in breastfeeding.
- Newborns who do not awaken to feed should be aroused to feed at least every 4 hours.
- Discourage use of pacifiers and discuss potential risks.
- Review normal breastfeeding patterns.
- Review normal elimination patterns.

Breastfeeding Interventions
- Supportive, nondisruptive care is important during first 24 to 48 hours.
- Attempt to identify signs of inadequate milk supply or intake, and address potential contributing factors.
- Maintain lactation if mother and newborn are separated.
- Consider referral to lactation specialist if problems are ongoing.

Discharge Visit
- Congratulate parents on decision to breastfeed their baby.
- Review some of the benefits of breastfeeding.
- Remind mother to eat when hungry and drink when thirsty.
- Arrange for follow-up in office at 3 to 5 days of age or sooner if indicated.

Adapted from *Checklists for Breastfeeding Health Supervision.* Elk Grove Village, IL: American Academy of Pediatrics; 1999.

Weight Changes

The most accurate appraisal of the adequacy of breastfeeding is the serial measurement of the infant's naked weight. Nearly all infants lose weight for the first 2 to 4 days after birth. Infants who are feeding well should not continue to lose weight after lactogenesis stage 2. A weight loss greater than 8% to 10% of birth weight may be excessive even if lactogenesis and milk transfer seem to be proceeding normally. In such a situation, milk production and transfer should be assessed. Once lactogenesis stage 2 is completed, an infant who did not lose excessive weight and who is nursing effectively should obtain enough milk to begin gaining weight by day 4 or 5 at a rate of approximately 15 to 30 g per day (0.5–1 oz per day). At this rate, most breastfed infants will exceed their birth weight by 10 to 14 days, and gain 150 to 210 g per week (5–7 oz per week) for the first 2 months. A breastfed infant who weighs less than his or her birth weight at 2 weeks requires careful evaluation and intervention. Refer to Table 8-2 for overall mean weight gains for breastfed boys and girls.

Elimination Patterns

Urine output usually exceeds fluid intake for the first 3 to 4 days after birth, a physiologic response to contract the extracellular fluid space. Stooling and voiding patterns after the first few days are good indicators of adequate milk intake (Table 7-4). A journal kept by the mother recording feeding and elimination by the infant in the first few weeks can be helpful.

Urine Output

By 5 to 7 days (usually a day or 2 after lactogenesis stage 2 is completed), the breastfed newborn should be voiding colorless, dilute urine 6 or more times per day.

Stool Output and Character

Both stool output and character are particularly useful indicators of adequate milk intake. The normal green-black meconium stool should change to transitional green, then to soft, seedy, yellow stool by day 4 or 5 after birth. By 5 to 7 days of age, well-nourished breastfed infants usually pass a medium-sized yellow stool at least 3 to 4 times a day. Some infants stool after most feedings. After the first month, the volume of each stool increases and the frequency decreases. Anticipatory guidance is essential because normal human milk stools are quite loose and may be confused with diarrhea if parents are accustomed to seeing the firm brown stools typical of formula-fed infants. Insufficient milk intake in an infant older than 5 days may be signaled by the presence of meconium stools, green-brown transitional stools, infrequent (<3 per day) stools, or scant stools.

Hypoglycemia

One of physicians' most commonly cited concerns regarding breastfed infants is hypoglycemia. The risk for hypoglycemia may be reduced by immediate and sustained mother-infant skin-to-skin contact and early initiation of breastfeeding. Infant energy expenditure and, therefore, glucose utilization can be decreased by early skin-to-skin contact. Blood glucose concentrations reach a nadir 1 to 2 hours after birth. An adaptive response to low blood glucose concentrations in breastfed infants is an increased concentration of ketone bodies and other substrates, which act as alternate fuels for the infant until breastfeeding is established. Infant energy expenditure and, therefore, glucose utilization, can be decreased by early skin-to-skin contact.

Signs and Symptoms: The clinical signs of hypoglycemia may be nonexistent, nonspecific, or include changes in the level of behavior (irritability, lethargy, stupor, coma), apnea, tachypnea, cyanotic episodes, hypothermia, hypotonia, tremor, seizures, temperature instability, and change in feeding patterns/responses.

Causes: In general, healthy term breastfed neonates do not experience symptomatic hypoglycemia. If symptomatic hypoglycemia develops, an underlying illness must be excluded. Infants of diabetic mothers, infants who are small for gestational age, and preterm infants are among the common groups of infants at risk for hypoglycemia.

Evaluation: Routine monitoring of blood glucose in asymptomatic, not at-risk, term neonates is unnecessary. Blood glucose concentrations should be measured in at-risk infants and/or those with clinical signs suggestive of hypoglycemia. Bedside screening tests should be confirmed by laboratory blood glucose measurements. At-risk infants and those with abnormal blood glucose concentrations should be monitored before each feeding and require continued monitoring until several normal prefeeding blood glucose concentrations are obtained. Serial monitoring does not preclude routine breastfeeding.

Management: Hypoglycemia can be reduced by early skin-to-skin contact and initiation of breastfeeding within the first hour after delivery. Early breastfeeding is not precluded even though an infant meets the at-risk criteria for glucose monitoring. The intervention in an asymptomatic breastfed infant is to increase the frequency of breastfeeding to every 1 to 2 hours and to recheck the blood glucose before the next feeding. If breastfeeding alone cannot correct and maintain an appropriate blood glucose concentration, expressed human milk or formula should be offered. Symptomatic hypoglycemia requires treatment with intravenous glucose. As long as the infant is clinically stable, breastfeeding should continue, even if intravenous glucose is provided.

Feeding at the Breast Versus the Bottle

General

A distinct difference exists between tongue and jaw movements of breastfeeding and bottle-feeding infants. In breastfeeding, breathing is coordinated with sucking and swallowing, usually in a 1:1:1 pattern. The rapid flow from a bottle may result in respiratory pause and shortened expiration. It is often assumed that breastfed infants who have difficulty obtaining milk will be more likely to prefer bottle-feeding if given the opportunity. Some infants may simply prefer the more rapid, gravity-induced flow from a bottle. Because the introduction of a bottle has the potential to disrupt the development of effective breastfeeding behavior, its use should be minimized until breastfeeding is well established.

Pacifiers

Pacifier use is best avoided during the initiation of breastfeeding and used only after breastfeeding is well established. In some infants, early pacifier use may interfere with establishment of good breastfeeding practices, whereas in others, it may indicate the presence of a breastfeeding problem that requires intervention.

Assessment of the Mother

Nipple Pain

Nipple soreness is the most common complaint of breastfeeding mothers in the immediate postpartum period. Actual nipple pain should not be considered normal. Nipple pain beyond mere soreness or discomfort or even soreness that continues beyond the beginning of a nursing episode or after letdown should be investigated immediately. If ignored, it can lead to other problems, such as engorgement, mastitis, or early cessation of breastfeeding (see Chapter 9).

Signs and Symptoms: Early mild nipple discomfort is common among breastfeeding women. Transient nipple pain attributed to suction injury of the skin usually begins on the second postpartum day, increases between days 3 and 5, and then improves. Severe nipple pain, or even discomfort that continues throughout a feeding or that does not improve at the end of the first week, should not be considered a normal part of breastfeeding.

Causes: Some potential sources of sore nipples in the immediate postpartum period include:

- Improper breastfeeding technique, specifically poor position and improper latch, is the most common cause of nipple pain in the immediate postpartum period. Limited milk transfer occurs when the infant is attached incorrectly, resulting in poor infant weight gain and impaired milk production. Mothers with abdominal incisions from a cesarean delivery or other surgery should find comfortable positions, such as the football (or clutch) hold, to feed the infant.
- Trauma that produce cracking, such as from overzealous breast cleansing, failing to release suction before removing the infant from the breast, climate variables, and unique skin sensitivity, are other potential causes of nipple pain. There is no need for nipple cleansing other than routine bathing. Counsel the mother to avoid using soap on the nipples because it can be irritating.

Evaluation: A feeding history, examination of the mother's breasts and nipples, and an oral-motor examination of the infant should accompany the observation of a feeding. The latch-on technique and infant positioning should be evaluated carefully. Infant suck also should be assessed. The mother should be asked about use of cleansers, abrasives, or any creams or ointments on the breast. Rarely are bacterial or fungal cultures indicated (see Chapter 9).

Management: Limiting the time at the breast, even with the intention of gradually increasing nursing time, will not prevent nipple pain. Treatment for nipple pain depends on the underlying etiology. Skilled help with position and latch-on are primary interventions. Specific infections and dermatoses require directed therapy. Some creams and lotions can be irritating and result in allergic manifestations. Wound care specialists now suggest moisture-retaining occlusive dressings instead of dry heat for optimal healing. Pain may be helped by taking a pain reliever such as ibuprofen or acetaminophen a half hour before nursing. If severe trauma exists, it may be necessary to either manually or mechanically express milk until the tissue has healed well enough to resume breastfeeding. Nipple healing might be hastened if a small amount of milk is applied to the area after a feeding.

Different breastfeeding positions also may be helpful in avoiding more sensitive or traumatized areas. If only one breast is affected, nursing should begin on the unaffected breast to achieve the letdown reflex and the infant moved to the affected breast when suckling may be less vigorous. Nipple pain also may be lessened by the use of a silicone nipple shield (see Chapter 11).

Engorgement

Normal breast fullness occurs because of vascular congestion during lactogenesis stage 2. Engorgement is the firm, diffuse, and painful overfilling and edema of breasts usually because of infrequent or ineffective milk removal. The woman may notice a low-grade fever. Therefore, the best treatment of engorgement is prevention by frequent breastfeeding. If left untreated, engorgement may lead to difficulties in latch and to mastitis. Engorgement should not be confused with a plugged milk duct, which can result in a localized lump in one area of the breast (see Table 9-1). Engorgement also may occur later in the course of breastfeeding related to a missed feeding or an abrupt change in feeding frequency.

Signs and Symptoms: Engorgement usually occurs around the time of increased milk production on days 3 to 7 and can be most severe in primiparous women. The breasts become swollen, warm, and tender. In severe cases, the nipples can become flattened to the point the baby cannot grasp them. Engorgement is sometimes confused with mastitis, but with engorgement the temperature will rarely be higher than 38°C, systemic symptoms are absent, and the white blood cell count is normal. The swelling and tenderness of engorged breasts are bilateral, generalized, and not unilateral or localized as in an infection (see Table 9-1).

Causes: Engorgement may be the result of infrequent or ineffective nursing from such causes as sore nipples, a sleepy baby, or mother-baby separation. Engorgement is potentiated by vascular congestion, either caused by hormonal responses or obstructed lymphatic drainage.

Evaluation: Examination of the breasts should be undertaken visually and by palpation of all aspects of both breasts, particularly noting redness, induration, tenderness, and asymmetry.

Management: The treatment for engorgement is frequent and effective milk removal (Box 7-7). Once the engorgement is relieved, the mother needs to take steps to prevent its recurrence. Mothers should have ready access to an efficient pump or be trained in manual expression if separated from their infants.

Box 7-7. Management of Breast Engorgement

- Moist, warm packs for 20 minutes or a warm shower before feeding to encourage milk flow
- Gentle massage of the breast with hand expression to ease attachment of the infant to the breast
- Frequent and effective feedings every 1 to 3 hours
- Frequent and effective draining of the breast by hand or pump if mother and infant are separated, or if the breast is so tense that latch is not possible
- Cold packs for 20 minutes after feeding
- Supportive bra to provide comfort to the heavy breasts
- Analgesics (ibuprofen or acetaminophen; see Chapter 6)

Discharge Planning

Education/Anticipatory Guidance

The success of breastfeeding is measured in the duration of breastfeeding and of exclusive breastfeeding, not in the initiation of breastfeeding alone. Anticipatory attention to the needs of the mother and newborn at the time of discharge from the hospital facilitates successful, long-term breastfeeding. It is assumed that the family had adequate preparation for breastfeeding during prenatal education sessions. Building on this, the patient should again receive basic education regarding breastfeeding. The education should be simple, targeted, and culturally sensitive, and recognize that hormonal factors and maternal fatigue may precipitate information overload.

General Education

This should include information about infant positioning, latch-on, expected feeding and elimination patterns, jaundice, and signs that warrant physician notification, which can be communicated in infant care classes given before discharge and individual instruction, and with the use of noncommercial literature or video presentations. Mothers should be given information on reputable local breastfeeding support groups. Short hospitalizations and limited extended family assistance heighten the need for adequate support after hospital discharge. Support groups increase women's confidence in their breastfeeding abilities. Strategies that provide face-to-face contact seem to be most effective, but providing a 24-hour telephone source for assistance is also valuable. Breastfeeding mothers should receive instruction on manual and mechanical milk expression methods so that they can maintain their milk supply and obtain milk for feeding if the mother and infant are separated. Discharge packs containing infant formula, pacifiers, and/or commercial advertising materials should not be given to a breastfeeding mother. The spouse and other family members should also be encouraged to provide assistance for the new mother in a way that is supportive of breastfeeding. They may assist with the evaluation of breastfeeding, burping, cuddling, carrying, and bathing the infant, as well as helping the mother with other household chores.

Basic Breast Care

Information regarding basic breast care should also be given to the mother. She should be instructed that little special care is required outside of avoiding the use of harsh soaps and detergents directly on the nipple and areola. The use of a comfortable, nonconstraining nursing bra during lactation is advised. If an underwire-type bra is used, care should be taken to ensure that it fits properly and does not compress any tissue, which could lead to poor drainage and the potential for plugged ducts. The woman should also be counseled regarding the use of breast pads to absorb leakage. These can either be reusable pads made of cloth or disposable pads. If disposable pads are chosen, those backed with plastic liners should be avoided to reduce the possibility of inducing sore nipples from constantly being moist. Reusable pads should be changed frequently (when moist) and laundered.

Maternal Nutrition

Recommendations for healthy eating should also be given to the new mother. Care should be taken to avoid implying that her milk will not be adequate if her diet is not perfectly balanced (see Chapter 9).

Contraception

The new mother should be asked about plans for contraception prior to hospital discharge. This should be addressed again at the postpartum visit. The patient should be counseled that she might require the use of a vaginal lubricant to treat vaginal dryness during lactation. Various contraceptive options affect lactation in different ways (see Chapter 13).

Follow-up

General Support

Every breastfeeding mother should be provided with names and phone numbers of individuals who can provide advice on a 24-hour-a-day basis, as well as on a less intensive basis. Although the primary physicians' offices provide general support to the breastfeeding mother, other community-based resources exist, such as WIC (Special Supplemental Nutrition Program for Women, Infants, and Children) and peer support groups (eg, La Leche League). Contact information should be shared, and mothers should be encouraged to participate.

Pediatric Follow-up

Before discharge, an appointment should be made for an office visit. A newborn discharged before 72 hours should be seen within 2 days of discharge. If the mother is ready for discharge but the infant is not, every effort should be made to allow the mother to remain in the hospital either as a continuing patient or as a "mother-in-residence" with access to the infant for continued exclusive breastfeeding.

Maternal Follow-up

Assessment of breastfeeding should be an integral part of the postpartum obstetric evaluation. If the woman has undergone cesarean delivery, she may be seen at 1 to 2 weeks after delivery (see Chapter 9). At the routine 4- to 6-week postpartum visit, the obstetric care professional should assess breastfeeding and provide support for the patient's decision to breastfeed (see Chapter 9).

Return to Work

The physician can discuss plans with the new mother who intends soon after delivery to return to work outside the home or to attend school. The timing of the return to work and a plan to adjust the infant's feedings and the milk supply should be discussed well before the anticipated date of return (see Chapters 8, 10, and 11).

Continued Communication Among Caregivers

Any issues that are brought up regarding breastfeeding that could affect the breastfed child should be communicated from the obstetric care professional to the pediatric care professional (and vice versa, as appropriate).

Selected References

1. American Academy of Pediatrics. *Bright Futures Tool and Resource Kit [CD-ROM].* Elk Grove Village, IL: American Academy of Pediatrics; 2009
2. American Academy of Pediatrics Quality Improvement Innovation Network. *Safe & Healthy Beginnings: A Resource Toolkit for Hospitals and Physicians' Offices [CD-ROM].* Elk Grove Village, IL: American Academy of Pediatrics; 2009
3. American Academy of Pediatrics Subcommittee on Hyperbilirubinemia. Management of hyperbilirubinemia in the newborn infant 35 or more weeks of gestation. *Pediatrics.* 2004;114:297–316
4. American College of Obstetricians and Gynecologists. *Breastfeeding Your Baby.* Washington, DC: American College of Obstetricians and Gynecologists; 2001. ACOG Patient Education Pamphlet AP029
5. Chantry CJ, Nommsen-Rivers LA, Peerson JM, Cohen RJ, Dewey KG. Excessive weight loss in first-born breastfed newborns relates to maternal intrapartum fluid balance. *Pediatrics.* 2011;127:e171–e179
6. Committee on Fetus and Newborn; Adamkin DH. Clinical report—postnatal glucose homeostasis in late-preterm and term infants. *Pediatrics.* 2011;127:575–579
7. Dewey KG, Nommsen-Rivers LA, Heinig MJ, Cohen RJ. Risk factors for suboptimal infant breastfeeding behavior, delayed onset of lactation, and excess neonatal weight loss. *Pediatrics.* 2003;112:607–619
8. Eidelman AI. Hypoglycemia and the breastfed neonate. *Pediatr Clin North Am.* 2001;48:377–387
9. Eidelman AI, Schanler RJ, Johnston M, et al. Breastfeeding and the use of human milk. *Pediatrics.* 2012;129:e827–e841
10. Holmes AV. Establishing successful breastfeeding in the newborn period. *Pediatr Clin North Am.* 2013;60:147–168
11. Howard CR, Howard FM, Lanphear B, deBliecki EA, Eberly S, Lawrence RA. The effects of early pacifier use on breastfeeding duration. *Pediatrics.* 1999;103:e33
12. Howard CR, Howard FM, Lanphear B, et al. Randomized clinical trial of pacifier use and bottle-feeding or cupfeeding and their effect on breastfeeding. *Pediatrics.* 2003;111:511–518
13. Mass S. Breast pain: engorgement, nipple pain and mastitis. *Clin Obstet Gynecol.* 2004;47:676–682
14. Merewood A, Philipp BL. Implementing change: Becoming baby-friendly in an inner city hospital. *Birth.* 2001;28:36–40
15. Neifert MR. Early assessment of the breastfeeding infant. *Contemp Pediatr.* 1996;13:142–166
16. Neifert MR. Clinical aspects of lactation. *Clin Perinatol.* 1999;26:281–306
17. Neifert MR. Prevention of breastfeeding tragedies. *Pediatr Clin North Am.* 2001;48:273–297
18. Szucs KA, Miracle DJ, Rosenman MB. Breastfeeding knowledge, attitudes, and practices among providers in a medical home. *Breastfeed Med.* 2009;4:31–42
19. Wight NE. Management of common breastfeeding issues. *Pediatr Clin North Am.* 2001;48:321–344
20. Wolfberg AJ, Michels KB, Shields W, O'Campo P, Bronner Y, Bienstock J. Dads as breastfeeding advocates: results from a randomized controlled trial of an educational intervention. *Am J Obstet Gynecol.* 2004;191:708–712

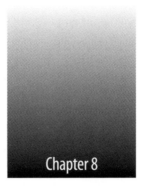

Chapter 8

Maintenance of Breastfeeding—The Infant

Skilled anticipatory guidance and positive support are critical to the maintenance of lactation. A good understanding by the physician of common breastfeeding issues can help foster a growing, healthy infant and a mother who is comfortable and confident with breastfeeding. Issues common to breastfeeding maintenance in the infant are addressed in this chapter.

Insufficient Milk Syndrome

The lack of milk, either real or perceived, is a common reason for discontinuing breastfeeding. Insufficient milk syndrome is an imprecise term because it refers to failure of mother's milk production, either primary or secondary, or failure of the infant to extract milk. Because most infants leave the hospital between 24 and 72 hours of age, insufficient intake and dehydration are problems that may be seen in follow-up. However, problems that arise from insufficient intake usually can be prevented with appropriate interventions. Formal evaluation of breastfeeding before hospital discharge is important to assure appropriate technique.

Signs and Symptoms: Insufficient intake in the infant includes delayed or infrequent bowel movements, decreased urinary output, early jaundice, an inconsolably hungry baby, lethargy, and/or a loss of more than 8% to 10% of birth weight. Generally, there are noticeable abnormalities in milk supply (see Table 7-3), feeding, and elimination patterns (see Table 7-4).

Causes: Insufficient milk intake may either be related to failure of the mother to produce milk or failure of the infant to extract milk (see Boxes 7-1, 7-2, and 8-1). Although primary lactation failure is rare (and often heralded by a lack of breast growth during pregnancy), delayed lactogenesis stage 2 may occur with retained placental fragments, primary pituitary insufficiency, diabetes, or certain maternal medications. Mothers who have had breast surgery are also at risk for insufficient milk production and/or inability to transfer the milk, especially if nerves and ducts have been severed. Insufficient milk supply more commonly is caused by inappropriate early feeding routines, including the use of formula supplements. Occasionally, an infant may not be able to extract milk effectively, leading to a gradual decrease in milk supply. Such is the case with orally fed late preterm infants (34–36 weeks) and some infants with neurologic problems or oral anomalies. Any factor that limits milk removal may result in diminished milk synthesis because local factors in the breast govern milk production (see Chapter 4).

Evaluation: A review of the perinatal history (see Boxes 7-1 and 7-2) will often identify maternal or infant factors, or both, to be addressed. A mother whose breasts did not enlarge during pregnancy or did not become full by 5 days postpartum may have structural or hormonal problems resulting in inadequate milk supply. Direct observation of breastfeeding may reveal improper latch, positioning, or inadequate infant effort. Objective measures of infant growth should be performed before beginning any intervention. Significant weight loss usually indicates a problem with milk supply, transfer of milk to the infant, or both. Infant birth weight may also be falsely elevated

---

Box 8-1. Potential Causes of Primary Insufficient Milk Syndrome

Anatomic variants of the breast
- Breast hypoplasia
- Tubular breasts
- Marked breast asymmetry

Breast surgery
- Reduction
- Augmentation
- Breast abscess
- Breast cancer
- Radiation therapy

Endocrine abnormalities
- Pituitary insufficiency

as a function of peripartum intravenous (IV) fluids administered to the mother during prolonged labor. The subsequent diuresis of the infant after delivery may make weight loss more notable. Inquiring about peripartum IV fluid administration may be helpful in investigating excessive weight loss in the newborn in the first postpartum days. Also, apparent excessive weight loss may be an artifact of the scale, especially when there are separate scales in the delivery area and in the postpartum area.

Electronic infant scales calibrated to ±2 g are available that can accurately measure prefeeding and postfeeding weights to estimate the volume of milk ingested (see Chapter 11). Some clinicians found a high predictability of maternal lactation insufficiency if the change in weight for infants in the first few weeks from before to after the feeding was less than 45 g. Manual milk expression or mechanical milk expression techniques may be needed to ascertain total milk volume before feeding or residual milk volume in the breast after a feeding. If the residual milk volume is high (>30 mL), this may be a reason for concern. Less invasive procedures, such as observing a feeding or performing a physical examination, should be undertaken before performing prefeeding and postfeeding weights or milk expression after feeding to determine residual milk volume. These extra measures may contribute to the mother's feeling of inadequacy, and breastfeeding success correlates with maternal confidence in feeding efficacy.

Management: The major goal in management is to increase milk production and milk transfer. Regardless of cause, consultation with a certified lactation specialist should be considered.

- *Primary management* depends on the cause but usually involves increasing the frequency and effectiveness of breastfeeding. Mothers also may need to mechanically express milk after each breastfeeding to increase stimulation and breast drainage.
- *Supplementation* adversely affects establishing a full milk supply by decreasing the frequency and completeness of breast draining, leading to milk stasis and reduced milk supply. However, supplementation may be necessary if milk production does not increase with increased frequency of breastfeeding with the infant properly latched on, milk supply is markedly inadequate, or signs of dehydration and/or malnutrition already are present.
- *Supplements* are given when there is inadequate milk intake. Fluids preferred for supplementation are expressed mother's own milk, pasteurized donor human milk from a bank following the protocols of the HMBABA

(if available), or infant formula. Some clinicians recommend protein hydrolysate-based formulas for this purpose. Glucose water is not a preferred fluid. Glucose water provides significantly fewer calories and no alternate substrates and does not stimulate intestinal motility as does human milk or formula. Depending on the circumstances, if dehydration and/or malnutrition are present, the infant should be given enough supplemental milk to produce improved weight gain. Breastfeeding should continue with the addition of the supplemental milk after nursing. Sometimes as little as 1 or 2 oz of supplemental milk is needed per feeding. At the same time, the mother should continue milk expression techniques to increase milk production. As milk production increases, the need for supplemental fluids will diminish.

- *Perceived inadequate milk supply.* If the objective evaluation reveals that milk supply is adequate, it is important to reassure the mother that her milk supply is adequate and provide her with the knowledge to assess its adequacy. Even with appropriate prenatal education, many women and many cultures do not appreciate that colostrum is milk and that the volumes produced in the first 2 to 5 days (2–20 mL per feeding) are adequate for the infant.

Jaundice

The association between breastfeeding and jaundice is observed in 2 distinct entities: breastfeeding jaundice and breastmilk jaundice.

Breastfeeding Jaundice

Hyperbilirubinemia is the most frequent reason for readmission of term and late preterm infants. Many of these infants are breastfed. Inadequate breastfeeding management is often a contributing factor. Jaundice may be part of the clinical picture of the dehydrated, malnourished breastfed infant in the first week after birth (see earlier Insufficient Milk Syndrome section). Markedly increased levels of unconjugated serum bilirubin may cause acute bilirubin encephalopathy manifest as lethargy, hypotonia, and poor feeding that progresses to chronic encephalopathy, known as kernicterus, with permanent brain injury manifest by athetoid cerebral palsy, auditory dysfunction, and paralysis of upward gaze. In recent years, approximately 75% of infants who had kernicterus were breastfed. This almost always is a preventable outcome.

Signs and Symptoms: In their first week, these infants have increasing serum unconjugated bilirubin levels and poor milk intake. Usually a history is obtained of decreased maternal milk production and/or poor milk intake by the infant. Dehydration, weight loss, failure to gain weight, and/or hypernatremia also may be observed (see Boxes 7-1 and 7-2). Late preterm infants are at risk for development of kernicterus, especially if breastfeeding. Clinicians cannot assume that these infants will feed like term infants. In the hospital, late preterm infants may appear to feed well. However, once home, they may not have the stamina required to ingest larger volumes. They may struggle to achieve an adequate intake but demonstrate a slow rate of weight gain. In addition, milk removal may be suboptimal and inadequately stimulate maternal milk supply. Close observation of late preterm infants is essential.

Causes: Breastfed infants who have an insufficient milk intake during the early days may have an increase in serum unconjugated bilirubin because of an exaggerated enterohepatic circulation of bilirubin. Although this entity is called breastfeeding jaundice, a more appropriate term would be breast non-feeding jaundice because of lack of human milk intake.

Evaluation: Similar to that for insufficient milk syndrome, evaluation should include the monitoring of serum total, unconjugated, and conjugated bilirubin initially, then followed by total serum bilirubin serially. Other causes of jaundice (hemolytic, infection, metabolic) should be considered to ensure optimal overall management.

Management: Breastfeeding jaundice management includes the following strategies:

- *Establishment of good breastfeeding practices* that ensure adequate milk production and adequate intake of milk by the infant will prevent breastfeeding jaundice.
- *Objective measurement of bilirubin,* either with a reliable transcutaneous bilimeter or total serum bilirubin, is encouraged before discharge from the birth hospital. Plotting serum bilirubin on a bilirubin nomogram is helpful to predict future risk.
- *Follow up* of all breastfed infants should occur at 3 to 5 days after birth to assess general health, percent weight loss from birth, and breastfeeding efficacy, as well as for the presence of jaundice. Early detection of jaundice will allow for prompt attention to the issue, as well as address any breastfeeding issues that may contribute to the jaundice. This plan tends to support breastfeeding success.

- *Close monitoring of serum bilirubin* is necessary to determine when to initiate phototherapy and/or perform an exchange transfusion. Breastfed infants should follow the same criteria for intervention as formula-fed infants. AAP recommendations have been published on evaluation and management of hyperbilirubinemia.
- *Phototherapy,* if initiated, warrants thought on infant feeding. The infant can receive expressed breast milk, and depending on the circumstances, some clinicians permit breastfeeding. In severe hyperbilirubinemia, intensive phototherapy should be applied continuously to treat the infant in the shortest time interval, which is the least time for mother-baby separation. As soon as the bilirubin level declines, breastfeeding should continue. In the interim, the mother should be shown how to express her milk.

Breastmilk Jaundice

In many breastfed infants, serum unconjugated bilirubin concentrations will remain elevated, and in a few infants, this may last for as long as 6 to 12 weeks. In formula-fed infants, serum bilirubin levels decline, reaching values of less than 1.5 mg/dL by the 11th or 12th day after birth. In contrast, by week 3, 65% of normal, thriving breastfed infants have serum bilirubin concentrations greater than 1.5 mg/dL, and 30% will be clinically jaundiced. It has been suggested that the elevation in serum bilirubin may be protective against oxidative injury because bilirubin has been shown to be an effective antioxidant in vitro.

Signs and Symptoms: Because this is a normal response to breastfeeding, other than jaundice, the infants appear healthy and are thriving. The infants are growing normally and manifest no abnormal clinical signs suggesting hemolysis, infection, or metabolic disease.

Causes: Mature human milk contains an unidentified factor that enhances the intestinal absorption of bilirubin, resulting in breastmilk jaundice. As infant responses to the factor and/or maternal production of the factor probably diminishes over time and the infant's liver matures, serum bilirubin concentrations eventually return to normal.

Evaluation: The infant should be evaluated clinically. Total serum bilirubin or transcutaneous bilirubin measurement should be performed if clinically indicated. Unconjugated and conjugated bilirubin should be checked if jaundice persists. Other causes of prolonged unconjugated hyperbilirubinemia (including galactosemia, hypothyroidism, urinary tract infection, pyloric stenosis, low-grade hemolysis) should be considered in the appropriate clinical circumstances.

Management: Breastfeeding should be continued and encouraged, and parents should be reassured. Persistently increasing serum bilirubin levels may necessitate a diagnostic challenge by interrupting breastfeeding for 24 to 48 hours. Following interruption of breastfeeding, the serum bilirubin will decline markedly and not increase to prior levels with resumption of breastfeeding. If breastfeeding is interrupted, the mother should be encouraged and helped to maintain her milk supply. The mother may be reluctant to resume breastfeeding because of the association between breastfeeding and jaundice. Because of this, a positive attitude on the part of the health care professionals and assurance that this will not recur later may avoid termination of breastfeeding.

Appetite and/or Growth Spurts

Both appetite and growth spurts are common, but they may be interpreted as "transient lactational crises."

Signs and Symptoms: The infant acts hungrier than usual and may not be satisfied, leading the mother to believe her milk supply is insufficient and that she should start supplemental fluids or introduce complementary foods to satisfy her infant's appetite.

Causes: Approximately one third of breastfeeding mothers experience these "spurts" 1 or more times during lactation; most occur during the first 3 months of lactation (typically around 2–3 weeks, 6 weeks, and 3 months) and are of short duration.

Evaluation: History and physical examination are unchanged. Verify that no new medications that might diminish milk production have been introduced, such as oral contraceptives.

Management: Extra breastfeeding over a few days will stimulate an increased milk supply to enable the infant to resume a more normal feeding pattern. Anticipatory guidance regarding infant feeding patterns often prevents unnecessary supplementation and premature weaning. If the problem persists more than 3 or 4 days, the nursing dyad should be evaluated to determine the adequacy of the mother's milk supply and the infant's weight gain.

Nursing Refusal

Signs and Symptoms: An infant's sudden refusal to nurse, often called a nursing strike, can occur at any time and is often perceived by the mother as a personal rejection or rejection of the breastfeeding relationship, or as evidence that her milk is bad or inadequate. The mother frequently responds by weaning.

Causes: Nursing strikes are patterns of infant behavior that may be associated with the onset of the mother's menses; change in maternal diet; a change in maternal soap, perfume, or deodorant; or maternal stress. Infant nasal obstruction, gastroesophageal reflux, and teething also can cause nursing strikes. The older breastfeeding infant might suddenly refuse to nurse when the mother goes back to work, the infant is offered a bottle, or there is separation of the dyad. Occasionally, infants will refuse to feed from one breast. Sometimes this occurs after an episode of mastitis when the milk tastes slightly saltier. If the reason can be identified and changed, nursing will usually resume quickly.

Evaluation: History and physical examination are unchanged.

Management: When a baby refuses the breast, efforts to restore breastfeeding may take several days or longer. Infants may nurse more willingly when they are sleepy or just awakening. Other methods to reestablish the nursing relationship include making feeding special and quiet with no distractions; increasing the amount of cuddling and stroking, including skin-to-skin care; and using cobathing as a relaxation, reattachment strategy. Avoiding the bottle and using other methods of feeding, such as cup feeding, are often successful in overcoming breast refusal. Mothers should be advised to maintain their milk supply by manual or mechanical expression techniques so breast refusal is not compounded by insufficient maternal milk supply.

Ankyloglossia

Commonly known as tongue-tie, ankyloglossia is a congenital oral anomaly that may result in difficulty with suckling and could lead to sore nipples, low milk supply, poor weight gain, maternal fatigue, and frustration. It may affect breastfeeding more than bottle-feeding because of the differences in tongue movements between the feeding modalities.

Signs and Symptoms: The infant is unable to extend the tongue forward beyond the gum line, preventing compression of the nipple and areola, and reducing the effectiveness of the suckling effort. Milk intake may be low and the infant may become frustrated. Frantic suckling may traumatize the nipple. Maternal pain may lead to withdrawal of the breast and/or inhibition of milk letdown.

Cause: The cause of ankyloglossia is abnormally short and/or thick lingual frenulum.

Evaluation: Careful oral evaluation of the infant is needed, assessing the ability to extend the tongue beyond the lower gum border, observing for restriction of tongue mobility, and especially the ability to elevate the tongue. Digital oral assessment, including a finger sweep under the tongue, may be helpful in palpating the tight frenulum. The mother should be evaluated for nipple pain or evidence of nipple trauma. If impending lactation failure or maternal pain is present, a frenotomy should be performed in the hospital or office setting.

Management: The anterior portion of a tight or thick frenulum may be divided with scissors in a procedure called frenotomy. Anesthesia is not usually required and suturing is not necessary. The infant should be observed for bleeding from the site of division, although this is usually minimal or absent because the ligament binding the tongue is relatively avascular. The infant can be put to the breast right after the procedure.

Growth Patterns of Breastfed Infants

The conclusions drawn from plotting the growth of a breastfed infant may be erroneous if the growth chart does not adequately reflect the normal growth of the breastfeeding infant (Table 8-2).

Growth Charts

In 2010, the World Health Organization growth standards were adopted as the growth curves for children through the first 2 years of age by the Centers for Disease Control and Prevention and their use is endorsed by the AAP. The curves were derived from a multinational, multicultural prospective study of infants who were healthy and optimally breastfed. These curves are available on the Centers for Disease Control and Prevention Web site, and their use is considered standard of care for assessing the growth of all infants.

Growth Faltering

Concern should arise when the weight-for-age (or weight-for-length) changes by more than 2 standard deviations below the median (~5th percentile), or

Table 8-2. Average of Mean Values for Published Gains in Weight for Healthy Exclusively Breastfed Infants

Interval (mo)	Girls (g/d)	Boys (g/d)
0–1	30	33
1–2	28	34
2–3	22	23
3–4	19	20
4–5	15	16
5–6	13	14
6–7	12	11
7–8	10	12
8–9	8	9
9–10	11	10
10–11	8	6
11–12	7	9

Adapted with permission from Krebs NF, Reidinger CJ, Robertson AD, Hambidge KM. Growth and intakes of energy and zinc in infants fed human milk. *J Pediatr.* 1994;124:32–39; and Dewey KG, Heinig MJ, Nommsen LA, Peerson JM, Lönnerdal B. Growth of breast-fed and formula-fed infants from 0 to 18 months: the DARLING Study. *Pediatrics.* 1992;89:1035–1041.

the weight-for-age crosses more than 2 percentile channels downward on the growth chart. Nutritional assessment of the infant with slow weight gain or faltering linear growth includes an evaluation of milk supply and infant intake, appropriateness of complementary foods, intake of micronutrients (eg, zinc, vitamin D), and the feeding environment. The principles in the assessment of insufficient milk syndrome also should be considered for these infants.

Vitamin and Mineral Supplementation

Fat-Soluble Vitamins

Vitamin K
Deficiencies in vitamin K result in blood clotting difficulties and may cause early-, classic-, or late-onset neonatal hemorrhage in sites such as skin, mucous membrane, gastrointestinal tract, or brain. Vitamin K sufficiency depends on production by the intestinal flora. The intestinal flora of the breastfed infant produces relatively little vitamin K in the early weeks. The content of vitamin K in human milk is low. Vitamin K is supplemented

in infant formula. To ensure vitamin sufficiency and prevent hemorrhagic disease of the newborn, a single dose of vitamin K (0.5–1.0 mg intramuscularly) is given to all newborns near the time of delivery (see Chapter 2).

Vitamin D

Requirements for vitamin D can be met by sunlight exposure, but it is not possible to define what adequate sunlight exposure is for a given infant, and there is wide geographic and ethnic variation in endogenous vitamin D production. Furthermore, in recent years, concern about the risk for later skin cancer has led to the recommendation against sunlight exposure in all children and encouraging the use of sunscreen, which also reduces vitamin D production. An adequate intake of vitamin D for infants (400 IU/day) is not met with human milk alone or an intake of less than 1 L of infant formula. Cases of rickets in infants caused by inadequate vitamin D intake and limited exposure to sunlight have been reported. Thus, these infants, without supplemental vitamin D, are at increased risk for rickets. A dosage of 400 IU/day of vitamin D should be started by hospital discharge in all infants.

This should be continued while the infant is breastfed. Supplementation may be discontinued if the infant is consuming either 1 L of infant formula or vitamin D–fortified cow milk (after age 12 months). Maternal dietary supplementation does not preclude the need for infant vitamin D supplementation. Note that there are differences in vitamin D content among commercial preparations, so it is advised that the dose is ordered in units (400 IU) rather than in volume (mL).

Multivitamins

Multivitamins should be given to human milk-fed preterm infants. Routine multivitamin supplementation is not needed in breastfed term infants in most areas of the world. In many developing countries, vitamin A deficiency has been found in breastfed infants and children, and programs for periodic supplementation are recommended. Vitamin concentrations in human milk may be affected by maternal diet. Maternal malnutrition and alcoholism are situations where nutritional rehabilitation should include a multivitamin supplement for the mother. Mothers who follow a vegan diet do not receive adequate vitamin B_{12} from their diet, and this may result in low B_{12} concentrations in their milk. Their infants may present with vitamin B_{12} deficiency without obvious symptoms in the mother. Therefore, vegan mothers should receive a multivitamin supplement to ensure adequate availability of micronutrients. If the mother is supplemented, then water-soluble vitamin supplements do not need to be given to the infant.

Iron

Iron reserves at birth are a critical factor determining the risk for anemia during infancy. In normal full-term infants, who generally have adequate iron reserves, there is little risk for anemia with exclusive breastfeeding before 9 months of age, although biochemical indices of low iron status may occur in some between 6 and 9 months. Some infants may require supplementation with oral iron drops before 6 months to support iron stores. At about 6 months, iron should be given in the form of iron-containing or iron-fortified complementary foods, or iron drops can be given (1 mg/kg/day). Pureed meats are good sources of heme iron. Iron-fortified infant cereals contain less bioavailable iron but are still a moderate source of iron. The risk for iron deficiency, including anemia, is much greater in preterm or low-birth-weight infants because the iron stores at birth are smaller, because placental iron transfer occurs predominantly during the last trimester of pregnancy. Iron needs for such infants are likely to be best met by an iron supplement (2 mg/kg/day) beginning by 2 weeks of age, or when the infant is tolerating all feeds enterally. The dose of iron provided by liquid multivitamin preparations containing iron is not likely to meet the needs of the breastfed preterm infant. Treatment of iron deficiency should be undertaken with iron drops at a dosage of 2 to 4 mg/kg/day.

Fluoride

Supplementation of breastfed infants with fluoride is not recommended during the first 6 months. Thereafter, if the local water supply is less than 0.3 ppm, a supplement of 0.25 mg/day is recommended. Maternal fluoride intake does not affect the fluoride content of human milk.

Zinc

Zinc intake from human milk is marginally adequate by about 6 months of age, and infants are reliant on complementary foods or supplements. Preterm or low-birth-weight infants are at increased risk for development of zinc deficiency, typically manifest only by growth faltering.

More severe deficiency is associated with a characteristic peri-orificial dermatitis. Zinc is not included in liquid multivitamin preparations for infants. A liquid supplement can be compounded to provide 10 mg/mL elemental zinc; the dosage for supplementation is 1 mg/kg/day. Pureed meats or multiple-micronutrient–fortified infant cereals are excellent sources of zinc for the older infant receiving complementary foods.

Duration of Exclusive Breastfeeding

The AAP recommends that the preferred duration of exclusive breastfeeding is 6 months, a recommendation concurred to by the World Health Organization and the Institute of Medicine. Support for this recommendation is found in the differences in health outcomes of infants breastfed exclusively for 4 versus 6 months (see Table 2-2). The PROBIT study documented a reduction in gastrointestinal tract disease and improved cognitive outcomes in infants exclusively breastfed for 6 months compared with those exclusively breastfed for 3 to 4 months. A reduction in asthma and childhood leukemia has also been noted in infants breastfed exclusively for 6 months. Data on acute otitis media indicate greater protection with 6 months of exclusive breastfeeding.

Compared with infants who never breastfed, infants who were exclusively breastfed for 4 months and partially thereafter had a 35% lower risk for infection, whereas infants exclusively breastfed for 6 months had a 64% lower risk for infection. When compared with infants who exclusively breastfed for 6 months or longer, those exclusively breastfed for 4 to 6 months had a 4-fold increase in the risk for pneumonia. Furthermore, exclusively breastfeeding for 6 months extends the period of lactational amenorrhea, and thus may improve child spacing.

Complementary Feeding

The AAP is cognizant that for some infants, because of family and medical history, individual developmental status, and/or social and cultural dynamics, complementary feeding, including gluten-containing grains, is begun between 4 and 6 months of age. Breastfeeding is thought to be immunoprotective against the development of celiac disease, wheat allergy, islet cell autoimmune processes, and diabetes. Thus, when such complementary foods are introduced, it is advised that this be done while the infant is feeding only breast milk and not being exposed to cow milk protein in any form. Mothers should be encouraged to continue breastfeeding through the first year and beyond as more and varied complementary foods are introduced.

The timing of introduction of complementary foods into the diet of the breastfed infant is difficult to define with precision, and indeed there may not be a single optimal age for all infants. Most authorities recognize that many infants are developmentally ready to accept complementary foods before 6 months, but delaying introduction of solid food may be of benefit. Decisions about the introduction of complementary foods for individual infants need to be based on a number of considerations, including birth weight, postnatal growth rate, and developmental readiness. Infants who were born prematurely or small for gestational age may need micronutrients provided by complementary foods earlier, especially iron and zinc. Delaying the introduction of complementary foods beyond 6 months is not recommended because of increasing risk for micronutrient deficiencies and potentially increased risk for atopic disease.

Sleep Patterns

Lack of sleep, in mother and infant, is a frequent parental concern. Parent and physician expectations regarding sleep are shaped by cultural norms, which may not be based on normal physiology.

Mother

In early stages of establishing breastfeeding, it is important that the infant nurse at least 8 to 12 times per 24 hours, which implies feedings at least every 1.5 to 3 hours, including during the night. Mothers with continuous rooming-in during hospitalization sleep for the same duration as mothers whose infants are taken to the nursery. Once a mother's milk supply is well established, a single, longer sleep interval of about 4 hours may be possible for some term infants, but it is not the norm for exclusively breastfed infants in the first 2 to 3 months. The mother should be encouraged to sleep when the infant is sleeping.

Co-sleeping

The concern of nighttime feedings can be lessened by allowing the infant to co-sleep in close proximity, ideally on a separate sleep surface than the mother. This facilitates intermittent nursing throughout the night while leaving the mother's sleep relatively undisturbed. Some families may prefer a co-sleeper attachment to the bed or a bedside bassinet. Bed sharing, or sharing the same sleep surface with an infant, is a common sleeping arrangement for most of the world, including developed countries, and has beneficial effects on the success of breastfeeding. The AAP does not endorse such a sleeping arrangement because of concern for sudden infant death syndrome or sudden unexplained infant death (SUID). Families who choose to bed share should be made aware of the risks and recognize it may be hazardous under certain conditions. If a mother chooses to have her infant sleep in her bed to breastfeed, care should be taken to use a supine sleep position, avoid soft surfaces or loose covers, avoid waterbeds, and ensure that no entrapment possibilities exist. Adults (other than parents), children, or other siblings should avoid sharing a bed with an infant. Parents who choose to share a bed with their infant should not smoke or use substances which may impair arousal, such as alcohol or drugs (over the counter, prescription, or substances of abuse). Sleeping on a sofa or chair with an infant is dangerous and should be discouraged.

Dental Health

The risk for dental decay exists for the breastfed child as it does for the bottle-fed child. Early childhood dental caries results from a complicated combination of factors including genetics, general nutrition, preventive dental care, and the presence or absence of Streptococcus mutans, which usually is acquired from the mother or another adult through close oral contact. Breastfeeding has been implicated in the disease, but population-based studies do not support a definitive link between prolonged breast-feeding and dental caries. Children should see a dentist as early as 6 months and no later than 6 months after the first tooth erupts or 12 months of age (whichever comes first). Good dental hygiene is important for the breastfed infant, as it is for the formula-fed infant.

Infant Illness

Infant illness, such as upper or lower respiratory infection, otitis media, and gastroenteritis, is reduced overall if breastfeeding is maintained. Because of its low solute load, human milk enables the ill infant to maintain hydration despite fever, diarrhea, or other increased fluid losses. Continued breastfeed-ing helps lessen the severity and duration of the diarrhea and helps preserve gut mucosal integrity. With significant respiratory symptoms, an infant may feed better at the breast than with a bottle because the infant has more con-trol over the milk flow. Human milk can be expressed and fed through a syringe, small cup, or through a feeding tube if the infant is unable to suckle. In addition to the appropriateness of human milk for a sick infant, there is the added comfort of nursing because of the closeness with the mother.

Readmission to the Hospital

As breastfeeding rates have increased, so have readmissions for excessive weight loss, dehydration, hyperbilirubinemia, and hypernatremia that result from inappropriate breastfeeding routines and inadequate follow-up. During any hospitalization, efforts should be made to continue breastfeeding while supplying appropriate supplemental nutrition to the infant and providing lactation evaluation and interventions to recover successful breastfeeding. The milk supply should be increased through appropriate feeding routines and, if indicated, mechanical breast pumping or hand expression. Every effort should be made to keep the mother and infant together. When the breast-feeding mother requires hospitalization, efforts should also be made to continue the breastfeeding relationship either by having the newborn stay with the mother through the hospitalization or by bringing the newborn to the mother one or more times per day to complement mechanical milk expression (see Chapter 10).

Breastfeeding Guidance During Preventive Pediatric Health Care Visits

Lactation is a dynamic process, as is growth and development, so the practitioner should be mindful of the changing agenda at each follow-up visit. Incorporation of breastfeeding assessments, encouragement, and anticipatory guidance may enhance successful breastfeeding outcomes. A summary of key points for each follow-up visit from the first newborn office visit to 12 months of age is provided in Boxes 8-3 through 8-10.

Breastfeeding in the Second Year and Beyond

Breastfeeding should be continued, with appropriate complementary foods, for as long as the mother and infant mutually desire. In societies where children are allowed to nurse as long as they wish, they usually self-wean, without emotional trauma, between 3 and 4 years of age. Physicians may be surprised to discover that their patients are actually nursing much longer than they believe. Mothers may fail to disclose that they are continuing to nurse an older infant or child because they perceive that their physician may not approve of or support their continued breastfeeding.

The studies demonstrating advantages of breastfeeding for infants and mothers suggest that many of the benefits are directly related to the duration of breastfeeding. The composition of human milk does not change markedly from 12 to 24 months, including most nutrients and bioactive factors. Because the human immune system may not mature completely for several years, the constituents of human milk continue to support host defense of the infant. Breastfeeding also promotes comfort and caring. A strong attachment to the mother during the early years may have a positive neurobehavioral effect. Long-term breastfeeding seems to be a mutually positive experience for mother and child.

Box 8-3. Newborn Office Visit

Breastfeeding Assessment

- Review maternal prenatal and intrapartum records, and newborn recovery and transition records.
- Discuss timing and events of delivery and first feeding. Was it within 30 minutes of delivery?
- Has mother previously breastfed?
- How is mother doing and how is she feeling about breastfeeding?
- Have they been doing skin-to-skin care and cue-based feedings (often mothers prefer skin-to-skin continuously)?
- Is the newborn excessively sleepy and difficult to arouse for feedings?
- Does the newborn easily latch on to the breast and nurse eagerly?
- How many times has the newborn been to the breast within the first 24 to 48 hours?
- Is the newborn receiving any supplements?
- What is the number of wet diapers in the past 24 hours?
- What is the number of stools in the past 24 hours?
- Address any discomfort (or pain) mother may note.
- Is mother taking any medications?
- How do family members feel about breastfeeding?

Examination of the Newborn and Mother

- Obtain birth weight and gestational age.
- Evaluate neurobehavioral condition of the newborn.
- Calculate the newborn's weight gain or loss since birth.
- Perform newborn examination with attention to oral-motor examination.
- Assess state of hydration.
- Observe for jaundice and review objective values and risk zone of bilirubin.
- Observe breastfeeding.
- Teach mother techniques to hand express.
- Encourage mother to express concerns about breast changes during lactation; examine and refer as clinically necessary.

Anticipatory Guidance

- Explain normal newborn feeding behaviors.
- Review normal patterns of weight loss and gain using current growth standards.* (Older growth references may distort normal percentile.)
- Encourage breastfeeding on demand, approximately 8 to 12 times per 24 hours.
- Discuss the importance of exclusive human milk feedings until about 6 months of age.
- Discourage use of pacifiers and discuss potential risks.
- Review normal elimination patterns.
- Recommend baby receive 400 IU vitamin D daily as a supplement.

Box 8-3. Newborn Office Visit *(continued)*

Breastfeeding Interventions
- Supportive, nondisruptive care is important during the first 24 to 48 hours.
- Attempt to determine and treat the cause of inadequate milk supply before supplementing.
- Screen for maternal diabetes and other maternal illnesses that may affect milk production.
- Maintain lactation if mother and newborn are separated.
- Consider referral to lactation specialist if problems are ongoing.

Discharge Visit
- Validate parents on decision to breastfeed their baby.
- Review some of the benefits of exclusive breastfeeding.
- Remind mother to eat when hungry and drink when thirsty.
- Arrange for a pediatric follow-up visit in office or home within 48 hours after discharge or days 3 to 5 of life (sooner if indicated).
- Refer to community-based breastfeeding support groups or services.

*Centers for Disease Control and Prevention. WHO growth standards are recommended for use in U.S. for infants and children 0 to 2 years of age. Available at: http://www.cdc.gov/growthcharts/who_charts. htm. Updated September 9, 2010. Accessed December 3, 2012.

Adapted from Checklists for Breastfeeding Health Supervision. Elk Grove Village, IL: American Academy of Pediatrics; 2013.

Box 8-4. 48 to 72 Hours After Discharge

Breastfeeding Assessment
- What is the number of feedings in the past 24 hours?
- What is the number of wet diapers in the past 24 hours?
- What is the number and color of stools in the past 24 hours?
- Does the newborn need to be awakened to feed?
- Does the newborn easily latch on to the breast and nurse eagerly?
- Is the newborn receiving any supplements?
- How is mother doing and how is she feeling about breastfeeding?
- Address any discomfort (or pain) mother may note.
- Has mother experienced signs of increased milk production? If so, when? If not, explain the importance of monitoring mother and baby until this occurs.
- Is mother taking any medications?
- How is mother's nutrition?
- How do family members feel about breastfeeding?

Examination of the Newborn and Mother
- Calculate the newborn's weight gain or loss since birth (see Table 8-2).
- Observe breastfeeding.
- Encourage mother to express concerns about breast changes during lactation; examine and refer as clinically necessary.
- Perform routine newborn examination with attention to oral-motor examination.
- Assess state of hydration.
- Observe for jaundice and develop follow-up plan for bilirubin level in high- or intermediate-risk zone.

Anticipatory Guidance
- Discuss the importance of exclusive human milk feedings until about 6 months of age.
- Encourage breastfeeding on demand.
- Review normal breastfeeding patterns.
- Discourage use of pacifiers and discuss potential risks.
- Recommend sleeping within close proximity but avoid sharing same sleep surface.
- Avoid long nighttime intervals without feeding.
- Review normal elimination patterns.
- Reinforce the need to use vitamin D supplement.

Breastfeeding Interventions
- Attempt to determine and treat the cause of inadequate milk supply before supplementing.
- Consider referral to lactation specialist if problems are ongoing.
- Develop a support group or refer to an existing breastfeeding support group.

Closing the Visit
- Congratulate parents on decision to breastfeed their newborn.
- Review some of the benefits of breastfeeding.
- Remind mother to eat when hungry and drink when thirsty.
- Arrange for appropriate follow-up until weight gain is adequate and breastfeeding is going well.

Adapted from Checklists for Breastfeeding Health Supervision. Elk Grove Village, IL: American Academy of Pediatrics; 2013.

Box 8-5. 1-Month Office Visit

Breastfeeding Assessment
- What is the newborn's feeding pattern?
- What is the number of feedings per 24 hours?
- Is the newborn breastfeeding on demand?
- What is the number of wet diapers and stools per 24 hours?
- Is the newborn receiving any supplements?
- How is the mother feeling?
- How does the mother perceive her milk supply?
- Evaluate the mother's nutrition.
- How do family members feel about breastfeeding?

Examination of the Newborn and Mother
- Calculate the newborn's weight change since birth and previous visit (see Table 8-2).
- Newborn should be gaining 140 to 200 g (5–7 oz) per week.
- Observe breastfeeding if weight gain is inadequate or feeding is ineffective.
- Screen for maternal depression using standardized screening tools.
- Perform complete examination.

Anticipatory Guidance
- Discuss the importance of exclusive human milk feedings until about 6 months of age.
- Is the mother usually breastfeeding 8 to 12 times per 24 hours?
- Encourage unrestricted breastfeeding.
- Review normal patterns of nighttime feedings, typically 1 or 2 per night.
- Remind family about the importance of vitamin D supplementation.
- Discourage use of pacifiers and discuss potential risks.
- Explain change in normal stooling patterns.
- Review maternal nutrition.
- Discuss mother's plans to return to school or work.
- Explain techniques for expressing and storing human milk.
- Discuss common over-the-counter medications.

Breastfeeding Interventions
- Attempt to determine and treat the cause of inadequate milk supply before supplementing.
- Consider referral to lactation specialist if problems are ongoing.

Closing the Visit
- Commend mother on ongoing breastfeeding success.
- Review some of the benefits of breastfeeding.
- Encourage continued breastfeeding if baby is to be enrolled in a child care program (see Chapter 10).

Adapted from Checklists for Breastfeeding Health Supervision. Elk Grove Village, IL: American Academy of Pediatrics; 2013.

Box 8-6. 2-Month Office Visit

Breastfeeding Assessment
- What is baby's feeding pattern?
- Is baby content with feedings?
- Is baby breastfeeding on demand?
- Has baby had any feedings other than human milk?
- How does mother feel?
- How does mother perceive her milk supply?
- Is mother taking any medications?
- How is mother's nutrition?
- Is mother restricting any foods?
- How do family members feel about breastfeeding?

Examination of the Baby and Mother
- Calculate baby's weight change since birth and previous visit (see Table 8-2).
- Baby should be gaining 140 to 200 g (5–7 oz) per week.
- Observe breastfeeding if weight gain is inadequate or feeding is ineffective.
- Perform routine examination.

Anticipatory Guidance
- Discuss the importance of exclusive human milk feedings until about 6 months of age.
- Is mother usually breastfeeding 8 to 12 times per 24 hours?
- Encourage unrestricted breastfeeding.
- Review normal patterns of nighttime feedings, typically 1 or 2 per night.
- Stools may become less frequent in normally breastfeeding baby.
- Discuss breastfeeding baby who is teething.
- Review maternal nutrition.
- Discuss mother's plans to return to school or work.
- Explain techniques for expressing and storing human milk.
- Discuss common over-the-counter medications.

Breastfeeding Interventions
- Attempt to determine and treat the cause of inadequate milk supply before supplementing.
- Consider referral to lactation specialist if problems are ongoing.

Closing the Visit
- Commend mother on ongoing breastfeeding success.
- Review the benefits of continued exclusive breastfeeding for about 6 months.
- Encourage continued breastfeeding if baby is to be enrolled in a child care program (see Chapter 10).

Adapted from Checklists for Breastfeeding Health Supervision. Elk Grove Village, IL: American Academy of Pediatrics; 2013.

Box 8-7. 4-Month Office Visit

Breastfeeding Assessment
- What is baby's feeding pattern?
- Is baby content with feedings?
- Is baby breastfeeding on demand?
- Is baby's longest sleep period at night? If not, when?
- Has baby had any feedings other than human milk? If so, what?
- How does mother perceive her milk supply?
- Is mother taking any medications?
- How is mother's nutrition?
- How do family members feel about breastfeeding?

Examination of the Baby and Mother
- Calculate baby's weight change since birth and previous visit (see Table 8-2).
- Baby should be gaining 140 to 200 g (5–7 oz) per week.
- Observe breastfeeding if weight gain is inadequate, feeding is ineffective, or mother has concerns.
- Perform routine examination.
- Screen for maternal depression using standardized screening tools.

Anticipatory Guidance
- Is mother usually breastfeeding 6 to 12 times per day at 4 months of age?
- Discuss the importance of exclusive human milk feedings until about 6 months of age.
- Encourage unrestricted breastfeeding.
- Review normal patterns of nighttime feedings, typically 1 or 2 per night.
- Discuss potential for iron supplement.
- Stools may become less frequent in normally breastfeeding baby.
- Discuss breastfeeding baby during teething.
- Discuss the increasing distractibility of baby during feedings.
- Review maternal nutrition.
- Discuss mother's plans to return to school or work.
- Explain techniques for expressing and storing human milk.
- Discuss common over-the-counter medications.

Breastfeeding Interventions
- Attempt to determine and treat the cause of inadequate milk supply before supplementing.
- If baby is gaining weight and mother is satisfied with feeding behavior, interventions usually are not indicated.

Closing the Visit
- Commend mother on ongoing breastfeeding success.
- Review some of the benefits of breastfeeding.

Adapted from Checklists for Breastfeeding Health Supervision. Elk Grove Village, IL: American Academy of Pediatrics; 2013.

Box 8-8. 6-Month Office Visit

Breastfeeding Assessment
- What is baby's feeding pattern?
- Is baby content with feedings?
- Is baby's longest sleep period at night? If not, when?
- Has baby had any feedings other than human milk? If so, what?
- How does mother perceive her milk supply?
- Is mother taking any medications?
- How is mother's nutrition?
- How do family members feel about breastfeeding?

Examination of the Baby and Mother
- Calculate baby's weight change since birth and previous visit (see Table 8-2).
- Assess weight gain using current growth standards.
- Observe breastfeeding if weight gain is inadequate, feeding is ineffective, or mother has concerns.
- Complete examination.
- Screen for maternal depression using standardized screening tools.

Anticipatory Guidance
- Is mother usually breastfeeding 6 to 12 times per 24 hours?
- Review importance of continued breastfeeding.
- Discuss readiness for introduction of complementary foods.
- Discuss importance of iron-containing foods.
- Offer expressed human milk or supplemental fluids in a cup.
- Discuss the increasing distractibility of baby during feedings.
- Discuss breastfeeding baby during teething.
- Introduce fluoride supplement if indicated.
- Review maternal nutrition.
- Recommend that mother obtain routine breast examination from her physician.

Breastfeeding Interventions
- If baby is gaining weight and mother is satisfied with feeding behavior, interventions usually are not indicated.

Closing the Visit
- Commend mother on ongoing breastfeeding success, especially if baby was exclusively breastfed for 6 months.
- Review some of the benefits of continued breastfeeding for at least a year and beyond.

Adapted from Checklists for Breastfeeding Health Supervision. Elk Grove Village, IL: American Academy of Pediatrics; 2013.

Box 8-9. 9-Month Office Visit

Breastfeeding Assessment
- What is baby's feeding pattern?
- Is baby's longest sleep period at night? If not, when?
- What other foods does baby take?
- Is mother taking any medications?
- How is mother's nutrition?
- How do family members feel about breastfeeding?

Examination of the Baby and Mother
- Calculate baby's weight change since birth and previous visit (see Table 8-2).
- Assess weight gain using current growth standards.
- Observe breastfeeding if weight gain is inadequate, feeding is ineffective, or mother has concerns.
- Perform complete examination.
- Obtain hematocrit or hemoglobin measurement.

Anticipatory Guidance
- Is mother usually breastfeeding fewer than 6 to 8 times per 24 hours?
- Review importance of continued breastfeeding.
- Discuss importance of iron-containing foods.
- Offer expressed human milk or supplemental fluids in a cup.
- Discuss breastfeeding baby during teething.
- Discuss behavior of older breastfeeding baby, including nursing strikes.
- Discuss new communication skills that relate to breastfeeding behaviors.
- Discuss possible pressure to wean by family or friends.
- Discuss benefits of long-term breastfeeding.
- Review maternal nutrition.
- Recommend that mother obtain routine breast examination from her physician.

Breastfeeding Interventions
- If baby is gaining weight and mother is satisfied with feeding behavior, interventions usually are not indicated.

Closing the Visit
- Commend mother on ongoing breastfeeding success, especially if baby was exclusively breastfed for 6 months.
- Review the benefits of continued breastfeeding.

Adapted from Checklists for Breastfeeding Health Supervision. Elk Grove Village, IL: American Academy of Pediatrics; 2013.

Box 8-10. 12-Month Office Visit and Beyond

12-Month Office Visit

Breastfeeding Assessment
- What is baby's feeding pattern?
- Is baby's longest sleep period at night? If not, when?
- What other foods does baby take?
- Is mother taking any medications?
- How is mother's nutrition?
- How do family members feel about breastfeeding?

Examination of the Baby and Mother
- Calculate baby's weight change since birth and previous visit (see Table 8-2).
- Complete examination.
- Consider obtaining hematocrit or hemoglobin measurement, if indicated.
- Observe breastfeeding if weight gain is inadequate, feeding is ineffective, or mother has concerns.

Anticipatory Guidance
- Is mother usually breastfeeding 4 to 8 times per 24 hours?
- Review importance of continued breastfeeding.
- Discuss importance of iron-containing foods and introducing a wide variety of foods and flavors.
- Offer expressed human milk or supplemental fluids in a cup.
- Discuss breastfeeding baby during teething.
- Discuss behavior of older breastfeeding baby.
- Discuss new communication skills that relate to breastfeeding behaviors.
- Discuss possible pressure to wean by family or friends.
- If weaning is desired, discuss appropriate weaning techniques.
- Review maternal nutrition.
- Recommend that mother obtain routine breast examination from her physician.

Breastfeeding Interventions
- Provide indicated support or intervention.

Closing the Visit
- Commend mother on successfully breastfeeding for 12 months.
- Review some of the benefits of breastfeeding a toddler.

15 Months, 18 Months, 2 Years, and Older
- Breastfeeding support and anticipatory guidance should continue to be included in well-child visits as long as mother and child continue to breastfeed.

Adapted from Checklists for Breastfeeding Health Supervision. Elk Grove Village, IL: American Academy of Pediatrics; 2013.

Weaning

Weaning can mean either the beginning of a process of gradual introduction of complementary feedings and decreased breastfeeding or the complete cessation of breastfeeding. Weaning is a complex process involving nutritional, microbiological, immunologic, biochemical, and psychological adjustments.

Infant-Led Weaning

Easily confused with a nursing strike, the reasons commonly cited when infants attempt to wean from the breast include inadequate milk supply (eg, because of illness, return to work) and infant illness.

Mother-Led Weaning

Mother-led weaning should be done gradually by replacing one feeding at a time with solids, a bottle, or a cup, depending on the infant's age and stage of development. The bedtime breastfeeding is often the last to be eliminated. Occasionally, sudden weaning is necessary because of severe illness in the mother or prolonged separation of the mother and infant. Mothers should use manual or mechanical methods of milk expression to relieve breast fullness; wear a supportive, comfortable bra; and be alert to signs of a plugged duct or breast infection. Other measures, such as cold compresses, may help in reducing engorgement. Rapid weaning may increase the mother's risk for development of mastitis. The infant should receive extra cuddling and holding, as should the mother.

Selected References

1. American Academy of Pediatrics. Policy statement: SIDS and other sleep-related infant deaths: expansion of recommendations for a safe infant sleeping environment. *Pediatrics.* 2011;128:1030–1039

2. American Academy of Pediatrics Quality Improvement Innovation Network. *Safe & Healthy Beginnings: A Resource Toolkit for Hospitals and Physicians' Offices [CD-ROM].* Elk Grove Village, IL: American Academy of Pediatrics; 2009

3. American Academy of Pediatrics Committee on Fetus and Newborn. Controversies concerning vitamin K and the newborn. *Pediatrics.* 2003;112:191–192

4. American Academy of Pediatrics Section on Dentistry. Oral health risk assessment timing and establishment of the dental home. *Pediatrics.* 2003;111:1113–1116

5. American Academy of Pediatrics Section on Pediatric Dentistry and Oral Health. Preventive oral health intervention for pediatricians. *Pediatrics.* 2008;122:1387–1394

6. American Academy of Pediatrics Subcommittee on Hyperbilirubinemia. Management of hyperbilirubinemia in the newborn infant 35 or more weeks of gestation. *Pediatrics.* 2004;114:297–316

7. American Academy of Pediatrics Work Group on Breastfeeding. *Checklists for Breastfeeding Health Supervision: Breastfeeding Promotion in Pediatric Office Practices.* Elk Grove Village, IL: American Academy of Pediatrics; 1999

8. Baker RD, Greer FR; American Academy of Pediatrics Committee on Nutrition. Deficiency anemia in infants and young children (0–3 years of age). *Pediatrics.* 2010;126:1040–1050

9. Black LS. Incorporating breastfeeding care into daily newborn rounds and pediatric office practice. *Pediatr Clin North Am.* 2001;48:299–319

10. Chantry CJ, Nommsen-Rivers LA, Peerson JM, Cohen RJ, Dewey KG. Excess weight loss in first-born breastfed newborns relates to maternal intrapartum fluid balance. *Pediatrics.* 2011;127:e171–e179

11. Dewey KG. Nutrition, growth, and complementary feeding of the breastfed infant. *Pediatr Clin North Am.* 2001;48:87–104

12. Gartner LM, Herschel M. Jaundice and breastfeeding. *Pediatr Clin North Am.* 2001;48:389–399

13. Gartner LM, Greer FR; American Academy of Pediatrics Section on Breastfeeding and Committee on Nutrition. Prevention of rickets and vitamin D deficiency: new guidelines for vitamin D intake. *Pediatrics.* 2003;111:908–910

14. Grummer-Strawn LJ, Reinold C, Kreb NF, Centers for Disease Control and Prevention. Use of World Health Organization and CDC growth charts for children aged 0–59 months in the United States. *MMWR Recomm Rep.* 2010;59:RR-9

15. Hagan JF, Shaw JS, Duncan PM, eds. *Bright Futures: Guidelines for Health Supervision of Infants, Children, and Adolescents.* 3rd ed. Elk Grove Village, IL: American Academy of Pediatrics; 2008

16. Institute of Medicine. *Dietary Reference Intakes for Calcium, Phosphorus, Magnesium, Vitamin D, and Fluoride.* Washington, DC: National Academy Press; 1997

17. American Academy of Pediatrics Committee on Nutrition. *Pediatric Nutrition Handbook.* Kleinman RE, ed. 6th ed. Elk Grove Village, IL: American Academy of Pediatrics; 2009

18. Kramer MS, Guo T, Platt RW, et al. Infant growth and health outcomes associated with 3 compared with 6 mo of exclusive breastfeeding. *Am J Clin Nutr.* 2003;78:291–295

19. Kramer MS, Kakuma R. The optimal duration of exclusive breastfeeding: a systematic review. *Adv Exp Med Biol.* 2004;554:63–77

20. Kreiter SR, Schwartz RP, Kirkman HN Jr, Charlton PA, Calikoglu AS, Davenport ML. Nutritional rickets in African American breast-fed infants. *J Pediatr.* 2000;137:153–157

21. Neifert MR. Prevention of breastfeeding tragedies. *Pediatr Clin North Am.* 2001;48:273–297

22. Neifert M, Bunik M. Overcoming clinical barriers to exclusive breastfeeding. *Pediatr Clin North Am.* 2013;60:115–145

23. Noel-Weiss J, Woodend AK, Peterson WE, Gibb W, Groll DL. An observational study of associations among maternal fluids during parturition, neonatal output, and breastfed newborn weight loss. *Int Breastfeed J.* 2011;6:9

24. Powers NG. How to assess slow growth in the breastfed infant. Birth to 3 months. *Pediatr Clin North Am.* 2001;48:345–363

25. Quillan SI, Glenn LL. Interaction between feeding method and co-sleeping on maternal-newborn sleep. *J Obstet Gynecol Neonatal Nurs.* 2004;33:580–588

26. Valentine CJ, Wagner CL. Nutritional management of the breastfeeding dyad. *Pediatr Clin North Am.* 2013;60:261–274

27. Wagner CL, Greer FR; American Academy of Pediatrics Section on Breastfeeding and Committee on Nutrition. Prevention of rickets and vitamin D deficiency in infants, children, and adolescents. *Pediatrics.* 2008;122:1142–1152

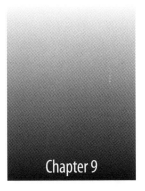

Chapter 9

Maintenance of Breastfeeding—The Mother

Support for the breastfeeding mother continues beyond the immediate postpartum period. The obstetric care professional should assess the breasts at various postpartum visits and be aware of the evaluation and management of various maternal problems and complications related to lactation.

Postpartum Visits

Routine Obstetric Visit

The mother's routine follow-up visit to her obstetric care professional is typically scheduled for 4 to 6 weeks postpartum. Obstetric care professionals should encourage the mother to bring the baby to this visit.

Assess Breastfeeding

Information about perceived breastfeeding problems or concerns of the mother can be elicited. This visit is an ideal time to observe the infant breastfeeding, specifically assessing position, latch, and milk transfer.

Provide Support

Obstetric support for the patient's decision to breastfeed has been shown to improve breastfeeding continuation. This is an ideal time to praise the success of her breastfeeding experience and allow the patient to explore any of her concerns.

Breast Examination

The provider should perform a breast examination to evaluate any signs of trauma, infection, or breast masses. It may be helpful to have the mother nurse her infant prior to the examination to decrease engorgement of tissue that could obscure physical examination findings. The obstetric care professional *should* also encourage continuation of breastfeeding and point out *benefits* of exclusive breastfeeding *during the first 6 months*. The patient also should be advised to continue her regular breast self-examinations and report any unusual findings to her health care professional.

Plans for Return to Work

The provider should discuss plans for the new mother to return to work outside the home at this visit, including options for feeding and milk expression. Milk expression should begin before return to work so that there is an adequate supply of stored milk to allow for daily variations in the amount of milk consumed by the infant (see Chapter 10). It should be noted that in 2010, the Patient Protection and Affordable Care Act ("Affordable Care Act") amended section 7 of the Fair Labor Standards Act (FLSA) to require employers to provide reasonable break time for an employee to express human milk for her nursing child for 1 year after the child's birth. Employers are also required to provide a place, other than a bathroom, that is shielded from view and free from intrusion from coworkers and the public.

Resources

Mothers should be provided names and phone numbers of local resources who can provide lactation advice on a 24-hour-a-day basis. Mothers also should know of peer support groups with contact information and be encouraged to participate (see the Appendix).

Postcesarean Delivery

If the mother has undergone a cesarean delivery, she may have an earlier visit than the typical 4- to 6-week postpartum interval. Although this visit is primarily focused on detecting surgical complications, it is well timed to assist with any early breastfeeding complaints, especially because mothers with cesarean deliveries may have more difficulty establishing and sustaining lactation.

Maternal Breastfeeding Issues—Short Term

Nipple pain and engorgement are the most frequent complaints of lactating women and may present early in the immediate postpartum period but also may arise at any time in lactation.

Nipple Pain

Assessment of breastfeeding technique and latch is the most important part of prevention and early management of nipple pain and skin breakdown. A detailed history of the onset of pain, location, and timing is important. Differential diagnosis includes simple irritation, abrasion, chapping, contact dermatitis, infection, and nipple vasospasm. No specific topical agent has been shown to provide relief superior to expressed breast milk applied to the nipple after feeding.

Nipple Bacterial Infections

Infection is one cause of nipple pain beyond the immediate postpartum period. As with any defect in the skin, a nipple crack or abrasion is likely to grow *Staphylococcus aureus*. Treatment with topical antibiotic ointment as well as local wound care often bring relief in a matter of days.

Nipple Candida Infections

A usual source of nipple infections is thrush in the infant.

Symptoms: Superficial nipple/skin infections caused by *Candida* may present with nipple pain, itching, or pinkness of the skin.

Causes: Predisposing factors for *Candida* infections of the breast include nipple trauma, antibiotic use, diabetes, steroid use, and immune deficiency. Some experts have noted the association of *Candida* with the use of plastic-lined breast pads, which keep the nipples moist.

Evaluation: *Candida* nipple infections can be treated based on clinical symptomatology alone if no other diagnosis is apparent. It is difficult to prove that *Candida* is the causative organism in many situations. Because yeast is ubiquitous, cultures of skin surfaces may represent skin flora and be positive even in asymptomatic mothers. Milk or skin surface cultures for *Candida*, therefore, are not helpful and are not performed routinely.

Management: Treatment of superficial nipple infections caused by *Candida* should be undertaken by treating the mother and infant simultaneously when either of them is symptomatic. The mother's partner also may need treatment. Therapies include:

- *Antifungal therapy.* A variety of effective antifungal agents are available. Typically, mothers are treated with a topical antifungal agent, such as ketoconazole, nystatin, or miconazole. The antifungal cream is applied to the mother's breast after feeding. An antifungal solution, such as Nystatin suspension, is swabbed on the inside of the infant's inner cheeks and tongue after feeding. The infant's diaper area also may need treatment. This therapy is usually continued for 14 days or at least several days after symptoms have resolved.
- *Gentian violet.* Other topical treatment options include the use of 0.25% to 1% gentian violet swabbed on the affected areas for up to 3 days. Gentian violet may cause permanent staining of clothing, temporary violet discoloration of the infant's mouth, and occasionally irritation, oral ulceration, stomatitis, nausea, vomiting, or diarrhea.
- *Oral fluconazole* may be prescribed for the mother if the nipples are not significantly better after several days of topical treatment or if symptoms persist or worsen. The infant may also require oral fluconazole in cases of recurrent or intractable oral candidiasis.
- *Additional management.* Any objects in contact with the infant's mouth (pacifiers, nipples) or the mother's breast (breast pump equipment) should be washed in hot, soapy water and boiled daily. Clothing, such as bras and blouses, should be laundered using a dilute bleach solution or dried in sunlight daily. If used, disposable nursing pads are preferred. Leaving the breasts exposed to air and applying good wound care principles may assist with rapid healing. Other sites of yeast infection also should be checked, such as yeast vaginitis or tinea cruris in her partner and diaper rash in the infant. Regardless of the treatment regimen used, the mother should be instructed on appropriate hygiene to prevent reinfection.

Engorgement

Swelling and distention that results from ineffective drainage of the breast, engorgement usually occurs around the time milk production increases, approximately 3 to 7 days postpartum (see Chapter 7). Engorgement also may occur later in the course of breastfeeding related to a missed feeding or an abrupt change in feeding frequency. Engorgement should not be confused with a plugged duct, which can result in a localized lump or cord in one area of the breast, or with mastitis, which can result in fever, systemic flu-like symptoms, and an elevated white blood cell count (see Table 9-1). Engorgement may be the result of infrequent or ineffective nursing from causes such as sore nipples, a sleepy infant, or mother-infant separation.

The breast must be examined to rule out related problems such as plugged ducts or mastitis. If left untreated, engorgement can lead to difficulties in properly latching the infant to the breast and to mastitis. The best treatment of engorgement is prevention. Frequent breastfeeding or pumping of the breasts (8–12 times per day from both breasts) is the best way to prevent engorgement.

Plugged Ducts (Milk Stasis)

Symptoms: A plugged duct is a localized blockage of milk, frequently presenting as a painful knot in the breast. This lump may decrease in size with nursing.

Causes: This condition may be caused by an abrupt change in the feeding schedule, inadequate draining of the breast, failure to vary nursing positions, wearing of tight and constricting clothing (eg, a poorly fitting underwire bra), or sleep position. Especially when the condition recurs in the same breast segment, the cause may be anatomic variations leading to plugged ducts. Rarely, what is considered a plugged duct may be a tumor, benign or malignant, that is blocking the duct.

Evaluation: Plugged ducts are easily differentiated from engorgement and mastitis because blockage is not associated with fever or other signs of

Table 9-1. Comparison of Findings of Engorgement, Plugged Duct, and Mastitis

Characteristics	Engorgement	Plugged Duct	Mastitis
Onset	Gradual, immediately postpartum	Gradual, after feedings	Sudden, after 10 days
Site	Bilateral	Unilateral	Usually unilateral
Swelling and heat	Generalized	May shift; little or no heat	Localized, red, hot, swollen
Pain	Generalized	Mild, but localized	Intense, but localized
Body temperature	<38.4°C (101°F)	<38.4°C	>38.4°C
Systemic symptoms	Feels well	Feels well	Flu-like symptoms

Adapted with permission from *Breastfeeding: A Guide for the Medical Professional.* 6th ed. Lawrence RA, Lawrence RM. Elsevier, Mosby, Philadelphia, PA; 2005:563..

systemic illness (see Table 9-1). If the plugged duct does not resolve within 48 to 72 hours or if fever develops, the patient should be seen and evaluated by a health care professional.

Management: The treatment for plugged ducts is to apply moist heat prior to feeding and massage the affected area before and during nursing. If possible, start feedings with the affected breast first. Attempt different positions to allow better drainage of the particular part of the breast that is affected, pointing the infant's nose in the direction of the blockage. Ensure that the breast tissue is not being compressed, such as indenting the breast with the finger(s) to provide an airway space for the infant.

Mastitis

Typically defined as a unilateral bacterial infection of the breast, mastitis occurs in 2% to 3% of lactating women.

Symptoms: Mastitis most commonly presents as a single area of localized warmth, tenderness, edema, and erythema in one breast more than 10 days after delivery. The highest incidence occurs in the second and third weeks postpartum. Depending on the severity of the infection, the area of inflammation can range from a few centimeters to almost the entire breast. Mastitis may present with a sudden onset of breast pain, myalgia, and fever that can be dramatic. Sometimes mastitis presents with flu-like symptoms such as fatigue, nausea, vomiting, fever, and headache.

Causes: The infection commonly enters through a break in the skin, usually a cracked nipple. However, milk stasis and congestion resulting from engorgement, or plugged ducts, also can lead to mastitis. Fifty percent of causative organisms are penicillin-resistant *S aureus*. Other organisms seen are *Escherichia coli*, Group A *streptococcus, Peptostreptococcus, Haemophilus influenzae, Klebsiella pneumoniae,* and *Bacteroides.*

Evaluation: Perform a careful examination of the breast to verify the diagnosis and to rule out abscess formation. Clinicians should be aware of resistant organisms in their community and should order a human milk culture and antibiotic sensitivities when women with mastitis are unresponsive to first-line treatment.

Management: Mastitis needs to be treated as soon as it is discovered. The following steps should be taken:

* *Prescribe an antibiotic* that is effective against penicillin-resistant Staphylococcus and administer a 10- to 14-day course. Safe antibiotics

for therapy include first-generation cephalosporins or dicloxacillin. If the patient is allergic to penicillin, erythromycin and its derivatives are also effective. Choose alternative therapies if methicillin-resistant *S aureus* is suspected.

- *Instruct the mother to continue nursing* because the milk is not harmful to the infant. Frequent feeding is recommended. If the mother can tolerate feeding on the affected breast first, this is preferable. However, if this is too painful, the mother may begin on the unaffected breast until symptoms subside. The affected breast should be drained at each feeding by nursing, pumping, or both. In an occasional circumstance, manual expression or a breast pump may be needed to remove the milk from the breast because of more severe pain prohibiting breastfeeding. Weaning should not be recommended during mastitis and may predispose the mother to developing a breast abscess.
- *Encourage fluid intake* to ensure hydration.
- *Recommend bed rest* until the mother's fever has subsided for at least 24 hours. She can have the baby with her and should seek help from family members.
- *Analgesics.* Symptomatic relief can be achieved with mild analgesics (acetaminophen or ibuprofen), warm or cold packs (whatever works best), and a supportive bra.

Severe cases of mastitis that do not respond rapidly to outpatient therapy will require admission to the hospital and parenteral therapy.

Recurrent and/or Chronic Mastitis

Symptoms: Recurrent or chronic mastitis share the same symptoms as acute mastitis but persist beyond treatment.

Causes: Recurrent or chronic mastitis usually results from incomplete treatment of mastitis or the use of an ineffective antibiotic. Patients with mastitis typically feel improved after only a short course of antibiotics and should be counseled to comply with the entire duration of therapy. Another cause of recurrent mastitis is a failure to treat underlying predisposing factors such as persistent nipple trauma and fissuring or an obstructive lesion.

Evaluation: In cases of recurrent infection, a thorough breast examination should be performed after resolution of infection to rule out any underlying solid or cystic masses. An ultrasound examination also may be useful.

Management: A midstream culture of expressed milk may prove helpful for diagnosis and management, particularly for recurrent cases due to uncommon pathogens or antibiotic resistance. Generally, midstream milk cultures do not grow pathogens. The patient should be counseled on compliance with a full 2-week course of therapy, and any potential predisposing factors should be addressed. In some circumstances, a longer course of antibiotics may be needed.

Breast Abscess

A breast abscess is a walled-off area of the breast that contains purulent material; it occurs in 5% to 11% of women with mastitis.

Symptoms: The presenting signs and symptoms are similar to mastitis with the added finding of a defined tense or fluctuant mass in the breast. Persistent symptoms of mastitis after 48 to 72 hours of therapy should prompt investigation for a possible underlying abscess.

Causes: If mastitis is not promptly treated or treatment is not adequate, abscess formation is possible.

Evaluation: The breast should be carefully evaluated to rule out other causes of a breast mass.

Management: Prompt treatment with incision and drainage, antibiotics, and complete draining of the breast every few hours is required. In these cases, the abscess fluid should be cultured so that the appropriate antibiotic can be prescribed. In some cases, hospitalization and parenteral antibiotics will be necessary. Feeding from the contralateral breast can be continued with the term healthy infant. Feeding from the affected breast will depend on practical considerations. If the incision can be made far enough from the areola to allow successful latch, then breastfeeding on the affected breast can be undertaken. If there is no breastfeeding, milk must be emptied via mechanical or manual methods. Sometimes applying pressure over the incision with sterile dressing during feeding or pumping helps avoid a fistula.

Postpartum Mood Changes— Postpartum Blues and Depression

Postpartum blues or mild depression is a common condition following childbirth, estimated to occur in up to 85% of new mothers. From 10% to 15% of women experience moderate to severe postpartum depression. Postpartum psychosis is less common, occurring in 0.1% to 0.2% of women. Because these conditions may affect not only the health of the woman but also the care of her child(ren), including breastfeeding, their acknowledgment and treatment are important.

Symptoms: Postpartum blues are transient and are characterized by mild sadness or weepiness. Symptoms of postpartum depression mimic other types of depression and may include changes in sleep patterns, appetite changes, fatigue, sadness, hopelessness, apathy, or persistent crying. In rare cases, symptoms may be severe and involve thoughts of harming self or infant, or an inability to care for self or infant, signaling postpartum psychosis.

Causes: Postpartum mood changes may be caused by sudden hormonal changes, fatigue, stress, sleep deprivation, or a combination of these factors. Risk factors for the development of depression include prior history of depression, prior postpartum depression, positive family history, and adjustment difficulties related to childbirth. Medical problems, such as hypothyroidism, should be considered.

Evaluation: Symptoms and coping mechanisms should be discussed with the patient.

Management: Transient or mild mood changes require support. If the new mother's symptoms do not resolve rapidly, she should be referred to her mental health care professional for further assistance. Depending on the severity of the condition, pharmacologic therapy may be required. If pharmacologic therapy is needed, antidepressants and selective serotonin reuptake inhibitors can be used during lactation (see Chapter 12).

Maternal Breastfeeding Issues—Long Term

Maternal Illness

A breastfeeding mother with an illness, whether it is acute or chronic, often finds that advice regarding breastfeeding during illness is inconsistent among medical professionals. Factors to consider include whether lactation worsens the mother's illness, whether milk composition or supply will be affected, and whether the infant will be affected by the mother's illness or medication use. The answer to all these questions is usually no, and breastfeeding may proceed. The providers involved in the mother's care should communicate fully to ensure the best and most consistent advice and management.

Acute Illness

During an immediate postpartum illness the infant should be allowed to room-in with the mother, or at least be brought to her for breastfeeding at frequent intervals. The mother's milk supply should be established and maintained through continued breastfeeding or breast pumping. Most acute illnesses (ie, maternal respiratory infections, gastroenteritis) are compatible with breastfeeding, and breastfeeding can provide the infant with protective antibodies. Interruption of breastfeeding at the time of onset of maternal symptoms may increase the risk of the child developing the infection.

Chronic Illness

A chronic illness may have a greater effect on a mother's ability to breastfeed because of changes in her own functioning, changes in milk supply, and the possible adverse effects of her medications on the infant. Mothers should be given information regarding the risks and benefits of breastfeeding to herself and her infant. Most chronic illnesses are compatible with breastfeeding, and breastfeeding can be one activity that helps normalize the mother's experience with her infant (see Chapter 16).

Diagnostic Studies

Tests performed to aid in diagnosis, especially those that require radioisotopes, may necessitate temporary "pump and dump" strategies to protect the infant (see Chapter 16).

Surgery and Anesthesia

When a nursing mother is required to have surgery, either urgently or electively, the patient and her health care professional should consider options for anesthesia and postoperative analgesia that meet the mother's health and comfort needs and have little effect on the breastfeeding infant (see Chapters 6 and 12). Hospital policies and support should encourage and be compatible with lactation maintenance, particularly if the procedure dictates a prolonged hospital stay. When possible, arrangements should be made for pumping and storage of milk before and after the procedure in the case of a prolonged separation. Postoperatively, the mother should pump or feed at least every 3 hours to maintain her milk supply and avoid engorgement.

Maternal Nutrition During Lactation

The assessment of maternal nutritional status is important to ensure the adequacy of the diet. In adequately nourished women, additional caloric intake and fluid intake do not enhance milk volume. Overall, the quality of milk is maintained over a wide spectrum of maternal diet, although specific components may be affected by maternal intake and nutritional status.

Fluid Intake

Milk volume is not affected by the amount of fluid intake during lactation. Breastfeeding women should drink to satisfy their thirst. Mothers are encouraged to drink fluids and to note whether their urine is pale yellow, indicative of adequate fluid intake. Inadequate fluid intake also may be associated with constipation.

Energy Intake

The Dietary Reference Intake for energy during the first 6 months of lactation is an additional 500 kcal per day above the usual diet appropriate for the woman's height, normal weight, and level of activity. From 7 to 9 months of lactation, the energy intake declines to an additional 400 kcal per day. When sufficient calories are not consumed, the mother's own nutrient reserves are affected. Intakes less than 1,500 kcal per day may cause maternal fatigue and lower milk volume.

Nutrient Intake

Specific nutrient needs generally are higher in lactation than in pregnancy (see Table 9-2). The milk contents for many nutrients are unrelated to maternal intake. Milk concentrations of water-soluble vitamins, however, reflect maternal intake, and a normal diet provides adequate vitamin levels. Strict vegetarians (vegans) who avoid all animal products are at risk for vitamin B_{12} deficiency and should be advised to take a vitamin B_{12} supplement. If the mother's vitamin B_{12} stores are depleted, her milk will also be low in this nutrient, and vitamin B_{12} deficiency may develop in the infant. Maternal intakes of some nutrients (vitamin B_6, vitamin D, iodine, selenium) are directly associated with their concentration in milk. For mothers at risk for vitamin D deficiency, those living in northern climates, and those not exposed to external sources of vitamin D, additional supplementation may be beneficial to improve maternal vitamin D status. The contents of some nutrients in milk may be maintained at a satisfactory level at the expense of maternal stores, especially folate and calcium. For this reason, folic acid supplementation (400 μg per day) should continue. There are no recommendations for calcium supplementation if Dietary Reference Intakes are met. Calcium losses occur from maternal skeleton in early lactation, but these losses are restored after weaning. Milk concentrations of calcium, iron, and zinc are essentially independent of maternal intake. High maternal dietary fat intake and obesity are associated with higher milk fat content. Some studies also suggest that maternal body fat stores are correlated with milk fat content. The pattern of fatty acids is affected by maternal diet. A maternal diet high in polyunsaturated fatty acids increases the proportion of these fatty acids in the milk. Most practitioners encourage the continued intake of prenatal vitamins during lactation.

Table 9-2. Dietary Reference Intakes for Lactating Women

Nutrient	Adult Women[b]	Pregnancy	Lactation	Percentage Increase During Lactation Over Nonreproducing Adult Women — Lactation %
		Dietary Reference Intakes[a]		
Energy,[c] kcal	19–50 yr	↑340 kcal/d 2nd trimester ↑452 kcal/d 3rd trimester	↑500 kcal/d 0–6 mo ↑400 kcal/d 7–9 mo	↑
Protein,[d] g	46	71	71	54
Vitamin C,[d] mg	75	85	120	60
Thiamin,[d] mg	1.1	1.4	1.4	27
Riboflavin,[d] mg	1.1	1.4	1.6	45
Niacin,[d] ng NE	14	18	17	21
Vitamin B_6,[d] mg	1.3	1.9	2	54
Folate,[d] µg DFE	400	600	500	25
Vitamin B_{12},[d] µg	2.4	2.6	2.8	17
Pantothenic acid,[e] mg	5	6	7	40
Biotin,[e] µg	30	30	35	17
Choline,[e] mg	425	450	550	29
Vitamin A,[d] µg RE	700	770	1300	86
Vitamin D,[e] µg	5	5	5	0
Vitamin E,[d] mg TE	15	15	19	27
Vitamin K,[e] µg	90	90	90	0
Calcium,[e] mg	1,000	1,000	1,000	0
Phosphorus,[e] mg	700	700	700	0
Magnesium,[d] mg	310	350	310	0
Iron,[d] mg	18	27	9	−50
Zinc,[d] mg	8	11	12	50
Iodine,[d] µg	150	220	290	93

| Selenium,[d] µg | 55 | 60 | 70 | 27 |
| Fluoride,[e] mg | 3 | 3 | 3 | 0 |

[a] Values are from the Institute of Medicine.
[b] Assumes age older than 19 years. Women younger than 19 years have greater nutrient needs for calcium (1,300 mg), phosphorus (1,240 mg), and zinc (13 mg).
[c] Calculations are based on recommended intakes per day, assuming 9 months is equivalent to 270 days.
[d] Recommended Dietary Allowance (RDA), the average daily dietary intake level that is sufficient to meet the nutrient requirements of nearly all (97% and 98%) individuals in a life stage and gender group, and based on the Estimated Average Requirement (EAR).
[e] Adequate Intake (AI), the value used instead of an RDA if sufficient scientific evidence is not available to calculate an EAR.
DFE = dietary folate equivalents; NE = niacin equivalents; RE = retinal equivalents; TE = tocopherol equivalents.
Adapted with permission from Picciano MF. Pregnancy and lactation: Physiological adjustments, nutritional requirements and the role of dietary supplements. *J Nutr.* 2003;133:1997S–2002S.

Weight Loss

Lactating women eating self-selected diets generally lose weight at the rate of 0.5 to 1 kg (approximately 1–2 lb) per month in the first 4 to 6 months of lactation. Approximately 20% of women, however, do not lose weight during this time. Women can lose as much as 1 lb per week without compromising milk volume. For the lactating woman who had an elevated body mass index before pregnancy or with excessive gestational weight gain who desires to lose weight more quickly, restriction in caloric intake has been shown to be more effective than exercise alone. Systematic reviews, however, conclude that maternal exercise has benefits for metabolic fitness and does not impair milk production or infant growth. Rapid weight loss should be discouraged because it can decrease milk volume. Weight loss drugs and liquid diets are not recommended during lactation, and a weight reduction diet in general is discouraged during the first 4 to 6 weeks postpartum. The average time to return to prepregnancy weight is 5 months. Mothers should be given sound nutritional advice to ensure adequate nutrient intake.

Breast Evaluation While Nursing

Screening for Breast Masses

The incidence of breast malignancy during pregnancy and lactation is estimated at 1:3,000 to 1:10,000 women. Approximately 3% of women diagnosed with breast cancer will be either pregnant or lactating. With increased childbearing in more advanced years, this number is expected to increase. Delay in diagnosis has been reported in pregnant and breastfeeding women. If a breastfeeding mother notices a lump in her breast that does not decrease with breastfeeding or one that increases in size, prompt evaluation should be pursued. If the mass persists, diagnostic tests should be performed (see Chapter 16).

Diagnostic Mammography

Mammograms are safe during lactation, but normal findings should not be completely reassuring in the presence of a palpable mass. If a mammogram is performed, the woman should either nurse her infant or express milk from her breasts immediately before the mammogram to allow optimal visualization.

Ultrasound

Further assistance in evaluating palpable breast masses (solid or fluid filled) during lactation can be provided by the use of ultrasounds.

Diagnostic Studies

Needle biopsy or fine needle aspiration, as well as other diagnostic studies, can be performed without significant interruption of lactation. Most breast masses identified and for which a biopsy is performed during pregnancy and lactation are benign (80%) and can undergo biopsy without harm to mother, fetus, or infant. About 30% have pathology specific to the lactating breast. Benign pathology specific to the lactating breast includes lactating adenoma, infarcted fibroadenoma, hypertrophied breast tissue, galactoceles, mastitis/ inflammatory lesions, and papillomas.

Bloody Nipple Discharge

A relatively frequent finding associated with nipple trauma and engorgement in early lactation, bloody nipple discharge typically occurs around days 3 to 7. Evaluation of the nipple for trauma and adjustment of problems associated with latching the infant may resolve the problem. Occasionally, women will complain of reddish brown milk as ducts become distended and capillaries leak (ductal ectasia or rusty pipe syndrome). This usually resolves within the first week. If the milk is blood-tinged, it is usually well tolerated by the infant, although occasionally it may be associated with vomiting and blood-tinged stools in the infant. If the bloody nipple discharge is persistent and from only a single milk duct, further evaluation is required. Most commonly, this will be caused by an intraductal papilloma. Intraductal carcinoma is rare and may also be associated with a mass in the affected breast.

Recommendations for Breast Evaluation During Lactation

- *Regular Breast Self-Examinations.* Although technically difficult, some women choose to continue to do regular breast self-examinations during lactation.
- *Clinical breast examinations* should be performed by a physician at the onset of pregnancy, in the postpartum period, and annually thereafter even while lactating.
- *Mammograms.* Routine screening mammograms in contrast with diagnostic mammograms as outlined earlier should be delayed until several months after weaning.
- *Biopsy,* if indicated, is safe during pregnancy and lactation.
- *Breast cancer* diagnosed during pregnancy and lactation generally has the same prognosis, stage for stage, as premenopausal breast cancer diagnosed outside of pregnancy and lactation. Early diagnosis is important and treatment should not be delayed. Early referral to a breast surgeon for further evaluation of a breast abnormality is indicated if there is any cause for concern.
- *Lactation* is possible (even if unilateral) after most breast surgeries and breast cancer treatments.

Selected References

1. Berens PD. Prenatal, intrapartum, and postpartum support of the lactating mother. *Pediatr Clin North Am.* 2001;48:365–375
2. Brent N, Rudy SJ, Redd B, Rudy TE, Roth LA. Sore nipples in breast-feeding women: a clinical trial of wound dressings vs conventional care. *Arch Pediatr Adolesc Med.* 1998;152:1077–1082
3. Committee on Nutritional Status During Pregnancy and Lactation. *Nutrition During Lactation.* Washington, DC: National Academies Press; 1991
4. Dewey K. Effects of maternal caloric restriction and exercise during lactation. *J Nutr.* 1998;128(suppl):386S–389S
5. Foxman B, D'Arcy H, Gillespie B, Bobo JK, Schwartz K. Lactation mastitis: occurrence and medical management among 946 breastfeeding women in the United States. *Am J Epidemiol.* 2002;155:103–114
6. Hartmann S, Reimer T, Gerber B. Management of early invasive breast cancer in very young women (<35 years). *Clin Breast Cancer.* 2011;11:196–203
7. Howard C, Howard F. Management of breastfeeding when the mother is ill. *Clin Obstet Gynecol.* 2004;47:683–695
8. Kalkwarf HJ. Hormonal and dietary regulation of changes in bone density during lactation and after weaning in women. *J Mammary Gland Biol Neoplasia.* 1999;4:319–329
9. Krebs NF, Reidinger CJ, Robertson AD, Brenner M. Bone mineral density changes during lactation: maternal, dietary, and biochemical correlates. *Am J Clin Nutr.* 1997;65:1738–1746
10. Labbok MH. Effects of breastfeeding on the mother. *Pediatr Clin North Am.* 2001;48:143–158

11. Lawrence RM, Lawrence RA. Breast milk and infection. *Clin Perinatol.* 2004;31:501–528
12. Mass S. Breast pain: engorgement, nipple pain and mastitis. *Clin Obstet Gynecol.* 2004;47: 672–682
13. Morland-Schultz K, Hill PD. Prevention and therapies for nipple pain: a systematic review. *J Obstet Gynecol Neonatal Nurs.* 2005;34:428–437
14. Picciano MF. Pregnancy and lactation: physiological adjustments, nutritional requirements and the role of dietary supplements. *J Nutr.* 2003;133:1997S–2002S
15. Section 7(r) of the Fair Labor Standards Act—Break Time for Nursing Mothers Provision. http://www.dol.gov/whd/nursingmothers/Sec7rFLSA_btnm.htm. Accessed August 30, 2013
16. Snyder R, Zahn C. Breast disease during pregnancy and lactation. In: Gilstrap LC 3rd, Cunningham FG, VanDorsten JP, editors. *Operative Obstetrics.* 2nd ed. New York, NY: McGraw-Hill; 2002
17. Valentine CJ, Wagner CL. Nutritional management of the breastfeeding dyad. *Pediatr Clin North Am.* 2013;60:261–274
18. Zemlickis D, Lishner M, Degendorfer P, et al. Maternal and fetal outcome after breast cancer in pregnancy. *Am J Obstet Gynecol.* 1992;166:781–787

Chapter 10

Supporting Breastfeeding During Mother-Infant Separation

There are circumstances, such as maternal hospitalization, return to work, or school attendance, in which an interruption in continuity of breastfeeding may occur by necessity. The physician can help the mother by providing guidance on specific strategies and appropriate plans for continued breast-feeding.

Maternal Employment and School Attendance

Attending work and school are often the most frequent reasons for consis-tent mother-infant separation during lactation and anticipatory guidance should be practiced so that health care professionals can discuss options for continued breastfeeding during these times. Counseling and discussion of strategies should begin prenatally, continue during visits to the office, and be included in the instruction provided in breastfeeding classes and other resources.

Support for Breastfeeding in the Workplace

On-site Child Care
Direct breastfeeding is preferable for continued milk supply. For mothers employed outside of the home, child care facilities on-site or close to the

workplace allow the mother to breastfeed during breaks. Alternatively, employees may be permitted to bring their young infant to the office, with or without a caregiver, during the day for breastfeeding. This may not be feasible in all work settings.

Off-site Child Care

Some employers offer lactation programs to encourage continued breast-feeding for mothers who return to work. These may include on-site lactation specialists, a contract with community or hospital lactation specialists, a designated space for breastfeeding women to breastfeed or express milk, and/or a fully equipped lactation room. In the absence of corporate on-site child care programs, at a minimum the breastfeeding mother should have access to appropriate facilities at work for milk expression (see Box 10-1). The creative use of scheduled breaks and lunchtime combined with strategies, such as a double pump kit that allows milk to be expressed from both breasts simultaneously, may facilitate maintenance of a milk supply. Milk expression should occur at least once every 3 to 4 hours during periods of separation, approximating the schedule for the infant's feedings. The off-site child care selected should be compatible with the parents' beliefs and the mother's desire to continue breastfeeding. Areas to be addressed when interviewing a prospective caregiver are listed in Box 10-2.

Box 10-1. Facilities Necessary to Support Breastfeeding in the Workplace

1. Private place for milk expression (office, break room, lounge), preferably with a lock on the door and an electrical outlet

2. Breast pump, either supplied by workplace or brought by mother

3. Sink for washing hands before handling pump equipment or milk and for rinsing equipment

4. Storage refrigerator, separate from that used for storing food in a common break area to avoid milk tampering or, alternatively, a cooler with ice packs for storing milk immediately after expression and used to transfer milk to the home or child care facility

5. Comfortable seating for milk expression or breastfeeding

Box 10-2. Questions for Parents to Ask a Prospective Child Care Professional

1. What has been your previous experience with breastfeeding and the use of expressed human milk?
2. Do you agree with our/my general philosophy and style of parenting?
3. Will you follow specific instructions in terms of feeding expressed human milk?
4. Will you be willing to attempt to soothe the baby or wait a brief period for the feeding if I am delayed at work?
5. Will you follow our/my plan for introducing cereal, solids, and juices?

Affordable Care Act

Section 4207 of the 2010 Patient Protection and Affordable Care Act amended the Fair Labor Standards Act of 1938 and currently provides hourly employees with workplace provisions:

- The employee must be provided reasonable break time to express breast milk for her child for 1 year after the child's birth each time such employee has a need to express the milk, and a place, other than a bathroom, that is shielded from view and free from intrusion from coworkers and the public, which may be used by an employee to express breast milk.
- Further guidance on this legislation is provided by the Department of Labor in its "Break Time for Nursing Mothers under the FLSA (Fair Labor Standards Act)."
- State legislation may provide more strict guidance on workplace support for breastfeeding mothers than the federal protection. In addition, breast pumps and other supplies to assist lactation are deductible medical expenses or can be reimbursed under flexible spending accounts or health savings accounts, according to the Internal Revenue Service.

Advocacy for Breastfeeding

Continued advocacy for breastfeeding in the workplace is needed.

Literature

Providing literature that discusses the benefits of breastfeeding and demonstrates the cost savings of breastfeeding to the employer may be helpful. Health care professionals may need to write letters or contact employers or school administrators in support of the health care interests of the infant and mother and the need for continued breastfeeding.

Professionals' Role

Health care professionals should advocate for insurance or managed care coverage for the cost of a pump to allow the mother to continue milk expression at work/school and for coverage for lactation services. In addition, health care professionals should advocate for supportive legislation and policies at the local, state, and national levels; these efforts may include paid maternity leave benefits.

The Business Case for Breastfeeding

The US Department of Health and Human Services Health Resources and Services Administration, Maternal Child Health Bureau, and Office on Women's Health offer guidance and toolkits for human resources personnel, business owners, managers, and employees to provide assistance to breastfeeding employees and their employers. These documents outline the business savings in terms of decreased employee absenteeism, lower health care costs, lower turnover rates, and higher productivity when employed women are supported in breastfeeding. The Business Case for Breastfeeding program has trained health care professionals in workplace support and also provides technical assistance and tools to businesses in developing worksite lactation programs.

Options for Continued Breastfeeding After Return to Work or School

All options for continued breastfeeding should be considered before the beginning of mother-baby separation. Ideally, the mother should discuss her desire to breastfeed, and continue breastfeeding or milk expression after return to work or school, with her supervisor, human resources director, school guidance counselor, and/or administrator prior to family planning, maternity leave, or childbirth. The physician also may need to advocate for breastfeeding or milk expression with the employer or school official.

Preparing for the Return to Work or School

Strategies

Strategies for the mother to prepare for separation are listed in Box 10-3.

Medical Students and Residents

Medical students and residents pose unique situations because of the schedule and workload demands. Residents who have had successful experiences breastfeeding, either personally or with their spouse or partner, are more

Box 10-3. Suggested Strategies for the Mother Who Is Returning to Work or School

A. **Preparation before the day of separation**
   1. Arrange as long a period of maternity leave as feasible.
   2. Make arrangements with the employer/school before the day of return,
   3. preferably before maternity leave begins.
   4. Practice using the breast pump at least 2 weeks before the planned separation.
   5. Begin milk expression early to allow storage of a sufficient supply.
   6. Introduce alternative methods of feeding in advance.
   7. Experiment with different types of bottle nipples or cups to find one that the infant prefers.
   8. Encourage the father/partner, or other relatives or friends, to provide assistance with household chores or with the care of other children to ease the transition.
   9. Leave the infant or child with the caregiver for brief periods before the first day.
   10. Let the caregiver practice giving the baby a bottle or cup before the separation.

B. **Preparations at the work/school site**
   1. Enlist the support of coworkers (or teachers, principals, or guidance counselors) who are breastfeeding or who have breastfed in the past.
   2. Arrange gradual return to work schedule if possible, beginning with half days.
   3. If returning to work full time, consider starting on a Thursday or Friday to avoid having to work a full 5-day period the first week back at work.
   4. Breastfeed just before leaving the infant and as soon as mother and infant are reunited at the end of the day.
   5. Allow the infant to breastfeed as often as desired in the evening and overnight to encourage continued milk supply. Having baby close by at night may facilitate frequent feedings. Maximize skin-to-skin contact.
   6. Remember to clean and pack the breast pump, kit, bottles, and other equipment ahead of time.
   7. Take a cooler or bag with freezer packs for transporting expressed milk home or for storage while away.
   8. Take a picture of the infant (or consider having a blanket with the baby's smell or an audio or video file of the baby's coos, squeals, or cries) to use when expressing to facilitate the milk ejection reflex (letdown).
   9. Have a change of clothing available in case of milk leaks or spills.
   10. Wear clothing with a pattern or wear a jacket over a blouse or dress to conceal accidental leaks or spills.
   11. Wear 2-piece outfits or commercially available clothing designed for breastfeeding women that allows easy access to the breasts for feeding or expressing milk.

likely to be knowledgeable about breastfeeding and can potentially become strong advocates and role models for their peers and patients when they become practitioners. Medical school administrators and residency training program directors and faculty should support and encourage breastfeeding among their students and residency staff. Optimal support may involve flexibility in terms of work assignments or accommodation of part-time scheduling for a period.

Separation Because of Newborn or Infant Illness

Prematurity or neonatal illness may preclude continuous rooming-in or necessitate discharge of the mother before the infant's discharge. Strategies to promote continued bonding and stimulation of milk production include skin-to-skin contact and facilities that permit overnight stays of the mother to maximize the amount of time she can spend with the infant. These "mother-in-residence" programs also permit the infant to remain in the room with the mother either continuously or intermittently. Newer intensive care nurseries are designed with individual patient rooms with sleeping accommodations for parents. If physical separation of mother and infant is required, the mother should be provided with a hospital-grade electric pump and kit for double pumping, and she should be assisted with collection and storage of pumped milk. Strategies to assist breastfeeding if the infant is ill are addressed in Chapters 11 and 14.

Separation Because of Maternal Illness or Surgery

Acute Minor Maternal Illness

For acute minor illness in the mother, including fever, breastfeeding should not be interrupted. By the time maternal symptoms develop, the infant has already been exposed to the infectious agent. Continued breastfeeding is protective to the infant (see Chapters 8 and 9).

Planned Elective Surgery

If it cannot be postponed, elective surgery should prompt a discussion with the surgeon and anesthesiologist to select the most appropriate medications for anesthesia, pain control, and other therapies (see Chapters 6, 8, 9, and 12). Rooming-in for continued nursing or having the infant visit at intervals to breastfeed should be considered whenever possible. Family and/or friends should be encouraged to assist in caring for the infant during such visits. In some hospitals, breastfeeding infants may be kept with mothers in postoperative units. Milk should be expressed and stored in advance of the procedure, in case there is a longer than expected interruption in breastfeeding. In the event of a more serious maternal condition or emergency surgery, the mother should be provided an electric pump and assisted in the collection and storage of breast milk. This should occur even for those mothers in intensive care, in which case the nurses or lactation specialists may need to assist.

Milk Expression

Throughout the period of separation, milk expression should continue on a regular basis to maintain supply and prevent engorgement.

Unanticipated Separation

The frequency of milk expression should approximate the frequency at which the infant would be breastfeeding (every 2–3 hours for the newborn, every 4–5 hours for the older baby) to maintain an adequate milk supply.

Anticipated Separation

In situations in which there is elective surgery or return to work or school, milk should be expressed before the anticipated absence and stored for later use. Milk volume can be increased by increasing the frequency of milk expression 1 to 2 weeks before the anticipated date.

Bottle-feeding

If the mother desires that the baby learn to drink from a bottle, she should consider introduction of the bottle gradually, a few weeks before its anticipated need. Acceptance of a bottle is more likely if someone other than the mother offers it. The breastfed infant will typically accept expressed human milk from the bottle better than infant formula. If the bottle is not accepted on the first attempt, repeat introductions may be necessary, approximately once every day or two. Trying another style, size, or shape of nipple may be helpful. If the baby does use a pacifier, a nipple that is similar in size and shape to the pacifier may be helpful. Attempting the feeding when the infant is hungry, but not crying inconsolably, will enhance the chances for positive acceptance of the bottle. For older infants who continue to refuse bottles, a cup can be used to offer the feeding.

Selected References

1. Angeletti MA. Breastfeeding mothers returning to work: possibilities for information, anticipatory guidance and support from US health care professionals. *J Hum Lact.* 2009;25:226–232

2. Biagioli F. Returning to work while breastfeeding. *Am Fam Physician.* 2003;68:2201–2208

3. Bocar DL. Combining breastfeeding and employment: increasing success. *J Perinat Neonatal Nurs.* 1997;11:23–43

4. Cohen R, Mrtek MB, Mrtek RG. Comparison of maternal absenteeism and infant illness rates among breast-feeding and formula-feeding women in two corporations. *Am J Health Promot.* 1995;10:148–153

5. Corbett-Dick P, Bezek SK. Breastfeeding promotion for the employed mother. *J Pediatr Health Care.* 1997;11:12–19

6. Feldman-Winter LB, Schanler RJ, O'Connor KG, Lawrence RA. Pediatricians and the promotion and support of breastfeeding. *Arch Pediatr Adolesc Med.* 2008;162:1142–1149

7. Greenberg CS, Smith K. Anticipatory guidance for the employed breast-feeding mother. *J Pediatr Health Care.* 1991;5:204–209

8. American Academy of Pediatrics. Healthy Child Care America. http://www.healthychildcare. org. Accessed August 30, 2013

9. Jacknowitz A. The role of workplace characteristics in breastfeeding practices. *Women Health.* 2008;47:87–111

10. Meek JY. Breastfeeding in the workplace. *Pediatr Clin North Am.* 2001;48:461–474

11. Ortiz J, McGilligan K, Kelly P. Duration of breast milk expression among working mothers enrolled in an employer-sponsored lactation program. *Pediatr Nurs.* 2004;30:111–119

12. Pantazi M, Jaeger MC, Lawson M. Staff support for mothers to provide breast milk in pediatric hospitals and neonatal units. *J Hum Lact.* 1998;14:291–296

13. Rojjanasrirat W, Wambach KA. Maternal employment and breastfeeding. In: Riordan J, Wambach KA, eds. *Breastfeeding and Human Lactation.* 4th ed. Boston, MA: Jones and Bartlett Publishers; 2010

14. Shealy KR, Li R, Benton-Davis S, Grummer-Strawn LM. Support for breastfeeding in the workplace. In: *The CDC Guide to Breastfeeding Interventions.* Atlanta, GA: Centers for Disease Control and Prevention; 2005

15. Slusser WM, Lange L, Dickson V, Hawkes C, Cohen R. Breast milk expression in the workplace: a look at frequency and times. *J Hum Lact.* 2004;20:164–169

16. US Breastfeeding Committee. *Workplace Accommodations to Support and Protect Breastfeeding.* Washington, DC: US Breastfeeding Committee; 2010

17. US Department of Health and Human Services, Health Resources and Services Administration, Maternal and Child Health Bureau. *The Business Case for Breastfeeding.* 2008. http://www.womenshealth.gov/breastfeeding/government-in-action/ business-case-for-breastfeeding. Accessed August 30, 2013

18. US Department of Health and Human Services, Office of Women's Health, American Association of Health Plans. *Advancing Women's Health: Health Plans' Innovative Programs in Breastfeeding Promotion.* Washington, DC: US Government Printing Office; 2001

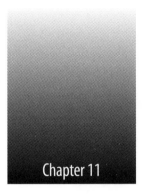

Chapter 11

Lactation Support Technology

Lactation support technology refers to the equipment and methods used to support successful breastfeeding. These include breast pumps, breast shells, nipple shields, feeding tube devices, weighing scales, and proper milk storage, any or all of which can be useful in supporting women to initiate and maintain their human milk supply, and ultimately to breastfeed.

Manual and Mechanical Milk Expression

Both expression techniques, manual and mechanical, are effective in helping initiate and maintain milk production during infant-mother separation, maternal or infant illness, inability of the infant to latch to the breast, and poor maternal milk production.

Manual Milk Expression

This technique works well during short-term separation and to alleviate engorgement or sore nipples (see Figure 11-1). These simple steps can be mastered by the mother after some practice (see Box 11-1). High-quality educational videos are available online for instructing mothers in this technique (http://newborns.stanford.edu/Breastfeeding/HandExpression.html).

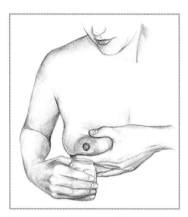

Figure 11-1. Manual milk expression.

Box 11-1. Manual Milk Expression Technique

1. Wash hands thoroughly.
2. Gently massage the breast from the outside quadrants toward the areola; avoid applying deep pressure or friction.
3. A washcloth with warm water may be placed on the breast about 5 minutes before milk expression.
4. Place the hand with the fingers below and the thumb above about 3 cm away from the nipple base. Press toward the chest wall and then compress the thumb and fingers together, rolling them toward the nipple. Move the hand around the areola to reach all of the areas that cover the pooled milk in the lactiferous sinuses. Use the free hand to massage the breast from the outer quadrants toward the nipple. Do not squeeze the nipple.
5. The manual method can take 20 to 30 minutes for adequate draining of both breasts.
6. For a video demonstrating this technique, see http://newborns.stanford.edu/Breastfeeding/HandExpression.html.

Mechanical Expression

Mechanical expression of milk can be accomplished using a manual, small, battery-operated or hospital-grade electric breast pump (see Figure 11-2). Mechanical expression works best for those planning to express their milk on a regular, ongoing basis, such as for a return to work or school, or in case of maternal or infant illness. See Box 11-2 for a list of common questions used to evaluate breast pumps before purchase.

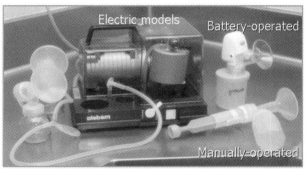

Figure 11-2A. Various styles of electric and manual breast pumps.

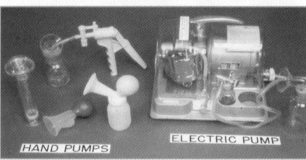

Figure 11-2B. Various styles of electric and manual breast pumps.

Box 11-2. Questions to Answer Before Obtaining a Breast Pump

1. Is the pump for short- or long-term use?
2. What will the pump cost?
3. How much does the pump weigh?
4. How comfortable is the pump?
5. Does it drain the breast efficiently?
6. How easy are the pump and collection kits to clean?
7. Are there clear written instructions on how to use the pump?
8. Can a standard bottle be used to collect milk with the pump?
9. How many suction cycles are there per minute?
10. Does the pump cycle on its own?
11. Are variable collection cup sizes available?
12. Are there mechanisms to prevent pump contamination?
13. How quiet is the pump?
14. How long are the electrical cords?
15. Can it pump both breasts at the same time?
16. Is the pump approved for use in the hospital, if applicable?
17. What is the manufacturer's warranty?
18. Is the pump meant for a single owner or for multiple users?
19. Does the pump come with a case or a tote bag?
20. Do you have to use 2 hands to operate the pump?
21. Is the pump efficient and effective?

Adapted from Slusser W, Frantz K. High-Technology Breastfeeding. *Pediatr Clin North Am.* 2001;48:505–516, copyright 2001, with permission from Elsevier.

Battery-Operated and Electric Pumps

These kinds of pumps generally are lightweight and have variable frequency (2–76 cycles/min), suction pressures (8–360 mm Hg), and capabilities for double pumping. The electric breast pump with automatic cycling yields milk that has a higher calorie content (secondary to increased fat concentration from complete breast drainage) compared with the milk expressed by manual methods. Guidelines for mechanical milk expression are listed in Box 11-3. Certain breast pumps and breast pump features appear to be superior or more acceptable to pump-dependent mothers, for example, mothers of preterm babies, than are other pumps. It is critical that neonatal intensive care unit (NICU) mothers receive the most effective, efficient, comfortable, and convenient electric breast pump available. A lactation specialist working in the NICU can be a valuable asset to mothers of the preterm infants and can assist in providing the best pump and training.

Box 11-3. General Guidelines for Mechanical Milk Expression

1. Wash hands before beginning to express milk.
2. To initiate and maintain milk supply for a hospitalized infant, begin as soon as possible after birth (preferably within the first 6 hours) and continue at a frequency of 8 times in 24 hours. After an adequate milk supply is established, the frequency can be reduced; this is generally 2 to 3 weeks after birth, or when milk production of 500 mL per 24 hours occurs. For other situations, the frequency can be less.
3. Ten minutes of pumping each breast is sufficient for maintenance of adequate milk production, preferably from both breasts simultaneously.
4. Develop relaxation techniques, such as sitting in a comfortable environment. Think about the infant, look at a photograph of the infant, or sit at the bedside of the hospitalized infant. Gently massage the breast before and during milk expression.
5. It is unnecessary to discard the first few milliliters of milk.
6. A pump collection kit should be used by only one mother unless it is sterilized between uses. Verify manufacturer's instructions before sterilizing.
7. Pumps categorized for in-home single users should be used by only one mother.
8. Routine microbiologic surveillance is costly and not indicated.
9. Review recommendations verbally and in written form for washing and cleaning of pump equipment. (Instructions usually accompany the pump.)

Breast Pump Maintenance

- *Assembly.* A knowledgeable person should demonstrate to the family how to assemble and disassemble a pump.
- *Cleaning.* Each mother should have her own collection kit and storage containers, which should be rinsed to remove milk residue; cleaned with hot, soapy water; and dried in the air after each use. Dishwasher cleaning also is adequate. Bottled or boiled water should be used for cleaning parts where the water supply is potentially contaminated. Manufacturer's instructions should be followed. When more than one mother is using the same breast pump, as in a hospital lactation room, hospital staff should be responsible for cleaning the pump daily, examining for milk backup, and regularly checking the suction settings.
- *Double pumping system.* Long-term mother-baby separation warrants a breast pump that is capable of simultaneous double (bilateral) pumping because of the time saved, higher amount of prolactin released, and potential for greater milk production (see Figure 11-3). Nursing bras that assist mothers with positioning of both flanges simultaneously are now available.
- *Fitting the flange.* The opening where the breast meets the collection kit needs to be wide enough to allow the nipple to easily move in and out without pain, but not so large that milk removal is impaired. Some collection kits have breast shield inserts to accommodate for different nipple sizes. A poorly fitted flange, used repeatedly, can cause nipple trauma and pain.

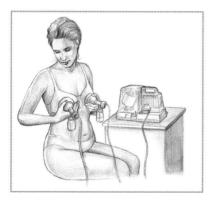

Figure 11-3A. An electric breast pump that allows collection of milk from both breasts simultaneously is best for mothers who express milk on a routine basis, especially if they have a hospitalized infant.

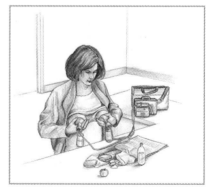

Figure 11-3B. Double pumping system.

Manual Breast Pumps

These pumps are available in 3 styles:

- Piston or cylinder pumps. For intermittent pumping, these are simple and effective devices; however, their use is unlikely to be adequate to increase milk production or maintain supply if there is prolonged mother-infant separation. Mothers who choose to use a hand pump need to be instructed on how to use it properly because lateral epicondylitis (tennis elbow) has been associated with the use of trombone action-style hand pumps.
- Squeeze-handle pumps are effective at removing milk, but some women develop fatigue in their hand after prolonged use.
- Rubber bulb (bicycle horn) pumps are not recommended because of the potential for bacteria buildup inside the rubber bulb and contamination of the milk.

Economics of Pump Purchase/Rental

If a physician prescribes a breast pump for a patient, some health insurance companies and the Special Supplemental Nutrition Program for Women, Infants, and Children (WIC) will cover the cost of a breast pump rental or purchase. In addition, many employee breastfeeding support programs support the cost of purchasing or renting the equipment. Physicians may be asked to write letters of medical necessity for breast pumps.

Nipple Shields and Breast Cups and Shells

Nipple Shields

Made of latex or silicone, nipple shields provide a thin protective barrier over the nipple and areola with holes at the tip to allow the transfer of milk (see Figure 11-4). Nipple shields are used to help an infant latch on to a flat or inverted nipple or an engorged breast, protect sore nipples, reduce an excessively rapid milk flow, and sometimes entice an infant to the breast who is accustomed to the nipple of a bottle. Ultrathin silicone nipple shields have been shown to improve milk transfer in preterm infants transitioning from tube or bottle feeding to breastfeeding. The use of the nipple shield for preterm infants may be advantageous in establishing and maintaining breastfeeding; however, nipple shield use should not be routine but should be considered when preterm or ill infants have demonstrated persistent difficulty with sustained breastfeeding and milk transfer.

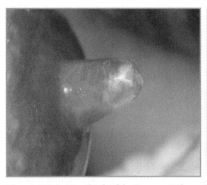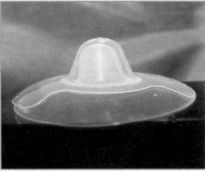

Figure 11-4. Nipple shields. Source: Wilson-Clay B, Hoover K. The Breastfeeding Atlas; 1999.

A review of 13 published reports of nipple shield use found little support for current practices regarding common nipple shield use and did not demonstrate safety in the long term for milk supply, infant weight gain, or duration of breastfeeding. Because of the potential to interfere with milk transfer and reduce stimulation of the areola, clinicians should monitor infant weight gain to ensure adequate milk intake while nipple shields are used. Health care providers should consider nipple shields an unknown risk and limit their duration of use whenever possible.

Breast Cups and Shells

Made of hard polypropylene, silicone, or other hard plastic, breast cups and shells are designed in a cup shape with air holes on one side and one larger hole on the other side for the nipple to protrude through the opening into the cup or shell. They help in the relief of sore nipples and in preventing milk from leaking onto clothes. The most important features of breast cups/shells are the air holes for ventilation, sufficient size to prevent overflow of milk onto the clothes, and a large enough nipple opening for comfort. They are worn inside the bra between breastfeeding episodes. Although they are sometimes used for correcting inverted nipples during the prenatal and postpartum period, there is no evidence that they are effective.

Supplemental Feeding Methods

For the infant who is unable or unwilling to suckle at the breast, there are other methods of providing expressed human milk, such as with feeding tube devices, cups, and bottles, and the finger-feeding technique. Unfortunately, there is little evidence about the safety or efficacy of most alternative feeding methods and their effect on breastfeeding. When selecting an alternative feeding method, clinicians should consider cost and availability, ease of use and cleaning, stress to the infant, whether adequate milk volume can be fed in 20 to 30 minutes, whether anticipated use is short or long term, maternal preference, and whether the method enhances development of breastfeeding skills.

Supplemental Nursing Systems

These are very thin, soft plastic feeding tubes that are attached to a milk container at one end, with the other end placed adjacent to the mother's nipple and fixed to the breast with a small piece of tape (see Figure 11-5). This device has the advantage of supplying appropriate supplement while simultaneously stimulating the breast to produce more milk and reinforcing the infant's feeding at the breast. It may be useful when the mother wishes to relactate or induce lactation. The use of feeding tube devices usually requires supervision by a certified lactation specialist. Most of these systems are awkward to use, difficult to clean, and expensive and require moderately complex learning. Although the feeding tube device improves stimulation at the breast so that a breast pump may not be needed, in some cases, mothers will use both the feeding tube device and the breast pump.

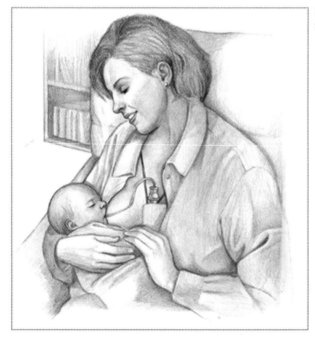

Figure 11-5. Feeding tube device.

Cup Feeding

Feeding by cup is an alternative method to bottle-feeding when breastfeeding is not an option or parents are opposed to the use of bottles (see Figure 11-6). Many clinicians are unaware that cup feeding has been compared with bottle-feeding in term babies in a controlled clinical trial. Cup feeding was found to be equivalent to bottle feeding in terms of duration of the feeding session, volume of milk ingested, and infant physiologic stability (heart rate, respiratory rate, and oxygen saturations). In addition, cup feedings may help preserve breastfeeding duration among those who require multiple supplemental feedings. Benefits of cup feeding for preterm infants also have been reported.

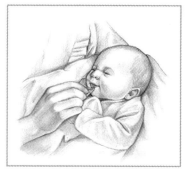

Figure 11-6. Cup feeding.

For some infants, bottle-feeding may interfere with the establishment of breastfeeding, so cup feeding is a reasonable alternative, provided an experienced provider is giving the cup feeding. It entails using a small plastic or glass medicine cup filled with milk. Infants are fed in a semi-upright position with head and upper back support. Infants can be stimulated to root by stroking the lower lip with the edge of the cup. The infant sips or laps the milk when the cup is placed against the infant's lower lip and tilted so that the milk is available, but not poured or dripped into the infant's mouth. Some infants may not be able to sustain the sipping or lapping effort to get an adequate volume or may lose significant amounts because of dribbling of milk.

Bottle-feeding

Although bottle-feeding is the most commonly used method of supplementation, it is of concern because of distinct differences in tongue and jaw movements, differences in milk flow, and possible long-term adverse consequences in the development of the mouth, jaw, and oral-motor structures. In general, bottles are not recommended for the first few weeks until breastfeeding is well established. Because the tongue, lips, and mouth are used differently for bottle-feeding and breastfeeding and because breastfed infants become accustomed to the soft, supple human nipple, bottle nipples may not be accepted readily. During a bottle-feeding, the infant should be held in a somewhat flexed position resting in the arms of the caregiver. The bottle should be introduced by touching the lower lip of the infant to elicit the rooting reflex, then slipping the bottle nipple in the mouth once the infant's mouth opens. In some infants, early introduction of bottles may lead to ineffective suckling at the breast or result in breast refusal. There may be a need to introduce bottles to infants whose mothers expect to be separated from them in the near future, such as return to work or school (see Chapter 10).

Other Temporary Feeding Methods

When breastfeeding is not possible, other temporary feeding methods to deliver milk to the infant include using a medicine spoon, dropper, or syringe, and finger feeds in which one holds a feeding tube with a finger near the junction of the hard and soft palates. These methods avoid delivering milk by bottle and artificial nipple. When using a syringe or a medicine dropper, avoid squeezing or pushing the milk into the baby's mouth. Allow the infant to suck the milk out by enticing the infant with a few drops placed on the infant's lip. No long-term studies have examined the risks and benefits of these alternative methods.

Intragastric (Orogastric, Nasogastric) Tube Feeding

These methods are usually used when an infant is preterm or too ill to suckle at the breast. There are 2 ways that milk can be fed by this method: intermittent bolus and continuous infusion. For the bolus technique, milk flows by gravity into the tube. A continuous infusion requires that the syringe of milk be placed on a syringe infusion pump and then attached to the feeding tube. Because the fat will separate from the milk on standing, efforts should be made to ensure that the separated fat is not left behind when the milk is fed. A single-syringe infusion pump with the shortest length of tubing is used to ensure the best delivery of fat with the continuous tube feeding method. The syringe should be oriented with the tip upright and the syringe emptied completely after each use (see Figure 11-7). With continuous feedings, syringe systems should be changed every 3 to 4 hours.

Test Weighing

Test weighing is a procedure to measure milk intake by weighing the infant before and after a feeding under identical conditions. The net intake in grams (closely approximating volume in milliliters) is obtained by subtracting the prefeed weight from the postfeed weight. Test weighing can be easily used both in the hospital and at home as a tool to assess the adequacy of milk

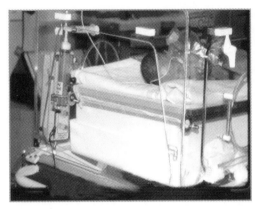

Figure 11-7. Orientation of syringe in continuous tube feeding system. Source: Schanler RJ. Special methods in feeding the preterm infant. In: Tsang R, Nichols BL, eds. Nutrition in Infancy. Philadelphia: Hanley & Belfus, Inc.; 1988:315–325

intake and evaluate milk production after changes in lactation performance. Short-term use of an electronic baby scale can be useful for estimating milk intake in the preterm infant during the transition from the hospital to the home. A sensitive scale (±2 g sensitivity) with a digital readout and computerized integration to correct for infant movement is recommended. Numerous controlled, blinded clinical trials have demonstrated that test weighing is accurate, acceptable to mothers, and superior to other tools or scoring systems previously used to "estimate" milk intake. However, test weighing on a nonelectronic scale is not reliable and not recommended. Although it has been used to estimate milk intake from a single feeding, for best estimates of milk intake, test weighing should be performed at each feeding for at least 24 hours because there is variation from feed to feed. The infant must wear the same clothing and diaper before and after the feeding to obtain an accurate reflection of intake.

Milk Storage

Human milk should be stored in a cool, safe place to maximize its preservation and minimize contamination. Human milk has significant immunologic protection that also protects it from contamination. However, when expressed into collection containers, some skin bacteria mix with the milk. Nevertheless, bacterial counts decrease in stored milk. See Table 11-4 for milk storage guidelines.

Table 11-4. Suggested Guidelines for Milk Storage and Use for All Infants

Storage Method and Temperature	Maximum Amount of Time for Storage
Room (25°C [77°F])	4 h*
Refrigerator (4°C [39°F])	96 h
Previously thawed refrigerated milk	24 h
Freezer (−20°C = 0°F)	3-9 mo

*Continuous milk infusions for tube-feeding neonates generally remain at room temperature for 3 to 4 hours.

General Storage Guidelines

Room Temperature (25°C [77°F])

The consensus is that fresh human milk can be maintained or used at room temperature for up to 4 hours. Continuous intragastric tube feeding syringes used in neonatal nurseries generally remain at room temperature for up to 4 hours.

Refrigeration (4°C [39°F])

Several studies have demonstrated the safety of refrigerating human milk either by evaluating the bactericidal capacity of stored milk as a marker for milk quality, milk constituents, or bacterial growth in the stored milk samples. Bactericidal capacity of stored refrigerated human milk declines significantly by 48 to 72 hours. However, studies of expressed human milk suggest that it can be stored at refrigerator temperature (4°C) in the NICU for as long as 96 hours. These data were obtained in refrigerators being opened several times a day with temperature verification daily.

Freezing (−20°C = 0°F)

The preferred method of storing milk that is not intended to be fed within 48 hours is freezing. Single milk expressions should be packaged separately. Unlike heat treatment, freezing preserves many of the nutritional and immunologic properties of human milk. When frozen appropriately, milk generally can be stored for at least 3 months before levels of free fatty acids increase (evidence for rancidity). Milk should not be stored in the door of the freezer. Milk bank freezers should have a thermometer and an alarm and should be opened only infrequently, especially if used for long-term storage. Under these conditions, long-term storage of human milk has been allowed for up to 9 months.

Thawing

Milk should be thawed using a waterless warmer or by holding the container of milk under running tepid (not hot) water. Milk should never be thawed in a microwave oven or left unattended in a beaker of water. After milk is fully thawed, it should not be refrozen but stored in a refrigerator until used. Thawed milk should be used within 24 hours or discarded. For hospitalized infants, expressed human milk remaining in a bottle after a feeding should be discarded.

Milk Identification

In the hospital setting, all containers for frozen expressed milk must carry a standardized label that includes the infant's name, medical record number, and date and time milk was expressed. Some hospitals request that mothers list medications and/or current illnesses on the label to ensure communication about the acceptability of the milk with hospital staff. Policies should be developed to avoid misadministration of human milk, that is, feeding one mother's milk to someone else's infant. In the child care setting, milk also must be labeled clearly.

Milk Storage Containers

Caps that provide an airtight seal should be used. Milk storage containers include:

- *Rigid plastic* storage containers made of polycarbonate (clear hard plastic), polypropylene (frosted hard plastic bottles), or other hard plastic are recommended for long-term storage of expressed human milk.
- *Glass* containers also can be used for long-term storage, but care must be taken to ensure they do not get overfilled and/or crack.
- *Soft plastic* (polyethylene) storage bags have potential for contamination from nicks in the bags, loss of nutrient properties (especially fat and fat-soluble vitamins), loss of milk because of spillage, and high cost. They are not recommended for hospitalized preterm infants, and some experts discourage their use for all infants. Polyethylene bags specifically designed for storing human milk, however, may be convenient for the workplace/school if mothers bring their milk home at the end of the day. If they are used, the milk should be poured into rigid containers before freezer storage.

Cleaning Collection/Storage Containers

Rinse to remove adherent milk, then wash with hot, soapy water and dry in the air. Dishwasher cleaning also is adequate.

Donor Human Milk

Donor human milk is milk contributed by lactating women other than the biological mother of the receiving infant. Donor milk generally is used as a replacement if a mother's milk is not available. The potent benefits of human milk are such that the AAP now recommends all preterm infants should receive human milk. Mother's own milk, fresh or frozen, should be the primary diet, and it should be fortified appropriately for the infant born weighing less than 1.5 kg. If mother's own milk is unavailable despite significant lactation support, then pasteurized donor milk should be used. In the United States, donor human milk must be collected and stored through a milk bank. Because of the risk for infectious disease transmission, banked donor human milk must be pasteurized. The AAP, the Centers for Disease Control and Prevention, and the US Food and Drug Administration all recommend against using donor human milk that is not pasteurized or is obtained freely via Internet access from unscreened donors and not via a milk bank following protocols of the Human Milk Banking Association of North America (HMBANA). Although pasteurization methods used by milk banks in the United States differ, methods currently used have been shown to effectively eradicate HIV, human T-cell lymphocytic virus, cytomegalovirus, hepatitis B virus, hepatitis C virus, and bacteria.

Use of banked donor milk should be preceded by a discussion of the potential benefits of pasteurized human milk versus the potential risks of its use, such as unknown exposure to drugs, medications, herbal products, or infectious agents. Some experts advocate obtaining written, informed consent for its use; others do not. The HMBANA is one source for information, policies, and procedures related to donor milk banking. All member banks of the HMBANA are required to follow established guidelines, such as carefully selecting and monitoring donors, following strict procedures for heat treatment and storage of donated milk, and evaluating processed milk for sterility after pasteurization. Health care professionals interested in potential uses of donor human milk should consult HMBANA (www.HMBANA.com) or one of its member milk banks. Alternatively, Prolacta Bioscience (www.prolacta.com) is another source of donor human milk and milk products.

Bacteriologic Surveillance of Mother's Own Milk

Human milk potentially can be a mode of transmission of infection. This particularly is a concern when breast pumps and other equipment are used. For example, the rubber bulb portion of the bicycle horn type of breast pump cannot be cleaned or sterilized properly, so its use is not recommended. Electric breast pumps that are disinfected inadequately also may serve as a potential source of infection in neonatal nurseries. Expressed milk samples commonly contain a diversity of bacteria.

Bacteriologic Cultures

Bacteriologic cultures of a mother's own milk may, under rare circumstances, be indicated to assess unexplained infections in infants. Some clinicians culture milk if an infant becomes infected with an unusual organism. There are reports of group B *Streptococcus, Staphylococcus aureus,* and other pathogenic infections occurring in NICU babies that were linked to colonization, mastitis, or both in the mother. Despite this possibility, routinely obtaining cultures of mother's own milk is costly, creates undue concern, and is not recommended. Indeed, a cause-and-effect relationship has not been proved in most case reports. Simultaneous exposure of mother and infant to pathogenic organisms may be more likely. Moreover, results from an initial milk culture do not correlate with subsequent milk cultures from the same mother.

Bacteriologic Screening Results

Bacteria found on screening usually are identical to that found on the mother's skin and nipples. A wide variety of bacteria contaminate human milk from donor mothers. These include both gram-positive organisms (usually $<10^5$ organisms/mL) and some gram-negative organisms. In the United States, milk banks uniformly culture pooled milk samples after pasteurization as a screening test of the adequacy of heat treatment.

How to Deal With a Positive Culture

If the organism is pathogenic and/or present in large quantities, the breast pump and the mother's equipment should be examined for contamination. The mother's milk expression technique also should be evaluated.

Selected References

1. Academy of Breastfeeding Medicine Protocol Committee. Clinical protocol #8: Human milk storage. Information for home use for full-term infants. *Breastfeed Med.* 2010;5:127–130

2. Academy of Breastfeeding Medicine Protocol Committee. Clinical protocol #3: Hospital guidelines for the use of supplementary feedings in the healthy term breastfed neonate. *Breastfeed Med.* 2009;4:175–182

3. Blaymore Bier JA, Ferguson AE, Morales Y, Liebling JA, Oh W, Vohr BR. Breastfeeding infants who were extremely low birth weight. *Pediatrics.* 1997;100:e3

4. Flaherman VJ, Lee HC. "Breastfeeding" by feeding expressed mother's milk. *Pediatr Clin North Am.* 2013;60:227–246

5. Hill PD, Aldag JC, Chatterton RT. Effects of pumping style on milk production in mothers of non-nursing preterm infants. *J Hum Lact.* 1999;15:209–216

6. Howard CR, de Blieck EA, ten Hoopen CB, Howard FM, Lanphear BP, Lawrence RA. Physiologic stability of newborns during cup- and bottle-feeding. *Pediatrics.* 1999;104:1204–1207

7. Howard CR, Howard FM, Lanphear B, et al. Randomized clinical trial of pacifier use and bottle-feeding or cupfeeding and their effect on breastfeeding. *Pediatrics.* 2003;111:511–518

8. Human Milk Banking Association of North America. *Best Practice for Expressing, Storing and Handling Human Milk in Hospitals, Homes, and Child Care Settings.* 3rd ed. West Hartford, CT: Human Milk Banking Association of North America; 2011. http://www.hmbana.org. Accessed August 30, 2013

9. Human Milk Banking Association of North America. *Guidelines for the Establishment and Operation of a Donor Human Milk Bank.* West Hartford, CT: Human Milk Banking Association of North America; 2011. http://www.hmbana.org. Accessed August 30, 2013

10. Landers S, Hartmann BT. Donor human milk banking and the emergence of milk sharing. *Pediatr Clin North Am.* 2013;60:247–260

11. Landers S, Updegrove K. Bacterial screening of donor human milk before and after Holder pasteurization. *Breastfeed Med.* 2010;5:117–121

12. Marinelli KA, Burke GS, Dodd VL. A comparison of the safety of cupfeedings and bottlefeedings in premature infants whose mothers intend to breastfeed. *J Perinatol.* 2001;21:350–355

13. McKechnie AC, Eglash A. Nipple shields: a review of the literature. *Breastfeed Med.* 2010;5:309–314

14. Meier PP. Breastfeeding in the special care nursery. Prematures and infants with medical problems. *Pediatr Clin North Am.* 2001;48:425–442

15. Meier PP, Engstrom JL, Patel AL, Jegier BJ, Bruns NE. Improving the use of human milk during and after the NICU stay. *Pediatr Clin North Am.* 2010;37:217–245

16. Robbins ST. *Infant Feedings: Guidelines for Preparation of Formula and Breastmilk in Health Care Facilities.* Chicago, IL: American Dietetic Association; 2004

17. Schanler RJ, Fraley JK, Lau C, Hurst NM, Horvath L, Rossmann SN. Breastmilk cultures and infection in extremely premature infants. *J Perinatol.* 2011;31:335–338

18. American Academy of Pediatrics Section on Breastfeeding. Breastfeeding and the use of human milk. *Pediatrics.* 2012;129:e827–e841

19. Slusser W, Frantz K. High-technology breastfeeding. *Pediatr Clin North Am.* 2001;48:505–516

20. Slutzah M, Codipilly CN, Potak D, Clark RM, Schanler RJ. Refrigerator storage of expressed human milk in the neonatal intensive care unit. *J Pediatr.* 2010;156:26–28

21. Zinaman MJ, Hughes V, Queenan JT, Labbok MH, Albertson B. Acute prolactin and oxytocin responses and milk yield to infant suckling and artificial methods of expression in lactating women. *Pediatrics.* 1992;89:437–440

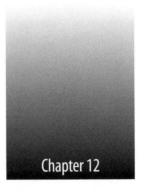

Chapter 12

Medications and Breastfeeding

The use of a medication by the breastfeeding mother continues to be a common reason for unnecessarily stopping breastfeeding. Usually this occurs because the mother gets misleading or confusing advice on the safety of the drug for the breastfed infant. The goal of successful maternal therapy during lactation is to provide the necessary medications to the breastfeeding mother while minimizing the amount of drug passed through the milk to the child, avoiding adverse effects on the infant or decreasing the milk supply. Decisions regarding the choice of a particular therapy for a nursing mother need to be individualized, based on the mother's condition, her tolerance of perceived risk, and the age and condition of her nursing infant.

Drug Passage Into Milk

During pregnancy, direct transplacental passage may result in similar serum concentration of a drug in both the fetus and mother. In a lactating woman, however, the steps of passage of a drug into human milk and then its absorption across the infant's gastrointestinal tract and possible metabolism almost always result in a peak infant serum level well below the maternal value. A factor that is often overlooked is that drugs can diffuse out of human milk over time. As the drug concentration in the mother's blood drops below the milk concentration because of maternal metabolism and excretion, the drug can pass from the milk back into the mother's plasma.

Small water-soluble nonelectrolytes (eg, alcohol, urea) pass into and out of human milk by simple diffusion through spaces between cells in the mammary epithelium. Equilibration between maternal plasma and human milk is rapid, and human milk levels of drugs approximate maternal plasma levels at all times. However, few drugs pass into milk in this way. For larger molecules, only the unbound, nonionized forms cross the mammary epithelium by passive diffusion driven by the concentration gradient between maternal plasma and human milk. Some physical and chemical factors such as low molecular weight, low protein binding, weak bases, and high lipid solubility favor higher passage into milk. However, none of these factors can always be applied in isolation to predict drug passage, because they interact with each other. For example, higher lipid solubility also results in higher plasma protein binding among beta-blockers, so the water-soluble beta-blockers attain higher concentrations in human milk than the lipid-soluble beta-blockers.

Extensive protein binding (>85%) and high molecular weight (>~800 daltons) are fairly reliable drug factors that predict poor passage into human milk, but some large molecules that are analogues of endogenous substances normally found in human milk (eg, synthetic insulins and interferons) have been found in the milk of mothers receiving them, possibly because of active transport. A few small molecules (eg, acyclovir, cimetidine, nitrofurantoin) are actively transported into milk. Pharmacokinetic investigation is the optimal method to ascertain the extent of drug passage into human milk.

The ratio of concentrations of a drug in milk and plasma (the milk/plasma, or M/P, ratio) can be used as a measure of a drug's passage into human milk. However, the M/P ratio has shortcomings that render it meaningless as a measure of drug safety. The currently accepted method of expressing drug passage into milk is the "weight-adjusted percentage of maternal dosage" or "relative infant dose," defined as follows:

$$\frac{\text{Daily infant dosage in breast milk (mg/infant weight in kg)}}{\text{Daily maternal dosage (mg/maternal weight in kg)}} \times 100$$

The relative infant dose has greater value than the M/P ratio in consideration of the safety of medication use during breastfeeding and is reported in well-designed pharmacokinetic studies and in some drug databases. In general, a relative infant dose less than 10% of the mother's dosage is usually considered acceptable for breastfeeding, and a relative infant dosage greater than 25% is considered unacceptable. About 90% of drugs fall below the 10% level, and only about 3% of drugs are passed to the infant in doses greater than 25%. Although this system works well for most drugs, a few exceptions can be made for drugs with very long half-lives (eg, diazepam, fluoxetine) which can accumulate in the infant. In addition, special consideration should apply to selected drugs (cancer chemotherapy, some radiopharmaceuticals) and in some cases to infants who have unusual genetic susceptibility.

Clinical Factors

The age of the infant is an extremely important factor in determining safety of maternal drug therapy. Most adverse reactions from drugs in human milk occur in the first 2 postpartum months, primarily during the first month. This increased susceptibility is probably related to neonates' slower metabolism and elimination of drugs, as well as factors such as red cell susceptibility to hemolysis, lower protein binding, and relatively permeable blood-brain barrier.

Medications taken by the mother during pregnancy can result in fetal exposures that have an impact on the newborn. Long-acting drugs can persist in the infant's circulation after birth and cause adverse effects. Conversely, newborns of mothers who took certain medications during pregnancy can experience drug withdrawal as neonatal serum levels decrease. Signs of neonatal abstinence that persist during breastfeeding result from low passage of the drug into human milk. However, enough drug may be passed into human milk to alleviate signs of withdrawal from some drugs (eg, anticonvulsants, antidepressants, methadone).

The risks of medication use during pregnancy have little to do with the drug's safety during breastfeeding because drug exposure of the fetus is usually much greater, often by 10-fold or more, than the exposure of the infant via human milk. This fact is sometimes not considered by clinicians who mistakenly apply pregnancy warnings or US Food and Drug Administration pregnancy categories (A, B, C, D, X) to breastfeeding. A mother who is concerned about exposing her nursing infant to a medication that she was taking during pregnancy can be comforted if her infant's exposure to the drug during breastfeeding is substantially less than fetal exposure during pregnancy.

During the colostral phase, the dosage of drugs the infant receives is low because of the small volume of colostrum the infant ingests. After lactogenesis 2, the dosage the infant receives increases in proportion to the milk volume. Because newborn infants often nurse every 2 to 3 hours around-the-clock, trying to time medication doses with respect to nursing to reduce infant drug exposure is not possible. Therefore, careful choice of maternal medications is critical during this time. Also, during the first postpartum month, interference with nursing, either by medications or inappropriate advice by health professionals regarding the risks of the medications to the infant, can have a profound impact on milk production and breastfeeding success. After that time, lactation is usually more resilient.

Once the infant begins to take a proportion of nourishment as formula or solid foods, the dosage of any medication via human milk declines proportionately and adverse reactions are rare. Some infants continue to nurse once or twice a day beyond the first year, often in the morning, before naps, or at bedtime. In this setting, the dosage of medication that the infant receives via human milk is also low, and timing maternal medication to occur after nursing can reduce infant drug exposure even further.

Information Resources

High-quality online resources include LactMed from the National Library of Medicine (http://lactmed.nlm.nih.gov) and Dr. Thomas Hale's Infant Risk Center (http://www.infantrisk.com). Most teratogen information services also answer questions on drug use during breastfeeding. They can be located via the Organization of Teratology Information Specialists Web site (http://www.otispregnancy.org). The Physician's Desk Reference and the package insert as they are currently configured do not necessarily contain all available information on the safety of medication exposure to the infant via human milk. The policy statement "The Transfer of Drugs and Therapeutics into Human Breast Milk" from the AAP Committee on Drugs has been included as an appendix to this publication.

Drug Categories

The following selected drugs frequently cause concerns in mothers.

Social Drugs

Cigarette Smoking

Infant are exposed to nicotine and other compounds, including heavy metals, cyanide, and carbon monoxide, from cigarette smoking both directly via milk and indirectly by secondhand smoke. Smokers have human milk with lower milkfat content, use formula supplements more often, and wean their infants from breastfeeding earlier than nonsmokers. Cigarette smoking during nursing increases the risk for sudden infant death syndrome to about the level of formula feeding in nonsmokers, reduces the antioxidant capacity of human milk, and may result in behavioral changes in the infant. Despite these concerns, breastfeeding should be encouraged because of its protection against respiratory illnesses, which are more common in the infant living in a home with smokers, and provides numerous other benefits to infants. Pregnancy and lactation are opportune times to counsel the mother on smoking cessation to protect her health, as well as her infant's. Nursing mothers should be advised to (1) cease or limit smoking to the greatest degree possible, (2) breastfeed before rather than after smoking, and (3) never smoke in the house, car, or in close proximity to the infant.

Smoking Cessation

Smokers may achieve smoking cessation through counseling with or without the use of pharmacologic aids. In general, all forms of replacement therapy are better than smoking.

- *Nicotine patches* deliver a constant amount of nicotine transdermally. With a 21 mg/day transdermal patch, nicotine passes into human milk in amounts equivalent to smoking 17 cigarettes daily. Lower patch strengths of 7 and 14 mg provide proportionately lower amounts of nicotine to the breastfed infant. Achievement of smoking cessation with the aid of serially decreasing strengths of nicotine patches is probably preferable to continued smoking, although data from animal studies indicate that nicotine exposure during nursing might interfere with normal infant lung development. Because nicotine appears in milk, there is a risk that the breastfed infant may exhibit signs of restlessness, jitteriness, poor feeding, and abnormal sleep patterns. Other forms of nicotine replacement (eg, gum, inhalers) may produce more variable plasma levels. Their use is not recommended during breastfeeding.
- *Bupropion* is an antidepressant that is also used to aid smoking cessation. Bupropion transfer to the infant via human milk seems to be low and usually well tolerated, although published data during nursing are limited. A seizure was reported in one infant that was questionably related to bupropion in stored human milk.
- *Varenicline* is a partial nicotine agonist used to assist smoking cessation. No information is available on the use of varenicline during breastfeeding, so other methods are preferred.

Alcohol

Alcohol (ethanol) consumption by the mother decreases the amount of milk ingested by the infant, disrupts infant sleep patterns, and interferes with maternal-infant interactions. Daily heavy use of alcohol (more than 2 drinks daily) may affect breastfed infants' development negatively. Binge drinking interferes with milk letdown. Alcohol rapidly equilibrates between maternal plasma and human milk, so waiting for maternal blood alcohol levels to decline will decrease the baby's exposure. It takes about 2 hours per drink (ie, 4–6 fluid ounces of wine, 1 beer, 1 mixed drink) for alcohol levels in milk to decrease to zero for women of average body weight. Mothers should be counseled to limit their alcoholic intake to 1 drink or less per day, preferable after a sufficient waiting period since the previous drink. The Institute of Medicine recommends lactating women limit alcohol intake to 0.5 g or less of alcohol per kilogram of maternal body weight per day, and to wait 4 hours after the last drink to breastfeed (see Chapter 16).

Caffeine

The negative side effects of caffeine in infants (eg, jitteriness, irritability, and poor sleep) appear only when mothers consume high amounts or in preterm or newborn infants with limited hepatic metabolism. The amount of caffeine in beverages and foods can vary widely depending on the product and the preparation. More important, the serving size of beverages has increased markedly in recent years. A maternal intake of 300 mg caffeine daily is a safe limit unlikely to affect the breastfed infant. Individualized assessment of caffeine intake may be necessary when consumption exceeds two 8-fluid ounce servings of coffee or two 16-fluid ounce servings of tea or soda.

Marijuana

Limited data suggest that the active ingredient, THC, in marijuana enters the infant's bloodstream in small amounts via maternal milk after maternal smoking of marijuana. Two 1-year studies found little effect on the breastfed infants of marijuana smokers, although a slight decrease in motor function was seen in 1 infant. The risk of smoke exposure to the infant's respiratory health cannot be overstated. Impairment of maternal judgment is a concern in mothers who use cannabis products during nursing.

Cocaine

Cocaine has not been studied in lactating women, but it is possibly the most dangerous street drug for mothers nursing newborns, because neonates metabolize cocaine poorly and can have convulsions with relatively small doses. Smoking "crack" cocaine in the presence of the infant is also very dangerous. The judgment of mothers with ongoing cocaine abuse may be impaired, indirectly affecting her infant adversely. Cocaine use is contraindicated during breastfeeding. Nursing mothers who use cocaine on a single occasion should withhold nursing for 24 hours after drug ingestion.

Anticoagulation

Unfractionated or low-molecular-weight heparins (eg, dalteparin, enoxaparin) given to the mother are safe for the breastfed infant, because the high molecular weight of these drugs prevents transfer into milk. Warfarin is also safe because high protein binding minimizes the concentration in milk. The newer anticoagulants (eg, dabigatran, rivaroxaban) and platelet aggregation inhibitors (eg, ticlopidine, clopidogrel) have not been studied during breastfeeding and are best avoided until data become available. All of the newer drugs are small molecules and theoretically enter milk more readily than the heparins or warfarin.

Asthma

Corticosteroids

Corticosteroids are transferred into milk in extremely small quantities, whether administered orally or by inhaler. The use of corticosteroids to treat asthma in the breastfeeding mother is safe for the infant. Exceptions are betamethasone and dexamethasone, which have not been studied and are much longer acting than other corticosteroids.

Beta-Agonists

Albuterol and other beta-agonists result in low serum levels after inhalation and appear to be safe.

Leukotriene Inhibitors

Manufacturers' data indicate low milk levels for zileuton and zafirlukast. No such data exist for montelukast. If essential for asthma control in mother, zafirlukast appears to be the preferred agent.

Maternal Depression

Maternal depression, often accompanied by anxiety, carries a risk for abnormal child development (see Chapter 9). Therapy should take into account individual benefits and risks. Mild depression may be best treated with psychological therapy. Antidepressants are indicated if the mother declines or fails psychological therapy and is moderately to severely depressed. If the mother was successfully treated for depression during pregnancy, treatment should generally continue postpartum with the same antidepressant (please see AGOG Practice Bulletin #92, April 2008 "Use of Psychiatric Medications During Pregnancy and Lactation"). Older antidepressants, such as the tricyclic antidepressants nortriptyline and amitriptyline, have a good safety profile in breastfeeding, including long-term infant neurodevelopmental outcomes. However, because of adverse effects associated with tricyclic antidepressants, selective serotonin reuptake inhibitors (SSRIs) are now the most widely prescribed antidepressants. Infant restlessness, irritability, colic, poor weight gain, and sleep disorders have been reported in association with maternal SSRI treatment, predominantly for SSRIs that have greater excretion into human milk (eg, citalopram, fluoxetine). Paroxetine and sertraline have lower milk levels and are the preferred SSRIs during breastfeeding, with careful monitoring for adverse effects. Long-term neurodevelopmental outcome data for infants exposed to SSRIs via human milk are relatively limited. Other antidepressants (eg, bupropion, mirtazapine, venlafaxine) have not been extensively studied and are not considered first-line therapy unless the patient responded well in the past.

Anxiety

Long-acting benzodiazepines (eg, diazepam) may accumulate in milk, especially with long-term use, and produce symptoms in the infant, such as lethargy, sedation, and poor suck. Sporadic use of long-acting drugs and the use of short-acting drugs (lorazepam, midazolam, oxazepam) pose a lower risk.

Diabetes

Insulin

Insulin is a normal component of human milk. Small amounts of the semi-synthetic insulins (eg, aspart, glargine) have been detected in the milk of some mothers using these drugs, but there appears to be no harm to the infant. Breastfeeding may reduce maternal insulin needs, so careful blood glucose monitoring is important during breastfeeding in insulin-dependent mothers.

Oral Diabetic Medications

The sulfonylureas, chlorpropamide, glipizide, glyburide, and tolbutamide, are minimally excreted in milk and are compatible with breastfeeding. Other hypoglycemics have not been studied. Although hypoglycemia has not been reported, infant blood glucose monitoring may be indicated. The alpha-glucosidase inhibitors (acarbose, miglitol) have almost no oral bioavailability and are acceptable to use. Substantial experience with metformin in nursing mothers with diabetes and polycystic ovary syndrome indicate that the drug is acceptable during breastfeeding.

Other Agents

The thiazolidinediones (pioglitazone, rosiglitazone), dipeptidyl peptidase-IV inhibitors (linagliptin, saxagliptin, sitagliptin), and various newer injectable antidiabetic agents (exenatide, liraglutide, pramlintide) have not been studied during breastfeeding.

Gastrointestinal Disorders

H_2 Receptor Blocking

Famotidine, ranitidine, and nizatidine and other H_2 receptor blocking agents appear to be safe during lactation. Cimetidine is not preferred because of potential hepatic enzyme inhibition. The proton pump inhibitors omeprazole and pantoprazole are minimally excreted into milk and are not expected to cause adverse effects in breastfed babies. Other proton pump inhibitors have not been studied during breastfeeding. Oral antacids (eg, calcium carbonate, magnesium hydroxide) are safe to use during breastfeeding.

Hypertension and Preeclampsia

The treatment of adult hypertension often involves combinations of drugs.

Diuretics

Diuretics appear to be safe during lactation with typical antihypertensive doses. Hydrochlorothiazide and chlorothiazide have been used for decades and no problems have been described in the breastfed infant. High doses of diuretics can suppress lactation.

Beta-Blocking Agents

The drugs within this class that seem to be safest for use during breastfeeding are propranolol, labetalol, and metoprolol. Atenolol and acebutolol may present problems to the breastfed infant because of the greater excretion in milk and slower elimination by the infant. It is prudent to avoid these drugs in the breastfeeding mother. The infant of a mother taking any beta-blocking agent should be monitored, especially for heart rate, feeding problems, respiratory pattern, and activity.

Angiotensin-Converting Enzyme Inhibitors

ACE inhibitors that have been studied include benazepril, captopril, enalapril, and quinapril and are excreted in limited quantities into milk. There are no reports of problems using these drugs. The related angiotensin receptor blockers (eg, losartan) have not been studied during breastfeeding.

Calcium Channel Blocking Agents
Calcium channel blocking agents that have been studied during breastfeeding include diltiazem, nifedipine, nitrendipine, and verapamil. Little drug is present in milk, and these agents appear to be acceptable during breastfeeding. Nifedipine 10 mg three times daily has been used successfully to treat nursing mothers with Raynaud phenomenon of the nipple. Other calcium channel blockers have not been studied during breastfeeding.

Magnesium Sulfate
Magnesium sulfate freely crosses the placenta and may affect the newborn's ability to nurse effectively. Intravenous administration for preeclampsia does not increase human milk magnesium levels, and magnesium has poor oral availability, so it is safe during breastfeeding.

Immunomodulating Agents

Anti-Tumor Necrosis Factor
These drugs are transmitted into milk in levels that are either undetectable (eg, adalimumab, certolizumab) or extremely low (etanercept, infliximab). Expert opinion holds that they are acceptable during breastfeeding.

Chloroquine and Hydroxychloroquine
Chloroquine and hydroxychloroquine have been studied in nursing mothers and their infants. Amounts in milk are low, and no adverse effects were seen with follow-up of the breastfed infants up to 1 year of age.

Immunosuppressants
A considerable amount of pharmacokinetic and clinical evidence indicates that cyclosporine usually does not affect the breastfed infant. Less evidence is available for tacrolimus, but it has not been detected in human milk or in the serum of breastfed infants. For both of these drugs, breastfed infants should be monitored carefully, possibly including measurement of serum levels to rule out toxicity if there is a concern. Safe use of azathioprine and its metabolite mercaptopurine during nursing has been reported in patients with inflammatory bowel disease, lupus, and organ transplants. Some professional organizations consider the above drugs to be acceptable during nursing but recommend monitoring exclusively breastfed infants with a complete blood cell count, differential, and liver function tests. Methotrexate should be avoided in dosages used for cancer treatment; however, limited data indicate that low levels are transferred into milk with single maternal doses up to 65 mg. Although less consensus is available, intermittent use of these low doses

may be acceptable, but the breastfed infant's complete blood cell count and differential should be monitored. Mycophenolate and sirolimus have not been studied and are best avoided during breastfeeding.

Intravenous Immunoglobulin
IVIG is considered safe, and it is the drug of choice for treating multiple sclerosis during breastfeeding.

Mesalamine
Mesalamine and its derivatives (eg, balsalazide) are acceptable to use during breastfeeding, although the infant should be monitored for diarrhea, which may occur rarely. Sulfasalazine is best avoided because of its sulfonamide component.

Antimicrobials
Almost all antimicrobials are transferred to milk. Many of them are also used for the treatment of infectious diseases in children. The doses received by the breastfed infant are always less than what would be given directly to the infant for therapy. Use of broad-spectrum antimicrobials, combinations of drugs, and long-term or repeated therapy of the mother, as for recurrent mastitis, increase the infant's risk for the development of diarrhea, thrush, or diaper rash.

Antifungal Agents
Nystatin and amphotericin B are not orally absorbed, so they pose no risk to the nursing infant. Maternal fluconazole is safe for the infant and has been used for direct infant therapy. Ketoconazole and itraconazole are less well studied and potentially more toxic, but they can be used with caution if no alternatives exist. Ketoconazole should not be used topically on the nipples because of possible direct ingestion by the infant. Clotrimazole and miconazole have poor bioavailability when ingested orally and are good choices for vaginal or topical use, including on the nipples.

Cephalosporins and Penicillins
These antibiotics appear in milk in minute quantities and are generally safe. There is a slight possibility of allergic reactions in the infant.

Clindamycin
Clindamycin is an option for the treatment of methicillin-resistant *Staphylococcus aureus* infections (eg, mastitis), but the infant should be observed for diarrhea and bloody stools.

Linezolid

An option for the treatment of methicillin-resistant *S aureus* infections, linezolid appears in milk at lower amounts than those used in infants.

Macrolides

Erythromycin, clarithromycin, azithromycin, and other macrolides are generally safe to use during breastfeeding, although there is a possibility that erythromycin might increase the risk for hypertrophic pyloric stenosis in breastfed infants, particularly in the first weeks.

Metronidazole

The caution against metronidazole is related to its in vitro ability to cause chromosomal damage leading to possible carcinogenesis. This has not been described in humans receiving the drug or in nursing infants of mothers treated with the drug, although a valid study would be almost impossible to perform. Metronidazole is occasionally used in infants for the treatment of *Giardia* and some anaerobic infections, and is used in pregnancy. Metronidazole seems to be safe for the breastfed infant in the short term, although there are reports of increased *Candida* colonization and poor feeding.

Fluoroquinolones

Fluoroquinolones (eg, ciprofloxacin, levofloxacin) appear in human milk in low levels. If there is no other choice for maternal therapy, a short (1- to 2-week) exposure to ciprofloxacin may be acceptable for the breastfed infant. No data are available on the safety of levofloxacin use in infants. Eyedrops or eardrops do not pose any risk for the breastfed infant.

Sulfonamides

Rarely indicated, sulfonamides should be avoided in breastfeeding mothers because of an increased risk for kernicterus in jaundiced infants and concerns of hemolysis in infants with a deficiency of glucose-6-phosphate dehydrogenase. Trimethoprim-sulfamethoxazole is an option for treatment of methicillin-resistant *S aureus* infections (eg, mastitis) while breastfeeding an older infant without glucose-6-phosphate dehydrogenase deficiency.

Tetracyclines

Short-term use of tetracyclines in nursing mothers is safe. The amount of tetracycline that appears in milk is low, and oral bioavailability is poor because of the calcium in milk. Long-term daily use (eg, for acne) is best avoided.

Migraine

Migraine headache treatment in adults is divided into prophylaxis of attacks and treatment of the acute episode. Drugs for migraine prophylaxis that are the best choices during breastfeeding are amitriptyline, gabapentin, metoprolol, nortriptyline, propranolol, sertraline, and valproic acid.

Initial Therapy for Acute Migraine Headache

The initial therapy for acute migraine headache may range from nonpharmacologic measures, such as rest, darkened room, and a wet cloth to the forehead, to some of the newest drugs. The use of acetaminophen and nonsteroidal anti-inflammatory drugs is acceptable during lactation because most are weak acids and highly protein bound, although short-acting drugs (eg, ibuprofen) are preferred while nursing a newborn. Products that contain a combination of acetaminophen with caffeine are considered safe during lactation (see Chapter 6).

Triptans

Data for sumatriptan and eletriptan demonstrate that the excretion in milk is low for these two drugs. Other triptans have not been studied.

Ergot Alkaloids

These alkaloids (ergotamine, dihydroergotamine) have not been studied. They may interfere with prolactin and adversely affect the breastfed infant. They are not recommended during lactation.

Pain Management

The breastfeeding mother can usually achieve pain management by appropriate doses of either acetaminophen or nonsteroidal anti-inflammatory drugs such as ibuprofen. Oral opiates (eg, hydrocodone, oxycodone) can be added in low doses for short courses or as needed when the nonopioid analgesia is inadequate. Oral codeine is falling out of favor because of excess sedation in some mothers and infants with pharmacogenomic variants. More severe pain, such as that occurring immediately after birth or after surgery, can be managed with the added use of short-acting intravenous or intramuscular narcotics such as fentanyl or dilaudid. Careful monitoring of newborn infants for sedation and respiratory depression is necessary whenever opiates are given to their mothers. See Chapter 6 for a discussion of pain management during lactation.

Seizure Management

There are numerous case reports of adverse effects in breastfed infants of mothers taking anticonvulsants, but most infants do not have noticeable effects. Given the widespread use of these agents over many years, it is uncertain that these effects were caused by exposure to human milk. Many of the reports were in infants whose mothers also took the drug during pregnancy or were taking more than one anticonvulsant or psychotropic. Older, sedating anticonvulsants (phenobarbital, primidone) have caused sedation in breastfed infants exposed to the drug through milk. Methemoglobinemia was reported in a neonate exposed to phenytoin during pregnancy and lactation. Reports of infant sedation and hepatic dysfunction have also been published with maternal carbamazepine use. Thrombocytopenia and anemia in 1 infant was possibly related to valproic acid in human milk. Lamotrigine and ethosuximide taken by the breastfeeding mother may result in near-therapeutic plasma levels in the infant. Zonisamide is also extensively excreted into human milk. Drugs that have relatively low excretion into human milk include gabapentin, pregabalin, topiramate, and vigabatrin. Follow-up of infants who were breastfed by mothers taking carbamazepine, lamotrigine, phenytoin, or valproate as a single agent found no difference in IQ scores at 3 years of age compared with the infants of mothers taking these drugs who did not breastfeed. Regardless of which drug or drugs the mother needs for the control of her epilepsy, it would be prudent not only to clinically observe the baby but also to measure drug concentrations in the infant's plasma if adverse effects are suspected, or to perform liver function tests if jaundice occurs, especially in the first 2 months.

Thyroid and Antithyroid Therapy

Levothyroxine is given at a dosage to replicate the normal serum levels of thyroid hormone in deficient individuals. With proper dosage adjustment, it will not affect the thyroid function of the infant. For women in the United States with hyperthyroidism, propylthiouracil had been the preferred drug because of low transfer into the milk and a lack of effect on infant thyroid function. Propylthiouracil can cause irreversible hepatic failure, although there are no reports in infants during breastfeeding. Therefore, methimazole is preferred despite its greater transfer into milk. Methimazole dosages of 20 mg/day do not affect the infant's thyroid function. Exposure can be minimized by waiting 3 hours after the dose before nursing. Topical iodine exposure (eg, povidone iodine), as well as ingestion of high doses of iodides, should be minimized because these agents may cause hypothyroidism in breastfed infants. Exceptions are low doses in iodine-deficient mothers and protection of the thyroid after radiation exposure, when potassium iodide should be given to both the mother and infant when indicated (see Chapter 18).

Diagnostic Agents

Currently used iodinated contrast media and gadolinium-based MRI contrast agents do not pose a risk to the breastfed infant after maternal administration because of low excretion into human milk and poor oral absorption. Mothers do not need to withhold breastfeeding after their use.

Radioactive Isotopes

Ideally, elective diagnostic nuclear medicine procedures should be delayed until the patient is no longer breastfeeding. If a diagnostic radioisotope is to be administered to a breastfeeding mother, an agent with a short half-life is preferred. She should be told how long she likely is to be unable to breast-feed, counseled to express and discard her milk during the time required for treatment, and told whether she should avoid holding her infant close to her body for a period of time after the examination. This information will allow her to express and refrigerate or freeze milk in advance for her infant's use while she is unable to breastfeed. The most concerning diagnostic isotope is iodine-131. The American Thyroid Association recommends using iodine-123 or technetium scans for diagnosis of hyperthyroidism in nursing mothers. Mothers who receive therapeutic radioactive isotopes will probably not be able to breastfeed for an extended period because the dose of radiation remains high for a sustained period. The US Nuclear Regulatory Agency has published guidelines on periods of abstinence from breastfeeding and close contact with the infant, including by the father or others in close proximity to the infant. Measurement of the radioactivity of pumped human milk can help determine the safe time to resume for a particular woman. A nuclear medi-cine physician should be consulted on individual patients.

Galactagogues

Drugs that stimulate the production of milk, galactagogues should be used only after usual efforts to increase milk production (eg, proper positioning, frequent breastfeeding, milk expression) are unsuccessful.Metoclopramide increases serum prolactin and might increase milk production in some women, although studies are equivocal. The duration of metoclopramide should not exceed 14 days, because it can cause maternal depression and tardive dyskinesia. The drug may also have short-term adverse effects in mothers, including tiredness, nausea, headache, diarrhea, dry mouth, breast discomfort, vertigo, restless legs, hair loss, and anxiety. Domperidone works in a similar manner to metoclopramide and is often used in Canada and other countries. Meta-analyses have found that it is effective as a galactagogue, although the total number of patients included in well-designed studies is small. Domperidone appears to have fewer central nervous system side effects than metoclopramide but can lengthen the QT interval, which generated warnings from the US Food and Drug Administration and Health Canada. It is not commercially available in the United States.

Other galactagogues, such as thyrotropin-releasing hormone and human growth hormone, may increase milk production through increasing prolactin secretion or working additively with prolactin to sustain normal lactation. There has been insufficient study of these hormones, and they are too expensive to be recommended for routine use to stimulate lactation. Oxytocin spray was commercially available in the past to improve milk ejection. Its efficacy as a galactagogue is questionable, and it is no longer marketed in most countries. A plethora of herbal products are claimed to be galactagogues, but none has been adequately studied.

Herbal Remedies

Herbal remedies are frequently used for a variety of conditions. Lactating women who ask about using herbal preparations should be informed that the composition, purity, and efficacy are not well regulated and that they should use caution when procuring them. There are few data on efficacy, but adverse effects have been reported in infants whose mothers took products containing arnica (neonatal hemolysis), seaweed (hypothyroidism from excess iodine), stinging nettle (urticaria), St. John's wort (possible colic, drowsiness, or lethargy), and an herbal tea mixture (hypotonia, lethargy, emesis, weak cry, poor sucking attributed to anethole in anise and fennel).

Environmental Agents

Environmental agents may affect breastfeeding and are as likely to be in the general food supply and infant formula as in human milk. An exception might be a mother who lives or works in a heavily contaminated area.

Lead Exposure and Breastfeeding
Women with elevated factors for lead exposure should be screened if they plan to breastfeed. A woman with a confirmed blood level of 40 micrograms/dl should not breastfeed (she may pump and discard her milk) until rescreening confirms a lower level and the source of exposure for mother and infant has been removed.

Selected References

1. Academy of Breastfeeding Medicine Protocol Committee. ABM clinical protocol #9: Use of galactogogues in initiating or augmenting the rate of maternal milk secretion (First revision January 2011). *Breastfeed Med.* 2011;6:41–49
2. American Academy of Pediatrics Committee on Drugs. The transfer of drugs and therapeutics into human breast milk: an update on selected topics. *Pediatrics.* 2013;132:e796–e809
3. American College of Obstetricians and Gynecologists. *Lead Screening During Pregnancy and Lactation.* Committee Opinion #533. August 2012
4. American College of Obstetricians and Gynecologists. *Use of Psychiatric Medications During Pregnancy and Lactation.* Practice Bulletin #92. April 2008
5. American College of Radiology Committee on Drugs and Contrast Media. Administration of contrast media to breast-feeding mothers. In: *ACR Manual on Contrast Media.* Version 8. 2012:79–80
6. Anderson GD. Using pharmacokinetics to predict the effects of pregnancy and maternal-infant transfer of drugs during lactation. *Expert Opin Drug Metab Toxicol.* 2006;2:947–960
7. Anderson PO, Pochop SL, Manoguerra AS. Adverse drug reactions in breastfed infants: less than imagined. *Clin Pediatr (Phila).* 2003;42:325–340
8. Anderson PO, Valdes V. A critical review of pharmaceutical galactagogues. *Breastfeed Med.* 2007;2:229–242
9. Bennett PN, ed. *Drugs and Human Lactation.* 2nd ed. Amsterdam, Netherlands: Elsevier; 1996
10. Berle JO, Spigset O. Antidepressant use during breastfeeding. *Curr Women's Health Rev.* 2011;7:28–34
11. Betzold CM. Galactogogues. *J Midwifery Womens Health.* 2004;49:151–154
12. Budzynska K, Gardner ZE, Duguoa JJ, Low Dog T, Gardiner P. Systematic review of breastfeeding and herbs. *Breastfeed Med.* 2012;7:489–503
13. Cressman AM, Koren G, Pupco A, Kim E, Ito S, Bozzo P. Maternal cocaine use during breastfeeding. *Can Fam Physician.* 2012;58:1218–1219
14. Donovan TJ, Buchanan K. Medications for increasing milk supply in mothers expressing breastmilk for their preterm hospitalised infants. *Cochrane Database Syst Rev.* 2012;3:CD005544
15. Hale TW. *Medications and Mother's Milk.* 12th ed. Amarillo, TX: Hale Publishing; 2006
16. Ho E, Collantes A, Kapur BM, Moretti M, Koren G. Alcohol and breast feeding: calculation of time to zero level in milk. *Biol Neonate.* 2001;80:219–222

17. Howe DB, Beardsley M, Bakhsh S. Appendix U. Model procedure for release of patients or human research subjects administered radioactive materials. In: NUREG-1556. *Consolidated Guidance About Materials Licenses. Program-specific Guidance About Medical Licenses. Final Report.* US Nuclear Regulatory Commission Office of Nuclear Material Safety and Safeguards. Vol. 9, Rev 2. 2008:9. http://www.nrc.gov/reading-rm/doc-collections/nuregs/staff/sr1556/v9/r2/. Accessed September 3, 2013

18. Ilett KF, Hale TW, Page-Sharp M, Kristensen JH, Kohan R, Hackett LP. Use of nicotine patches in breast-feeding mothers: transfer of nicotine and cotinine into human milk. *Clin Pharmacol Ther.* 2003;74:516–524

19. Ilett KF, Kristensen JH. Drug use and breastfeeding. *Expert Opin Drug Saf.* 2005;4:745–768

20. Ito S. Drug therapy for breast-feeding women. *N Engl J Med.* 2000;343:118–126

21. Lanza di Scalea T, Wisner KL. Pharmacotherapy of postpartum depression. *Expert Opin Pharmacother.* 2009;10:2593–2607

22. Mahadevan U, Cucchiara S, Hyams JS, et al. The London Position Statement of the World Congress of Gastroenterology on Biological Therapy for IBD With the European Crohn's and Colitis Organisation: pregnancy and pediatrics. *Am J Gastroenterol.* 2011;106:214–223

23. Meador KJ, Baker GA, Browning N, et al. Effects of breastfeeding in children of women on antiepileptic drugs. *Neurology.* 2010;74(suppl 2):A304–A305

24. Osadchy A, Moretti ME, Koren G. Effect of domperidone on insufficient lactation in puerperal women: a systematic review and meta-analysis of randomized controlled trials. *Obstet Gynecol Int.* 2012;2012:642893

25. Pringsheim T, Davenport WJ, Mackie G, et al. Canadian headache society guideline for migraine prophylaxis. *Can J Neurol Sci.* 2012;39:S1–S2

26. Rowe H, Baker T, Hale TW. Maternal medication, drug use, and breastfeeding. *Pediatr Clin North Am.* 2013;60:275–294

27. Stagnaro-Green A, Abalovich M, Alexander E, et al. Guidelines of the American Thyroid Association for the diagnosis and management of thyroid disease during pregnancy and postpartum. *Thyroid.* 2011;21:1081–1125

28. US Food and Drug Administration. *FDA Warns Against Using Unapproved Drug, Domperidone, to Increase Milk Production.* FDA talk paper. Rockville, MD: US Food and Drug Administration; 2004

29. van der Woude CJ, Kolacek S, Dotan I, et al. European evidenced-based consensus on reproduction in inflammatory bowel disease. *J Crohns Colitis.* 2010;4:493–510

30. Zapantis A, Steinberg JG, Schilit L. Use of herbals as galactagogues. *J Pharm Pract.* 2012;25:222–231

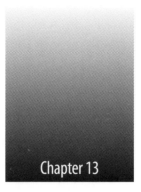

Chapter 13

Contraception and the Breastfeeding Mother

A woman should be encouraged to consider her future plans for child-bearing and desired birth spacing during prenatal care and should be given information and services that will help her meet her goals so that she can devote her time and energy to her new infant.

Contraceptive Counseling

Rationale

An unplanned pregnancy within a year after birth not only may cause nutritional and emotional stress, but it also may negatively affect a mother's commitment to ongoing breastfeeding.

Opportunities for Counseling

Frequent visits with a health care professional in the antepartum and post-partum periods provide many opportunities to discuss contraceptive plans.

Antepartum

An antepartum visit presents an opportunity to explore a mother's attitudes about contraception, her experience with different contraceptive methods, her preferred method(s), and her thoughts on birth spacing or, alternatively, sterilization. The advantages and disadvantages of different methods can be reviewed in relation to her health profile and her decision to breastfeed.

Immediate Postpartum

At the time of discharge counseling after birth, the mother's contraceptive plan can be reviewed and reinforced or revised. Consideration may be given to the potential risk for unintended pregnancy before a return visit if breastfeeding may not meet lactational amenorrhea criteria to ensure anovulation.

Postpartum Office Visit

The postpartum visit, typically 4 to 6 weeks after delivery, is an ideal time to assess the adequacy of breastfeeding frequency and duration in providing natural contraception. If the mother needs or wants more protection from unintended pregnancy, options can be discussed and initiated.

Contraceptive Options

Methods Not Using Exogenous Hormones

Intrauterine Devices (IUDs)

IUDs offer safe, effective long-term contraception and may be considered for all appropriate candidates who seek a reversible, effective, and coitally-independent birth control method. They offer long-term pregnancy protection (5–10 years depending on the product chosen). They may be conveniently inserted at the time of the postpartum visit. The main advantage to the use of IUDs is the long-term contraceptive effectiveness of 99% or greater. Additionally, they have no proven adverse effect on breastfeeding. It should be noted that some IUDs contain a progestin; characteristics of progestins in relation to breastfeeding are described below.

Barrier Methods

The advantage of barrier methods of contraception, including pre-lubricated latex condoms, the diaphragm, and spermicides, is the absence of any effect on breastfeeding. Condoms have additional, non-contraceptive advantages including effective protection against sexually transmitted diseases. The disadvantage of barrier methods is suboptimal effectiveness in typical use, with failure rates of approximately 10% to 20% across different barrier methods. These data are based on normally menstruating women and thus are likely applicable to the breastfeeding woman once menses resume. It is recommended that condoms be used at any time, but waiting until six weeks postpartum before using a contraceptive cap or diaphragm.

Lactational Amenorrhea Method

The lactational amenorrhea method (LAM) has been shown to be highly effective in a variety of cultural, health care, and socioeconomic settings and globally reduces prematurity because of increases in child spacing. The LAM is most appropriate for women who plan to exclusively breastfeed 6 months or longer. If the infant is breastfed exclusively (or is rarely given supplemental formula feedings) and if the mother has not experienced her first postpartum menses, breastfeeding provides more than 98% protection from pregnancy in the first 6 months after delivery. For optimal effectiveness, intervals between feedings should not exceed 4 hours during the day or 6 hours at night. Feeding practices other than direct breastfeeding, such as pumping, may reduce the vigor and frequency of suckling. This, in turn, may alter the maternal neuroendocrine response, and hence increase the probability that ovulation will resume. An alternative method of contraception should be used if the mother's description of the extent of her breastfeeding suggests it may not be adequate to suppress ovulation. It may be prudent to note plans for alternative contraception in the chart if the patient no longer meets criteria for suppression of ovulation from LAM. In addition, mothers using LAM should be provided standard counseling about strategies to prevent sexually transmitted diseases.

Methods Using Exogenous Hormones

Exogenous hormones are a readily accepted and highly effective means of preventing pregnancy. There are, however, potential disadvantages that relate to the postpartum state in general and to breastfeeding mothers in particular, and these disadvantages vary by hormonal method.

Progestin-Only Contraceptives

- *Advantages.* Compared with nonhormonal methods, progestin-only contraceptives, including progestin-only tablets ("minipills"), depot medroxyprogesterone acetate (DMPA), levonorgestrel implants, and levonorgestrel-containing IUDs, have no proven effect on the quality or volume of human milk. Progestin-only methods have traditionally been considered the hormonal contraceptive of choice for breastfeeding mothers.
- *Timing.* No scientific evidence proscribes the initiation of progestin-only contraception in the early postpartum period. However, the typical 2- to 3-day postdelivery decrease of progesterone is part of the physiologic process that initiates lactation. Thus, there is theoretical concern that giving progestins in the first few days before lactation is established could

interfere with optimal lactation. Contraception is not needed in the first 3 weeks postpartum because of a delay in return of ovulation in all women, and this delay is extended for women who breastfeed exclusively. Health care professionals should consider initiating progestin-only contraception at 6 weeks in those women who are breastfeeding exclusively and at 3 weeks in others. There may, however, be practical reasons for initiating contraception in the immediate postpartum period, such as uncertainty about the opportunities for follow-up visits.

Estrogen-Progestin–Containing Contraceptives

- *Disadvantages.* There are several disadvantages to the use of combination oral contraceptives in breastfeeding women. The first disadvantage, which applies to all postpartum women, is the potential contribution of the estrogen component to the known hypercoagulable state of the postpartum period. Furthermore, use of estrogen-containing contraceptives in the postpartum period can have negative effects on breastfeeding, including decreased milk production leading to a decreased duration of breastfeeding and an increase in supplementation. Estrogen also may be transferred into the milk.

- *Timing.* The most recent Centers for Disease Control and Prevention guidelines state that women should not use combined oral contraceptives in the first 21 days after delivery because of an unacceptable risk for venous thromboembolism. Women with no risk factors may—only with caution—use combined oral contraceptives in days 21 to 42 postpartum. The most conservative recommendation, that of delaying combined oral contraceptive use until at least 6 months after delivery in breastfeeding women, largely emanates from earlier studies of combination oral contraceptives that used higher doses of estrogen. Most contemporary formulations have 35 µg or less of estrogen, with some as low as 10 µg. Although progestin-only preparations remain the oral contraception of choice for breastfeeding women, combination oral contraceptives can be considered after 6 weeks postpartum if breastfeeding is well established and the infant's nutritional status is monitored.

Selected References

1. Abdulla KA, Elwan SI, Salem HS, Shaaban MM. Effect of early postpartum use of the contraceptive implants, NORPLANT, on the serum levels of immunoglobulins of the mothers and their breastfed infants. *Contraception.* 1985;32:261–266

2. American College of Obstetricians and Gynecologists. The intrauterine device. ACOG technical bulletin number 164—February 1992. *Int J Gynaecol Obstet.* 1993;41:189–193

3. American College of Obstetricians and Gynecologists. ACOG committee opinion. Condom availability for adolescents. Number 154-April 1995. Committee on Adolescent Health Care. American College of Obstetricians and Gynecologists. *Int J Gynaecol Obstet.* 1995;49:347–351

4. American College of Obstetricians and Gynecologists. Breastfeeding: maternal and infant aspects. ACOG educational bulletin number 258—July 2000. *Obstet Gynecol.* 1999;96

5. American College of Obstetricians and Gynecologists. ACOG practice bulletin. No. 73: use of hormonal contraception in women with coexisting medical conditions. *Obstet Gynecol.* 2006;107(6):1453–1472

6. Campbell OM, Gray RH. Characteristics and determinants of postpartum ovarian function in women in the United States. *Am J Obstet Gynecol.* 1993;169:55–60

7. Chen BA, Reeves MF, Creinin MD, Schwarz EB. Postplacental or delayed levonorgestrel intrauterine device insertion and breast-feeding duration. *Contraception.* 2011;84:499–504

8. Chi IC, Potts M, Wilkens LR, Champion CB. Performance of the copper T-380A intrauterine device in breastfeeding women. *Contraception.* 1989;39:603–618

9. Chi IC, Wilkens LR, Champion CB, Machemer RE, Rivera R. Insertional pain and other IUD insertion-related rare events for breastfeeding and non-breastfeeding women: a decade's experience in developing countries. *Adv Contracept.* 1989;5:101–119

10. Espey E, Ogburn T, Leeman L, Singh R, Schrader R. Effect of progestin compared with combined oral contraceptive pills on lactation: a randomized controlled trial. *Obstet Gynecol.* 2012;119:5–13

11. Gurtcheff SE, Turok DK, Stoddard G, Murphy PA, Gibson M, Jones KP. Lactogenesis after early post-partum use of the contraceptive implant. *Obstet Gynecol.* 2011;117:1114–1121

12. Tepper NK, Curtis KM, Jamieson DJ, Marchbanks PA. Update to CDC's U.S. medical eligibility criteria for contraceptive use, 2010: revised recommendations for the use of contraceptive methods during the postpartum period. *MMWR Morb Mortal Wkly Rep.* 2011;60:878–883

13. Trussell J, Hatcher RA, Cates W Jr, Stewart FH, Kost K. Contraceptive failure in the United States: an update. *Stud Fam Plann.* 1990;21:51–54

Chapter 14

Breastfeeding and Human Milk for Preterm Infants

The reported benefits of human milk for preterm infants include: reduced infection, less necrotizing enterocolitis, and decreased feeding intolerance. To enable human milk feeding, mothers of preterm infants require special assistance to establish and maintain their milk supply, collect and store their milk, and breastfeed their infants. The human milk-fed preterm infant also requires special considerations for tube feeding, nutrient supplements, and growth and development. When the delivery of a preterm infant is anticipated, it is recommended that discussions with the mother include the benefits of human milk (see Chapter 11). Breastfeeding issues are important for all preterm infants, but 2 subgroups will be discussed in this chapter: infants born weighing less than 1500 g (very low birth weight [VLBW]) and infants born between 34 and 36 weeks' gestation (late preterm infant).

Very Low Birth Weight Infants

When faced with the birth of a VLBW infant, many women who had intended to formula-feed their infants will often provide their own milk when encouraged by their health care professional, if only for short-term feedings, as a way of protecting her infant's health. The benefits of breastfeeding should be discussed with the mother, if possible, as soon as the birth of a VLBW infant is expected (see Box 14-1 and Chapter 2). Once a VLBW infant is born, trained staff should be readily available to provide to the mother instructions for milk expression and optimal milk production, as well as information on milk storage (see Chapter 11), and eventually assist the dyad with breastfeeding sessions. The goal should be the provision of an adequate supply of mother's milk when feasible. If there is inadequate mother's milk for all feedings, the use of pasteurized donor human milk from an approved milk bank should be encouraged (see Chapter 11). Preterm formula should only be used when human milk is unavailable or not indicated.

Colostrum and Early Feedings

Early trophic feedings of the VLBW infant are important to prevent intestinal mucosal and villous atrophy and to improve the development of the gastrointestinal tract by increasing intestinal trophic hormone release and improving intestinal motility. Human milk feeding of VLBW infants decreases the time to full enteral feeding and the length of hospitalization. Colostrum is ideal for trophic feeding because it is rich in proteins, minerals, and immunologic factors. Protective immune factors, including sIgA, are higher in the colostrum of women who deliver preterm than those who deliver at term, suggesting that preterm colostrum may be especially protective during the first days after birth. Some clinicians use colostrum as a means of oral care to the VLBW infant. Colostrum should be preferentially fed in the order it was pumped, even if frozen.

Box 14-1. Breastfeeding Lessens the Risk for these Health Issues in Preterm Infants

- Necrotizing enterocolitis
- Feeding intolerance
- Hospital-acquired infections
- Longer neonatal intensive care unit hospital stays
- Developmental delays
- Lower IQ on cognitive tests

Source: US Department of Health and Human Services, Agency for Healthcare Research and Quality. Breastfeeding & maternal & infant health outcomes in developed countries. Evidence Report/Technology Assessment 153. Available at: www.ahrq.gov

Fortification of Human Milk

Rationale
Delayed onset of enteral nutrition, volume restriction of enteral feedings, and variable composition of mother's milk are but a few of the factors that pose limitations to the use of unfortified human milk for VLBW infants. A rapid rate of postnatal growth is necessary to approximate intrauterine rates. Nutrient requirements to meet these growth needs are greater than at any other time. The nutrient content of preterm human milk cannot meet all the needs imposed by this rapid rate of growth in VLBW infants. Protein inadequacy (as evidenced by low blood urea nitrogen and albumin values) has been observed in VLBW infants fed unfortified human milk. Biochemical rickets, or osteopenia of prematurity (as evidenced by low serum phosphorus and high serum calcium concentrations and by high serum alkaline phosphatase activity), and radiologic rickets also are observed in VLBW infants fed unfortified human milk. Hyponatremia, as well as vitamin inadequacy, also are described in VLBW infants fed unfortified human milk. Severe zinc deficiency, with characteristic dermatitis and growth failure, continues to be reported in VLBW infants receiving unfortified human milk. The feeding of human milk fortified with protein, minerals, and vitamins is associated with improved growth (weight, length, and head circumference), bone mineralization, and nutrient balance compared with unfortified human milk. Importantly, the use of fortified human milk is not associated with significant changes in feeding tolerance or with increases in the incidence of necrotizing enterocolitis or sepsis.

Who Should Receive Human Milk Fortification?
All VLBW infants should receive fortified human milk until they achieve a body weight of approximately 2000 g if still hospitalized. Near the time of hospital discharge, an assessment should be made of infant growth, biochemical measurements, and oral feeding ability. If these parameters are optimal, then unfortified human milk and breastfeeding can be recommended. If any of these parameters are suboptimal, the diet of human milk should be supplemented with a preterm infant discharge formula or a human milk fortifier.

Approach to Fortification
In usual circumstances, fortifier is added to human milk once the infant has demonstrated no intolerance to feeding and has attained a feeding volume of approximately 80 to 100 mL/kg/d, although starting at a feeding volume of 40 mL/kg/d has been shown to be safe. The maximum concentration listed by manufacturers should be followed.

Milk Fat Content

The fat content is the most variable of all nutrients in human milk. The variance among women, through lactation and during the course of the day, probably is less than the variance from losses resulting from fat separation from the milk or its adherence to collection containers and feeding devices. The inability to predict milk fat content, and therefore energy content, is of concern because fat is the major determinant of milk calorie content. The creamatocrit, in which a capillary tube of human milk is centrifuged and the percentage of milk volume that is lipid is estimated, gives an approximation of the lipid (and caloric) content of the milk and should be considered by neonatal intensive care units (NICUs) to individualize optimal nutrition for VLBW infants.

Hindmilk

The fat content of human milk increases from the beginning to the end of a single milk expression. The terms foremilk and hindmilk refer to milk collected at the beginning and toward the end of a single milk expression, respectively. Hindmilk feedings have been shown to enhance growth by supplying 2- to 3-fold greater fat content, and therefore calorie content, than foremilk. Although differing in fat and energy contents, foremilk and hindmilk fractions have similar contents of protein and minerals. Mothers of VLBW infants who produce more milk than their infants require (approximately 130% of what is needed by the infant, or 500 mL/d) can be taught to fractionate their milk into foremilk and hindmilk. An arbitrary practice is to collect all milk produced in the first 3 to 5 minutes of pumping as foremilk and collect the remaining milk separately as hindmilk. Hindmilk usually is used in conjunction with human milk fortifiers to aid the lagging growth of some preterm infants. Hindmilk alone should be used with caution because it may result in an imbalanced protein/calorie ratio and a dilution of needed minerals and vitamins. This may occur because hindmilk has greater fat and calorie contents but similar protein and mineral contents when compared with foremilk.

Individualized Fortification

Despite the benefits of fortification, the fortified human milk diet using standard fortifiers is often not sufficient to cover the greater needs of the VLBW infant and to ensure an optimum rate of growth. This is thought to be related to variations in the lipid and protein content of expressed human milk. Researchers have recently developed methods using infrared laser technology to analyze milk for protein, lipid, and energy. If this becomes standard of care, individual fortification of human milk could then be performed by enriching with vegetable oil or medium-chain fatty acids to achieve a greater lipid composition and protein supplements to achieve a greater protein intake, although the expense of both equipment and labor make this unlikely at this time.

Exclusive Human Milk-Based Fortifier

Feeding VLBW infants an exclusively human milk-based diet has been associated with significantly lower rates of NEC when compared with a diet of human milk fortified with bovine milk-based products containing intact cow milk protein. Feeding VLBW infants exclusive human milk, however, is challenging because of the difficulty in pumping a sufficient volume of milk and the need to fortify the milk to meet nutritional needs. Many NICUs promote the use of mother's milk but fortify the milk with bovine fortifier and feed the infants preterm formula when the mother's milk supply is inadequate or not available. It is now possible to provide an exclusive human milk-based diet with the use of human milk-based fortifiers and banked donor human milk to supplement the mothers' milk supply. However, the feasibility of providing such a diet to the majority of VLBW infants warrants further investigation due to availability and cost considerations.

Oral Feeding Challenges

Many VLBW infants require tube feeding because they are medically unstable, developmentally unable to latch on to the breast, have uncoordinated swallowing and breathing patterns, and/or fatigue easily with oral feeding. Tube-feeding techniques should be modified to provide human milk without any nutrient losses (see Chapter 11). Infants who have been given bottle feedings may become accustomed to immediate milk flow, unlike the process of breastfeeding (which often requires 60–90 seconds of non-nutritive suckling before letdown and milk flow occurs). Oral feeding must be tailored to the specific needs of the VLBW infant. The following steps can be taken to progress from tube feeding to breastfeeding.

Skin-to-Skin Contact

The first step toward independent oral feeding is to allow skin-to-skin for VLBW infants. First established as a method to improve survival of preterm infants after hospital discharge in Bogota, Colombia, the technique of placing the infant skin-to-skin upright between the mother's breasts has gained much support in NICUs. Skin-to-skin or "kangaroo" care is associated with beneficial effects on thermoregulation, heart rate stability, oxygen saturation, periodic breathing, and weight gain. Skin-to-skin care provides psychological benefits to the mother and physical benefits to the infant. Mothers who practice kangaroo care have measurably increased milk production and enhanced confidence in their ability to actually breastfeed. Preterm infants held skin-to-skin have higher oxygen saturations and less apnea of prematurity. In addition, it is speculated that when the mother holds her infant skin-to-skin, she is exposed to the same skin and respiratory "environment" as her infant, and potentially might provide specific antibodies against nursery-acquired pathogens.

Pacifiers

Contrary to the advice given for healthy term infants, the use of pacifiers with preterm infants may be beneficial. Pacifiers facilitate the development and strengthening of muscles used for sucking, and the non-nutritive sucking provides a training effect for future oral feeding. Some studies suggest that when given a pacifier during tube feeding, preterm infants have better weight gain and reduced hospital length of stay.

Tube to Oral Feeding

The transition from tube to oral feeding usually begins with skin-to-skin contact. Eventually the infant can be encouraged to suckle at the mother's breast or smell or lick the milk on her nipple. The coordination of suck-swallow-breathe begins between 32 and 34 weeks' postmenstrual age, but considerable variability is observed in achieving this milestone. Some infants may begin to accept oral feeding much earlier. Preterm infants who are allowed to suckle at the breast after a mother just pumped or emptied her breasts (non-nutritive suckling) eventually may achieve oral feeding sooner than infants who began suckling to breastfeed. This suggests that non-nutritive breastfeeding encourages suck-swallow coordination.

Readiness to Breastfeed

Assessments of readiness to breastfeed should be performed serially and include signs of sucking, such as sucking on the hand, nipple, tube, or pacifier. In addition, signs of rooting behavior, ability of the infant to latch and stay on the breast, sucking ability, duration of suck, behavioral state, skin color changes, vital signs, and the infant's comfort level during the feeding are factors to be evaluated and documented. Corrected gestational age is an unreliable marker for readiness to breastfeed.

Early Breastfeeding

A mother who has a strong letdown reflex, with copious milk flow, may need to pump before an early breastfeeding session. This reduces the infant's risk for choking on high milk flow. Some preterm infants require feeding devices, such as a nipple shield, to optimize oral feeding (see Chapter 11). Use of a thin silicone nipple shield, as a temporary device, may increase milk transfer in preterm infants. Tube feeding (nasogastric) given during early attempts at breastfeeding is particularly helpful and allows supplementation without the introduction of a bottle after breastfeeding.

Weighing the baby before and after a breastfeeding has been shown to be accurate, if conducted on an electronic infant scale. The change in weight in grams approximates the amount of milk transferred in milliliters. If possible, bottle-feeding should be avoided until mother and infant have a secure, confident breastfeeding technique.

It is best to begin breastfeeding when the infant is alert and hungry, demonstrating appropriate cues, and not crying, frantic, or overly stimulated. The mother should be seated in a comfortable chair with an upright back with the infant on a nursing pillow, which allows the infant to be closer to the mother and at the level of her breast.

- Proper positioning of the infant is essential. The infant may be placed in the typical holds discussed in Chapter 6. Mothers commonly underestimate their preterm infant's weak neck muscles, positional airway challenges, and weak sucking efforts, and assistance should be provided to the mother-infant dyad by certified lactation specialists or others with experience doing so. The cross-cradle hold works best for most mothers of preterm infants, as this allows the mother to control her baby's head and breast simultaneously to ensure the best possible latch. The mother may have to modify her hold from a C-hold to a U-hold to ensure that the weight of her breast does not interfere with the infant's ability to suckle. In the latter hold, the hand can provide additional jaw support. The U-hold is achieved by placing the thumb on one side of the breast behind the areola, with other fingers placed on the opposite side.
- Behavioral cues should be used to identify times for feeding sessions when the infant is awake and alert. If the infant continually falls asleep during attempts at breastfeeding, the mother may try switching to the opposite breast or using a feeding device to reduce fatigue during suckling. If the infant does not initiate suckling, the mother can express some milk onto her nipple so that her infant tastes her milk when she places her nipple

and areola into the infant's mouth. Usually, if the infant suckles for a short period, the mother should pump afterward to drain her breasts and maintain her milk supply.

Nutritional Monitoring

Assessments of growth and biochemical indices of nutritional status are important in managing the human milk-fed VLBW infant. Growth parameters should be monitored serially (daily weight and weekly length and head circumference). Weight gain of approximately 20 g/kg/d (or 20–30 g/d if body weight is >2000 g) is a typical goal. Length and head circumference should increase by approximately 1 cm each week. Biochemical evaluation of nutritional status generally includes serial measurements of electrolytes (sodium declines through lactation and acidosis resulting from reduced buffering capacity of fortified human milk have been observed), urea nitrogen (to assess short-term protein adequacy), and phosphorus and alkaline phosphatase (to assess bone mineral status). These biochemical evaluations might be obtained every 2 to 3 weeks if abnormalities are observed.

Discharge Planning

Discharge planning must be ongoing, initiated well in advance of the actual date of hospital discharge, and include parent input. The projected date should be regularly updated at multidisciplinary caregiver discharge planning rounds. A certified lactation specialist with expertise in the care of preterm infants should have input whenever possible. Nutritional factors are prominent in the discharge plans (sustained pattern of weight gain of sufficient duration, nutritional risks assessed and treated, competent oral feeding without cardiopulmonary compromise). By discharge, it must be clear that the infant is capable of oral feeding ad libitum and continues to gain weight adequately. Abnormalities in biochemical measurements should be noted (eg, elevated alkaline phosphatase and decreased serum phosphorus and urea nitrogen) and treated.

Exclusive Breastfeeding

If there are no concerns with adequacy of intake, growth, or biochemical measurements, exclusive breastfeeding should be encouraged after discharge. Commonly, "exclusive" breastfeeding means a combination of breastfeeding and/or feedings of expressed human milk. After discharge, the use of expressed milk by bottle is often able to be reduced as breastfeeding sessions increase. It is a common misperception that every breastfed preterm infant will automatically need formula supplementation; this is not the case if babies are growing well on mother's milk exclusively.

Breastfeeding and Enriched Formula

A combination of breastfeeding and enriched formula some clinicians use (or human milk fortifier) should be fed after discharge if there are concerns of inadequate intake, poor weight gain, or persistent biochemical abnormalities. There are a variety of ways to provide multinutrient supplementation for the breastfeeding infant in the post- discharge period. One strategy is to add feedings of an enriched formula, providing a concentrated nutrient composition that ranges between a term and a preterm formula (from 22 to 30 kcal/oz), but the risk/benefit of using a powdered formulation requires discussion. Mothers should be encouraged to continue to breastfeed with the addition of 2 or 3 of the supplemental formula feedings per day. This plan allows nearly full breastfeeding. There are, however, no data to assess this practical approach for postdischarge breastfeeding with supplementation. If supplemental feedings are used, however, to obtain the best outcomes, some experts recommend continuing the supplementation for a minimum of 6 months after discharge.

Multivitamin and Iron Supplementation

If the preterm infant is exclusively breastfed or fed expressed human milk in the postdischarge period, multivitamin and iron supplementation is suggested. Multivitamins should be given as 1 mL/d orally. Ferrous sulfate should be dosed 2 mg/kg/d of elemental iron. If the infant is receiving formula or fortifier as a supplement to breastfeeding, the dosage of multivitamin and iron supplementation should be reduced based on the proportion of formula fed to the infant. There have been case reports suggesting a risk for zinc deficiency in exclusively breastfed preterm infants several months after hospital discharge. If growth is less than optimal, poor feeding is noted, and perioral or perianal rashes are present, zinc deficiency may be present and zinc supplementation of 1 to 2 mg/kg/d should be considered.

Monitoring

Growth and biochemical indices should be done 1 week after discharge and repeated at monthly intervals until normalized. This monitoring may help gauge when to add or withdraw some of the formula supplements. When growth parameters are plotted, the infant's age corrected for prematurity rather than the infant's chronological age should be used.

Late Preterm Infants

Late preterm infants, born between 34 0/7 and 36 6/7 weeks' gestation, account for nearly three fourths of preterm births in the United States. Despite appearances comparable with their term counterparts, late preterm infants lag behind in cardiorespiratory, metabolic, immunologic, neurologic, and motor development. In these infants, the development of jaundice, sepsis, respiratory distress, poor feeding, temperature instability, or hypoglycemia during the birth hospitalization is more likely; in addition, these infants are more likely to be readmitted to the hospital soon after discharge for jaundice, feeding difficulties, dehydration, sepsis, and apnea. Of particular concern, breastfeeding is the greatest risk factor for rehospitalization of the late preterm infant, especially for jaundice and/or dehydration, a finding largely attributed to insufficient human milk intake.

Given the known increased risk for medical problems of the late preterm infant as compared with the term infant, close observation and monitoring, especially in the first day after birth, is required. Although rooming-in to support breastfeeding is especially beneficial for these infants, delivery services need to determine the necessary level of care depending on the condition and gestational age of the infant. For the stable, more mature infant, breastfeeding within the first hour, rooming-in, and ad libitum breastfeeding should be encouraged. If the infant is admitted to the NICU, policies should be developed to support the mother-infant dyad and breastfeeding. Breastfeeding sessions should be evaluated for adequate milk transfer, and the infant should be followed for weight loss, dehydration, and jaundice. These infants need 2 mg/kg/d of iron to maintain iron sufficiency because of their rapid growth rates and their lack of iron accretion during the last part of gestation.

Discharge should not occur before 48 hours. Discharge criteria should be established and should include stable weight, with no greater than 7% to 8% loss from birth, stable temperature, mother with adequate supply of milk or plan for supplementation, documented effective milk transfer, a bilirubin level that has been assessed with follow-up planned, written postdischarge feeding plan, and scheduled outpatient visit within 24 to 48 hours. The outpatient visit should include a careful history with assessment of additional weight loss (<8%) or gain (goal of >20 g/d), voiding (goal of 6–8/d), stools (goal of yellow, seedy stools by day 4), jaundice, and breastfeeding ability. Breastfeeding problems and concerns should be addressed, and the need for nutritional supplements should be evaluated. Triple feeds are commonly needed for the late preterm infant who continues to lose weight or fails to gain weight. The "triple feed technique" consists of breastfeeding, bottle-feeding (human milk or formula), and expressing human milk to maintain the milk supply. Weighing an infant before and after breastfeeding may be helpful in assessing the adequacy of milk transfer during breastfeeding and to determine the amount of supplemental feeding that may be needed (see Figure 14-1).

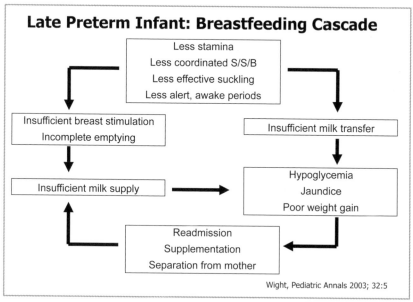

Figure 14-1. Increased Risks for the Late Preterm Infant
Source: Wight NE. Breastfeeding the borderline (near term) preterm infant. *Pediatr Ann.* 2003;32:329–336.

Selected References

1. Araujo ED, Goncalves AK, Cornetta M, et al. Evaluation of the secretory immunoglobulin A levels in the colostrum and milk of mothers of term and preterm infants. *Braz J Infect Dis.* 2005;9:357–362

2. Black RF, Jarman L, Simpson JB. *The Process of Breastfeeding. Lactation Specialist Self-Study Series.* Sudbury, MA: Jones and Bartlett Publishers, Inc; 1998:207–208

3. Bu'Lock F, Woolridge MW, Baum JD. Development of coordination of sucking, swallowing and breathing: ultrasound study of term and preterm infants. *Dev Med Child Neurol.* 1990;32:669–678

4. Engle WA, Tomashek KM, Wallman C; American Academy of Pediatrics Committee on Fetus and Newborn. Late-preterm infants: a population at risk. *Pediatrics.* 2007;120:1390

5. Ferber SG, Makhoul IR. The effect of skin-to-skin contact (kangaroo care) shortly after birth on the neurobehavioral responses of the term newborn: a randomized, controlled trial. *Pediatrics.* 2004;113:858–865

6. Field T, Ignatoff E, Stringer S, et al. Nonnutritive sucking during tube feedings: effects on preterm neonates in an intensive care unit. *Pediatrics.* 1982;70:381–384

7. Flaherman VJ, Lee HC. "Breastfeeding" by feeding expressed mother's milk. *Pediatr Clin North Am.* 2013;60:227–246

8. Ganapathy V, Hay JW, Kim JH. Costs of necrotizing enterocolitis and cost-effectiveness of exclusively human milk-based products in feeding extremely premature infants. *Breastfeed Med.* 2012;7:29–37

9. Lin HY, Hsieh HY, Chen HH, Chiu HY, Lin HC, Su BH. Efficacy of creamatocrit technique in evaluation of premature infants fed with breast milk. *Pediatr Neonatol.* 2011;52:130

10. Abrams SA, Hurst NM. Breastfeeding the preterm infant. http://www.uptodate.com/contents/breastfeeding-the-preterm-infant. Accessed September 3, 2013

11. Hurst NM, Valentine CJ, Renfro L, Burns P, Ferlic L. Skin-to-skin holding in the neonatal intensive care influences maternal milk volume. *J Perinatol.* 1997;17:213–217

12. Kirsten GF, Bergman NJ, Hann FM. Kangaroo mother care in the nursery. *Pediatr Clin North Am.* 2001;48:443–452

13. Kliethermes PA, et al. Transitioning preterm infants with nasogastric tube supplementation: increased likelihood of breastfeeding. *J Obstet Gynecol Neonatal Nurs.* 1999;28:264–273

14. Kuschel CA, Marding JE. Multicomponent fortified human milk for promoting growth in preterm infants. *The Cochrane Library.* 2005;1–36

15. Meier PP. Breastfeeding in the special care nursery: prematures and infants with medical problems. *Pediatr Clin North Am.* 2001;48:425–442

16. Meier PP, Engstrom JL, Murtaugh MA, Vasan U, Meier WA, Schanler RJ. Mothers' milk feedings in the neonatal intensive care unit: accuracy of the creamatocrit technique. *J Perinatol.* 2002;22:646–649

17. Meier PP, Patel AL, Bigger HR, Rossman B, Engstrom JL. Supporting breastfeeding in the neonatal intensive care unit: Rush Mother's Milk Club as a case study of evidence-based care. *Pediatr Clin North Am.* 2013;60:209–226

18. Morales Y, Schanler RJ. Human milk and clinical outcomes in VLBW infants: how compelling is the evidence of benefit? *Semin Perinatol.* 2007;31(2):83–88

19. Morgan JA, Young L, McCormick FM, McGuire W. Promoting growth for preterm infants following hospital discharge. *Arch Dis Child Fetal Neonatal Ed.* 2012;97:F295–F298

20. Narayanan I, Mehta R, Choudhury DK, Jain BK. Sucking on the 'emptied' breast: non-nutritive sucking with a difference. *Arch Dis Child.* 1991;66:241–244

21. Nyqvist KH, Rubertsson C, Ewald U, Sjoden PO. Development of the preterm infant breastfeeding behavior scale (PIBBS): a study of nurse-mother agreement. *J Hum Lact.* 1996;12:207–219

22. Ogechi AA, William O, Fidelia BT. Hindmilk and weight gain in preterm very low-birthweight infants. *Pediatr Int.* 2007;49:156–160

23. Powers NG. Slow weight gain and low milk supply in the breastfeeding dyad. *Clin Perinatol.* 1999;26:399–430

24. Quigley MA, Henderson G, Anthony MY, McGuire W. Formula milk versus donor breast milk for feeding preterm or low birth weight infants. *Cochrane Database Syst Rev.* 2007;(4):CD002971

25. Rodriguez NA, Meier PP, Groer MW, Zeller JM. Oropharyngeal administration of colostrum to extremely low birth weight infants: theoretical perspectives. *J Perinatol.* 2009;29:1–7

26. Schanler RJ, Lau C, Hurst NM, Smith EO. Randomized trial of donor human milk versus preterm formula as substitutes for mothers' own milk in the feeding of extremely premature infants. *Pediatrics.* 2005;116:400–406

27. Senterre T, Rigo J. Optimizing nutritional support based on early "aggressive" nutrition and recent recommendations allows abolishing postnatal growth restriction in VLBW infants. *J Pediatr Gastroenterol Nutr.* 2011;53:536–542

28. Shapiro-Mendoza CK, Tomashek KM, Kotelchuck M, et al. Effect of late-preterm birth and maternal medical conditions on newborn morbidity risk. *Pediatrics.* 2008;121:e223–e232

29. Simpson C, Schanler RJ, Lau C. Early introduction of oral feeding in preterm infants. *Pediatrics.* 2002;110:517–522

30. Sullivan S, Schanler RJ, Kim JH, et al. An exclusively human milk-based diet is associated with a lower rate of necrotizing enterocolitis than a diet of human milk and bovine milk-based products. *J Pediatr.* 2010;156:562–567

31. Tomashek KM, Shapiro-Mendoza CK, Weiss J, et al. Early discharge among late preterm and term newborns and risk of neonatal morbidity. *Semin Perinatol.* 2006;30:61–68

32. Underwood MA. Human milk for the premature infant. *Pediatr Clin North Am.* 2013;60:189–207

33. Wight NE. Breastfeeding the borderline (near term) preterm infant. *Pediatr Ann.* 2003;32:329–336

34. Zachariassen G, Faerk J, Grytter C, et al. Nutrient enrichment of mother's milk and growth of very preterm infants after hospital discharge. *Pediatrics.* 2011;127:e995–e1003

Chapter 15

Breastfeeding in Special Circumstances

Cleft Lip and Cleft Palate

Oral feeding is a major problem for infants with common congenital oral malformations. The cleft malformations prevent an effective seal around the nipple, which is needed to facilitate oral feeding.

Benefits of Breastfeeding

The breastfeeding of infants with cleft lip and/or palate has numerous benefits, including promotion of oral and facial muscular development, allowance for a better seal at the lip defect because of the pliability of the breast, reduced otitis media, and the provision of comfort and pleasure by non-nutritive sucking for the infant who cannot accomplish nutritive sucking. Mothers of infants ineffective at the breast should be instructed in milk expression techniques so that milk is still available.

Infants With Cleft Hard Palate

These infants are unable to generate negative sucking pressure in the oral cavity, resulting in an excessive intake of air. They commonly have nasal regurgitation of milk and often fatigue during prolonged attempts to breast-feed. These obstacles result in inadequate milk intake with subsequent poor weight gain during the first months after birth. If some negative pressure can be generated, breastfeeding may succeed; if not, then a soft artificial nipple with a large opening or direct delivery of milk into the mouth is used. Palatal prostheses are available to improve the ability to generate negative sucking pressure. Caution should be used with prostheses and nipples to prevent irritation or erosion of palatal edges.

Isolated Cleft Lip

This malformation is more likely to be associated with breastfeeding success. The infants are capable of generating negative pressure, providing occlusion of the lip is maintained. This can be accomplished by using the thumb of the hand supporting the breast in the C-hold to fill in the cleft and form a seal.

Infants With Cleft Lip and Palate

These infants are least likely to breastfeed because they cannot generate negative pressure and usually have poor oral-motor function. These infants usually require an individual feeding plan that uses a feeding device (see Chapter 11). Techniques to assist the mother in breastfeeding an infant with cleft palate and/or lip are outlined in Box 15-1. Meanwhile, the mother can express her milk to maintain an adequate supply.

Box 15-1. Breastfeeding Techniques for Infants With Cleft Lip and/or Palate

1. Feed frequently (every 2–3 hours) and know techniques to allow milk letdown and latch-on.

2. Hold the breast with the C-hold or palmar grasp technique (thumb above and fingers below areola). The U-hold from under the breast can also be used.

3. Hold the infant at breast level. For hypotonic infants, their trunk and head should be placed at the same level as the breast with pillows.

4. Use semi-upright positions such as the clutch, or football, hold to avoid nasal regurgitation and airway occlusion.

5. Use the straddle position (infant sits upright on the mother's lap and straddles her abdomen) for infants with bilateral cleft lip and palate to promote gravity delivery of milk and decreased nasal regurgitation and aspiration.

6. Position the breast toward the side of the palate that has the most intact bone and position the nipple down so that it is not pushed into the cleft.

7. Massage the breast rhythmically to enhance milk delivery. Mothers may need to manually express human milk into the baby's mouth to compensate for absent suction and to stimulate the letdown reflex.

Adapted from Wagner C. Personal communication.

Surgical Repair

Cleft lip is usually surgically repaired in the first few months after birth (1–4 months), whereas the palate is repaired at approximately 9 to 12 months. Historically, infants who underwent surgical repair of a cleft lip were fed with a cup, dropper, or spoon during post-operative recovery. Studies demonstrate enhanced recovery in infants allowed to breastfeed after cleft lip repair. One study found that six weeks after surgery, breastfed infants, when compared with device-fed infants, had better weight gain, shortened postoperative hospital stay, decreased use of analgesia and sedation, and less need for intravenous fluid. Thus, in some cases, breastfeeding should resume as soon as possible in the postoperative period.

Pierre Robin Sequence

The Pierre Robin sequence includes micrognathia, glossoptosis, and cleft palate, all of which may affect feeding ability and produce feeding problems. Infants with Pierre Robin sequence may have higher than average caloric needs as a result of increased breathing difficulties and chronic airway obstruction. Some will be able to achieve adequate caloric intake through modified breastfeeding and modified nipple-feeding techniques. Those who are unable to tolerate oral feedings will need tube feedings to provide adequate nutrition.

Sucking and swallowing dysfunction is a major cause of feeding difficulties in the initial newborn period. Micrognathia leads to problems with latch-on. The cleft palate creates sucking problems. The tongue is displaced posteriorly and infants are unable to stroke the nipple efficiently, so they have difficulty propelling the milk into the oropharynx. Other swallowing difficulties result from the tongue deformity (glossoptosis). The infants typically produce a few rapid sucks, then stop breathing. The coordination of simultaneous sucking and swallowing is difficult for these infants. During oral feeding, milk gets into the nasopharynx, which, together with swallowing dysfunction and abnormal tongue position, creates an increased risk for aspiration. In cases in which the tongue has been tacked down anteriorly (glossopexy) to prevent choking and aspiration, infants still encounter difficulty with latch and have tongue mobility problems and ongoing swallowing difficulties.

Human milk is advantageous for these infants because they have an increased risk for aspiration and associated respiratory infections. The use of human milk is associated with a decrease in otitis media and upper respiratory infection, which is a particular concern because these infants are at increased risk for otitis media and hearing deficits. Mothers should be encouraged to pump milk early to establish an adequate milk supply for those infants who are unable to breastfeed effectively.

Down Syndrome

Infants with Down syndrome often require special interventions to ensure successful breastfeeding. Their oral structures may include a variety of abnormalities that affect feeding: protruding tongue, furrowed tongue, narrow palate, and a small nose with a low nasal bridge. They may present with generalized hypotonia and may exhibit ineffective suckling or tongue thrusting, resulting in difficulty with latch-on. The infant cannot form a trough with the tongue around the areola which results in milk going down the side of the mouth instead of into the back of the mouth to be swallowed. Oral feeding competency usually improves as the generalized tone improves. See Box 15-2 for suggested techniques for breastfeeding the infant with Down syndrome.

Multiple Births

Including twins and triplets, multiple births can be breastfed successfully, and in many cases without the need for supplementation. Breastfeeding multiples, however, requires additional time and creates higher nutritional needs for the mother. Current recommendations for energy supplementation during breast-feeding are 500 to 600 kcal per baby per day. There are a variety of ways that a mother can nurse multiple infants. Twins may be breastfed in any of 3 modes: simultaneously, separately on an individual demand schedule, or separately on a modified demand schedule where one infant is fed on demand and then the other immediately afterward. Simultaneous breastfeeding saves time and also has a physiologic advantage in that the more vigorous baby on one side may stimulate the letdown reflex for the other twin. However, the most common practice is to start breastfeeding each baby individually because (1) it takes time for the mother to recover from the delivery, (2) infants do not necessarily have the same sucking ability, and (3) the new situation is often quite over-whelming for the parents. Encouraging the partner or extended family members to help with feedings alleviates some of the stress. Many mothers and infants adapt rapidly, and mothers can soon choose their preferred schedule. Some mothers breastfeed exclusively, others prefer a combination of breastfeeding, mechanical milk expression, and bottle-feeding or other device feeding.

Box 15-2. Breastfeeding Techniques for Infants With Down Syndrome

1. Feed at frequent, short intervals (every 2–3 hours).

2. Place the infant's trunk and head at the same level while supporting the head to facilitate head control.

3. Positioning:
   a. The C-hold with the thumb on top and fingers below the areola helps control the nipple.
   b. Support the infant's jaw from below with a finger. The index finger can be used to provide additional support for the jaw or to provide gentle downward pressure on the chin to open the baby's mouth wider.
   c. For hypotonic infants, the U-hold supports the breast and the infant's chin, allowing the mandible to rest within the interdigital space.

4. In cases of frequent choking and gulping air, place the back of the head superior to the nipple. The mother can lean back (such as in a recliner) so that the baby's throat is higher than the nipple. If this is effective, combine with frequent burping.

5. For infants with macroglossia, assist them in opening their mouths and latch. The C- and U-holds can be helpful.

6. To overcome the tongue thrusting:

   a. Breastfeed with infant's chin pointing downward, almost touching the infant's chest.
   b. Gently stroke the infant's cheek toward his or her mouth, brushing the lips a few times.
   c. Use a clean index finger with well-trimmed nail to massage the outside of the infant's gums. Begin at the midline of the gum and move toward the sides of the gum.
   d. As the infant's mouth opens, press down firmly on the tongue tip with the tip of the index finger and count 1-2-3.
   e. Release the pressure, and move back on the tongue repeating this 1 or 2 more times. Avoid gagging the infant.
   f. Repeat this procedure 3 or 4 times before each breastfeeding session.

7. A nipple shield may be useful in hypotonic or weak infants as a transition to breastfeeding (see Chapter 11).

Adapted from Wagner C. Personal communication.

Tandem Nursing

Tandem nursing refers to continuation of breastfeeding into the next pregnancy and after delivery of the next child. A normal pregnancy is not an indication for immediate weaning, but preterm labor usually precludes continued breastfeeding. Some cultures mandate weaning when pregnancy is confirmed based on cultural, religious, or social tenets. A review of breastfeeding during pregnancy practices found that only 43% of mothers continue breastfeeding throughout the pregnancy. Forty-eight percent of breastfeeding children wean spontaneously, most at the end of the second trimester, when most of the mothers reported a sharp decline in milk production. The main reason for mother-initiated weaning is breast and nipple pain, fatigue, and irritability. Only 7% of mothers reported uterine contractions during nursing. Psychological support of the weaning or weaned toddler is important.

Care must be taken to ensure that the new infant has priority at the breast and that milk intake and growth are not compromised. Often the previously breastfeeding older child will be nursing only for comfort and to assert a continuing claim on the mother. Some studies demonstrate slower weight gain in newborns whose mothers are tandem nursing, possibly due to qualitative longitudinal differences in the milk composition. The mother will produce milk at the same rate that it is removed; if she is nursing 2 or more infants, she will produce greater amounts of milk.

Adoptive Nursing

Breastfeeding an adopted infant is possible and may be accomplished following preparation of the breasts to induce milk production. The nonpregnant mammary gland may over a period undergo changes in response to the physical stimulation of suckling or pumping the breast. If the breast is stimulated, prolactin may be secreted and milk may be produced. The increase in prolactin and milk production, however, is variable. A key component to successful lactation is the letdown reflex, which is directly dependent on adequate levels of circulating oxytocin. Letdown may be facilitated by exogenous oxytocin. Milk production may take from 1 to 6 weeks, on average, about 4 weeks, after beginning pumping or nursing. Galactagogues often are used, but their efficacy is unproven (see Chapter 12). Clinicians advise beginning this process well before the arrival of the adopted baby because the adoption process can be stressful and may interfere with milk production. It is useful for the adoptive mother to use a supplemental feeding device and skin-to-skin contact. These techniques allow the infant to receive nutrition while suckling. Success varies with pregnancy history. Nulliparous women may have more difficulty.

Relactation

Relactation may be desired for mothers who initiated lactation but chose to stop because their infant was too sick to nurse or because they themselves were too sick to nurse. Compared with mothers who initiate lactation to nurse an adopted infant, mothers who have previously lactated have the psychological advantage that they previously made milk. With renewed stimulation to the nipple, the neuroendocrine loop is reactivated, and milk production ensues. Successful relactation occurs in about 75% of women who initiate the process.

Selected References

1. Academy of Breastfeeding Medicine Protocol Committee. ABM clinical protocol #9: use of galactogogues in initiating or augmenting the rate of maternal milk secretion. (First revision January 2011). *Breastfeed Med.* 2011;6:41–49
2. Betzold CM. Galactogogues. *J Midwifery Womens Health.* 2004;49:151–154
3. Cho SJ, Cho HK, Lee HS, Lee K. Factors related to success in relactation. *J Korean Soc Neonatol.* 2010;17:232–238
4. Clarren S, Anderson B, Wolf LS. Feeding infants with cleft lip, cleft palate, or cleft lip and palate. *Cleft Palate J.* 1987;24:244–249
5. Cruz MJ, Kerschner JE, Beste DJ, Conley SF. Pierre Robin sequence: secondary respiratory difficulties and intrinsic feeding abnormalities. *Laryngoscope.* 1999;109:1632–1636
6. Darzi MA, Chowdri NA, Bhat AN. Breast feeding or spoon feeding after cleft lip repair: a prospective randomised study. *Br J Plast Surg.* 1996;49:24–26
7. Flidel-Rimon O, Shinwell ES. Breast feeding twins and high multiples. *Arch Dis Child Fetal Neonatal Ed.* 2006;91:F377–F380
8. Habel A, Sell D, Mars M. Management of cleft lip and palate. *Arch Dis Child.* 1996;74:360–366
9. Kanamori G, Witter M, Brown J, Williams-Smith L. Otolaryngologic manifestations of Down syndrome. *Otolaryngol Clin North Am.* 2000;33:1285–1292
10. Kirschner E, LaRossa D. Cleft lip and palate. *Otolaryngol Clin North Am.* 2000;33:1191–1215
11. Lehman JA, Fishman JR, Neiman GS. Treatment of cleft palate associated with Robin sequence: appraisal of risk factors. *Cleft Palate Craniofac J.* 1995;32:25–30
12. Marquis GS, Penny ME, Diaz JM, Marín RM. Postpartum consequences of an overlap of breastfeeding and pregnancy: reduced breast milk intake and growth during early infancy. *Pediatrics.* 2002;109:e56
13. Moscone SR, Moore MJ. Breastfeeding during pregnancy. *J Hum Lact.* 1993;9:283–288
14. Skinner J, Arvedson JC, Jones G, Spinner C, Rockwood J. Post-operative feeding strategies for infants with cleft lip. *Int J Pediatr Otorhinolaryngol.* 1997;42:169–178
15. US Food and Drug Administration. *FDA Warns Against Using Unapproved Drug, Domperidone, to Increase Milk Production.* FDA talk paper. Rockville, MD: US Food and Drug Administration; 2004

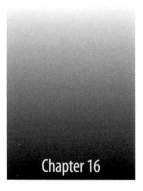

Chapter 16

Who Can and Who Cannot Breastfeed?

It is estimated that most women are able to establish and sustain breastfeeding for an extended period if they are motivated and if they have support from their families, employer, community, and the medical system. Despite motivation and support, however, women with certain medical and psychosocial conditions may not meet their breastfeeding goals, and there are rare situations when an infant should not be breastfed.

Physical Conditions of the Breast

Breast Size

Breast size is not an indicator of breastfeeding success. Because most breast mass is fat tissue, not glandular tissue, even small breasts may have enough glandular tissue to produce sufficient milk for breastfeeding. Small breast size, however, may limit the volume of milk that can be stored and may necessitate more frequent feeding to provide the infant with sufficient milk intake.

Hypoplastic/Tubular Breasts

Although uncommon, breast maldevelopment, sometimes characterized by a tubular shape, has been associated with a high risk for insufficient milk production.

Breast Enlargement During Pregnancy

Breast enlargement during pregnancy is an important factor in lactation success. If breasts do not enlarge during pregnancy, milk production may not occur and exclusive breastfeeding may not succeed. Hormonal or anatomic factors may be the cause. Regardless of the cause, breastfeeding, and especially measures of adequate milk intake, should be monitored closely (see Chapter 8).

Breast Injury and Breast Surgery

Whether because of reduction mammoplasty, implantation, or removal of a mass or as a result of trauma, breast injury or surgery may be a cause for breastfeeding difficulties. Generally, breastfeeding should be encouraged. Additional assistance, monitoring, and encouragement should be provided during the first few days and beyond to ensure sustained, successful milk production. The possibility of difficulty in establishing lactation should be discussed with the mother, and she should receive continuous encouragement and support and have access to experienced certified lactation counseling.

Reduction Mammoplasty

Women who have had reduction mammoplasty with repositioning of the areolae and nipples often have difficulty producing adequate milk. Periareolar incisions are likely to interrupt and block the flow of milk into the nipple ducts. The mother may still be able to produce some milk because of recannulization; however, exclusive breastfeeding is rare. Nevertheless, if the nipple and areola are left on a pedicle during surgery, the prognosis for successful lactation is improved.

Augmentation Mammoplasty

Breast augmentation surgery is compatible with successful breastfeeding, especially if the implant was placed behind the pectoral muscles for purely cosmetic reasons. However, excessively large implants may impinge on the capacity of the breast to enlarge during lactation, and thereby limit the volume of milk that the mother can store, as well as restrict blood flow to the mammary gland tissue, restricting milk production. The rationale for breast augmentation may need clarification. For example, augmentation may have been performed for abnormal shape or breast asymmetry, which may indicate inadequate breast tissue to support breastfeeding. Changes in the breast during pregnancy, and milk production during the immediate postpartum period, should be monitored closely.

Lumpectomy

The removal of a mass in the breast may affect breastfeeding if significant nerves and ducts have been severed or removed. Of greatest concern are incisions around the periphery of the areola. Milk production and infant weight gain should be monitored closely.

Previous Treatment for Breast Cancer

Pregnancy after breast cancer treatment has not been shown to increase recurrence and may confer a survival benefit. It has been recommended that women wait five years after treatment of breast cancer before attempting to conceive. If a woman does become pregnant sooner, she usually is able to breastfeed on the unaffected breast and, in some cases, on both breasts if surgery and/or radiation therapy did not interfere. Radiation therapy after lumpectomy may lead to insufficient lactation on the affected side.

Trauma and Burns

The effect of breast tissue trauma and burns on lactational performance varies depending on how much direct injury to the ducts and mammary gland tissue occurred. Even women who suffered severe burns to the chest in childhood that required extensive grafting have been able to breastfeed successfully.

Pierced Nipples

A history of pierced nipples has not been associated with breastfeeding difficulties unless there is infection or scarring. Nipple devices should be removed before feeding to avoid the risk for infant choking.

Absolute and Relative Maternal Contraindications to Breastfeeding

Infection Risk

Transmission of microorganisms from mother to milk has been shown to occur. The degree of infant risk varies.

HIV and T-Cell Lymphotropic Virus

Women in the United States who are infected with human immunodeficiency virus (HIV) and women with human T-cell lymphotropic virus 1 (HTLV, type I or type II) should not breastfeed because of the risk for transmission to the nursing infant. The Centers for Disease Control and Prevention also recommends not breastfeeding by women who are receiving antiretroviral (ARV) medications. In developing countries, where infectious diseases and malnutrition are the predominant causes of infant mortality, the health risks of not breastfeeding must be balanced with the risk for HIV acquisition. In 2010, the World Health Organization updated its recommendations for breastfeeding and HIV-positive women. Health authorities are encouraged to either counsel women to breastfeed and receive ARV therapy or avoid breastfeeding. Even when ARV drugs are not available, HIV-infected women should be encouraged to exclusively breastfeed for 6 months and to continue breastfeeding thereafter unless social and environmental factors are safe for and supportive of replacement feeding. All mothers should be specifically supported to appropriately feed their infants.

Tuberculosis

Because of the concern that tuberculosis could be transmitted by close contact with the mother, women with active pulmonary tuberculosis should not feed their infant themselves until they have received appropriate antibiotic treatment for approximately 2 weeks and are no longer contagious, as determined by their physician or public health official. The tubercle bacillus does not pass into the milk.

Varicella-Zoster Virus

Neonates should be given varicella-zoster immune globulin if their mothers develop varicella between the period beginning 5 days before delivery through 2 days after delivery. Varicella vaccine may be given to susceptible breastfeeding mothers if the risk of exposure to natural varicella is high. It is not known whether varicella virus is excreted in milk. Some clinicians recommend breastfeeding only after the exposed infant receives immune globulin. The infant should not have direct contact with lesions that have not crusted over.

Herpes Simplex Virus

Women with herpetic breast lesions should not breastfeed from the affected breast and should cover the lesions to prevent infant contact. Women with genital herpes, however, can breastfeed, although proper handwashing procedures should be strictly followed.

Cytomegalovirus

Cytomegalovirus (CMV) may be found in the milk of seropositive mothers.

In healthy term infants, symptomatic CMV disease from transmission through human milk is uncommon. There is some concern that preterm infants may be at greater risk for symptomatic disease that manifests as sepsis-like syndromes. Freezing at −20°C may decrease CMV infectivity. Clinicians should consider the benefits of human milk versus the risk for CMV transmission in preterm infants whose mothers are known to be CMV-positive or seroconvert during lactation.

Hepatitis B

Infants born to women who are hepatitis B surface antigen (HBsAg)–positive routinely receive hepatitis B immune globulin and hepatitis B vaccine, eliminating concerns of transmission through breastfeeding. There is no need to delay initiation of breastfeeding until after the infant is immunized because breastfeeding was not contraindicated, even before the vaccine was available.

Hepatitis C

Both hepatitis C virus and hepatitis C antibody have been detected in human milk; however, there are no reports of infant acquisition of the virus through breastfeeding. Maternal hepatitis C infection is not a contraindication to breastfeeding.

Influenza H1N1

For the H1N1 flu virus (sometimes called swine flu), the Centers for Disease Control and Prevention recommends that infected breastfeeding women express their milk and have someone who is not sick feed the infants expressed human milk. Breastfeeding during maternal treatment with antiviral medications for influenza is safe. Women who are taking medicines to prevent the flu because they have been exposed to the virus are encouraged to continue to feed the baby at the breast as long as they do not have symptoms of the flu such as fever, cough, or sore throat.

Substance Abuse

Women using drugs of abuse need counseling and should not breastfeed until they are free of the abused drugs that may harm the infant (see Chapter 12).

Alcohol

Changes in infant feeding patterns have been reported in infants soon after mothers have ingested large amounts of alcohol quickly. Mothers should be advised to limit alcohol consumption during lactation. Alcohol is one of the few substances ingested by the mother that achieves high concentrations in human milk. The Institute of Medicine recommends lactating women limit alcohol intake to 0.5 g or less of alcohol per kilogram maternal body weight per day. For a 60-kg woman, this represents the equivalent of 2 cans of beer, 2 glasses of table wine, or 2 oz of liquor (see Chapter 12). Breastfeeding is permissible 4 hours after the last drink.

Cigarette Smoking

Metabolites of cigarette smoke have been found in infants who live in an environment in which tobacco is smoked. Mothers should be discouraged from smoking during lactation. If they persist in smoking, breastfeeding should be encouraged for the protective effects in the infant, especially with respect to respiratory illnesses. Mothers and all others should be advised not to smoke in the presence of infants and children (see Chapter 12).

Medications

Most medications are compatible with breastfeeding, or if not compatible, a substitute medication may exist and should be sought (see Chapter 12).

Cancer Therapy

Women with breast cancer should not delay treatment so they can breastfeed. Depending on the therapy, women receiving antimetabolite chemotherapy may be able to breastfeed by pumping and discarding their milk after each treatment until the chemical has been cleared. Radiation therapy generally is compatible with breastfeeding. Radiation treatment of the breast, however, may significantly damage sensitive breast tissue and be detrimental to future lactation performance of the affected breast (see earlier Previous Treatment for Breast Cancer section).

Radiopharmaceuticals

Mothers receiving diagnostic or therapeutic radioactive isotopes or those who have had accidental exposure to radioactive materials should not breastfeed for as long as there is radioactivity in the milk (see Chapter 12).

Infant Contraindications to Breastfeeding

Galactosemia

Infants with classic galactosemia (galactose 1-phosphate uridyltransferase deficiency) cannot ingest lactose-containing milk. Therefore, because lactose is the principal carbohydrate in human and bovine milk, infants with classic galactosemia should not breastfeed or receive formula containing lactose. However, in some of the genetically milder forms of galactosemia, partial breastfeeding may be possible.

Inborn Errors of Metabolism

Infants with other inborn errors of metabolism may ingest some human milk, but this recommendation would depend on the desired protein intake and other factors. Phenylketonuria has been managed with a combination of partial breastfeeding and phenylalanine-free formula. Human milk contains relatively low levels of phenylalanine compared with formula.

Hyperbilirubinemia

For most newborns with jaundice and hyperbilirubinemia, breastfeeding can and should be continued without interruption. In rare circumstances of severe hyperbilirubinemia, breastfeeding may need to be interrupted for a brief period (see Chapter 8).

Primary Insufficient Milk Syndrome

Approximately 5% of women will not produce adequate milk. A history of minimal or no breast changes during pregnancy may be an important early sign of potential insufficient milk syndrome. A history of breast surgery or trauma also should alert caregivers to potential problems (see Chapter 8).

Selected References

1. American Academy of Pediatrics. *Red Book: 2012 Report of the Committee on Infectious Diseases.* 29th ed. Pickering LK, ed. Elk Grove Village, IL: American Academy of Pediatrics; 2012

2. American College of Obstetricians and Gynecologists. Committee opinion no. 471: smoking cessation during pregnancy. *Obstet Gynecol.* 2010;116(5):1241–1244

3. American College of Obstetricians and Gynecologists. ACOG practice bulletin: clinical management guidelines for obstetrician-gynecologists number 92, April 2008 (replaces practice bulletin number 87, November 2007). Use of psychiatric medications during pregnancy and lactation. *Obstet Gynecol.* 2008;111(4):1001–1020

4. Institute of Medicine Subcommittee on Nutrition During Lactation. *Nutrition During Lactation.* Washington, DC: National Academy Press; 1991

5. Lawrence RA, Lawrence RM. *Breastfeeding: A Guide for the Medical Profession.* 7th ed. Philadelphia, PA: Mosby-Elsevier; 2010

6. Lawrence RM. Circumstances when breastfeeding is contraindicated. *Pediatr Clin North Am.* 2013;60:295–318

7. Lawrence RM, Lawrence RA. Given the benefits of breastfeeding, what contraindications exist? *Pediatr Clin North Am.* 2001;48:235–251

8. Neifert MR. Prevention of breastfeeding tragedies. *Pediatr Clin North Am.* 2001;48:273–297

9. World Health Organization. *Guidelines on HIV and Infant Feeding 2010. Principles and Recommendations for Infant Feeding in the Context of HIV and a Summary of Evidence.* Geneva, Switzerland: World Health Organization; 2010

10. Zemlickis D, Lishner M, Degendorfer P, et al. Maternal and fetal outcome after breast cancer in pregnancy. *Am J Obstet Gynecol.* 1992;166:781–787

Chapter 17

The Breastfeeding-Friendly Medical Office

The medical home—whether a partnership between the family and pediatric, obstetric, or family health care professionals—should establish a breastfeeding-friendly environment that encourages breastfeeding in the office setting. Office medical practices should be directed to support the goals of Healthy People 2020 of increasing the percentage of mothers who breastfeed and the duration of breastfeeding. In addition, the entire office staff, professional and nonprofessional, should be educated about the value and implementation of breastfeeding, and how to support the breastfeeding dyad during the visit. Each visit is a valuable opportunity to provide that initial and ongoing support. Furthermore, incorporating breastfeeding management into the office can provide a resource to patients while offering a financial benefit to the practice.

A Breastfeeding-Friendly Environment

The medical office presents a valuable opportunity to demonstrate that health care staff believe breastfeeding is the normative form of nutrition for all babies. It is enlightening to walk through a clinical setting, critically observing the environment, and ask, "What message does the environment of this medical office convey to families?" The decor, advertising literature, and attention given to the needs of breastfeeding mothers reflect the values of the office. Transforming the physician's office into a setting where breastfeeding is the societal norm will create an influential educational experience for parents and children and will show that the practice enthusiastically promotes, supports, and protects breastfeeding.

Elements of a Breastfeeding-Friendly Environment

Posters or Enlarged Photographs
Pictures, posters, or enlarged photographs of breastfeeding mothers and babies from a variety of ethnic and cultural backgrounds should be displayed throughout the office to encourage breastfeeding mothers to nurse their babies.

Mother's Room and Waiting Room
A private area equipped with a comfortable chair, a changing table, an electric breast pump, and, ideally, a small refrigerator can become a breastfeeding room where mothers (including staff members) go to breastfeed in private or to express milk. The area will emphasize that breastfeeding is encouraged and supported in the practice. Breastfeeding in the waiting room itself should never be discouraged.

Discourage Formula Marketing
Prenatal packs containing formula undermine breastfeeding success. Gifts from formula companies reflect the beliefs and values of the staff and should be reviewed and discussed. If breastfeeding is important to the practice, accepting formula marketing and similar gifts is counterproductive and should be discouraged. Careful thought should be given to magazines and other materials in the waiting room. Prenatal or postnatal formula company gifts for mothers or sign-up forms for formula company-sponsored "new mothers clubs" should not be encouraged in the office practice. When women sign up for such clubs, they will probably receive free formula either before or after the baby's birth. In 2012, the AAP resolved that no formula industry advertising should be done in the medical office.

Track Breastfeeding Rates in the Practice
Breastfeeding rates in the practice should be tracked to determine the effectiveness of breastfeeding promotion, support, and optimal clinical management. This allows the practice to see how it measures up against national breastfeeding goals and impresses on parents and staff that breastfeeding is important. In addition, analyzing breastfeeding initiation and duration trends in the patient population can help pinpoint critical periods when more support for breastfeeding at well-child visits can make a significant difference

in breastfeeding success. Information can be gathered through the use of office surveys, periodic chart reviews, focus groups, and key informant interviews.

Give Encouragement

It should be assumed that all women are still breastfeeding at each visit and as such given the proper encouragement.

Staff Education

The key to providing breastfeeding care is effectively integrating relevant information and skills into existing daily routines without increasing the time required to provide a given service. Physicians and all staff should be educated in the basics of breastfeeding management to ensure that the practice communicates a consistent message and does not confuse families with conflicting information. Physicians and staff also should develop skills and comfort in evaluating breastfeeding through appropriate history and physical assessments. Excellent resources are available.

Physicians

Physicians need to be key leaders in promoting and supporting breastfeeding. Physician education should occur during medical school and residency training. Many myths and personal beliefs affect breastfeeding attitudes and advice. Unless they are educated, health care professionals frequently offer advice based on personal experience. Clinician education through reputable breastfeeding courses, conferences, and books and on the Internet can introduce the novice to the basics of breastfeeding and can expand knowledge of management and diagnosis for the more sophisticated physician. It is important that physicians provide age-appropriate breastfeeding intervention and anticipatory guidance as part of every routine health screening visit for mother and baby (see Chapter 8).

Nursing Staff

Nursing staff often can attend breastfeeding courses or conferences offering continuing education units or can be required to complete a course on breastfeeding competency. Shorter educational presentations can be offered to non-nursing staff on-site, such as a slide show covering the health benefits of breastfeeding and discussion of breastfeeding-related issues specific to the employees' type of patient interaction. It is important to emphasize that office breastfeeding facilities should also be available to all staff.

Support Staff

Nursing assistants, laboratory technicians, receptionists, housekeeping, administrative staff, and other support staff should be included in educational presentations because all individuals in the office setting interact with breast-feeding mothers. The staff also should be encouraged to use breastfeeding facilities within the office. Employees also may share a cultural or linguistic background with patients. Leadership should assess the educational gaps of staff and develop strategies to fill those gaps. Strategies may include holding in-house meetings or sending staff to conferences.

Lactation Specialists

Lactation specialists may be used in a practice. Some physicians prefer to select a lactation specialist who has been certified as an IBCLC by the International Board of Lactation Consultant Examiners. Certification involves meeting specific requirements and passing a written examination; it is open to physicians, registered nurses, and other qualified individuals who have experience helping breastfeeding women. Some practices may choose to hire lactation specialists to handle their breastfeeding educational needs. Another option is to hire a lactation specialist on a case-by-case basis or to choose one in private or hospital practice who can handle referrals on a regular basis. Physicians should be aware of appropriate resources in their community.

Patient Education

Most women make their feeding choice early. Nearly 3/4 of women make their feeding decision before the pregnancy or during the first trimester (see Chapter 5).

Prenatal Classes

Support groups for new mothers, breastfeeding classes for new mothers, and prenatal classes that incorporate breastfeeding will provide accurate information and social support for families.

Prenatal Visits

The routine prenatal visit offers an opportunity not only for the mother to express any questions or concerns she may have about breastfeeding but for the physician and staff as well to demonstrate a commitment to breastfeeding. Although optimal, prenatal visits with a pediatrician are infrequent, 11% in one study. Therefore, the early obstetric visits are important to set the stage for breastfeeding.

Telephone Support Lines

Support lines, either specifically dedicated to breastfeeding or incorporated within the practice telephone triage system, are beneficial as long as a health care professional with an appropriate level of breastfeeding knowledge handles the calls. The content of telephone calls should be recorded in the medical record. Although it is often tempting to give breastfeeding guidance over the phone or via e-mail, if there is a question regarding the adequacy of breastfeeding and milk supply, it is best to evaluate the infant and mother in person (see Chapter 8). The AAP publication *Breastfeeding Telephone Triage and Advice* is available to assist in telephone call advice.

Preventive Monitoring

Screening postpartum women for symptoms of depression along with other preventive monitoring should be provided (see Chapter 9).

Peer Counseling Services

La Leche League International, some Women, Infants, and Children Supplemental Nutrition Program (WIC) offices, and other breastfeeding support organizations offer peer counseling and should be available to breastfeeding women. Many women feel more comfortable exchanging breastfeeding information with mothers from similar ethnic and cultural backgrounds.

Community-Based Breastfeeding Groups

Good resources for information can be found in any number of community-based breastfeed groups. Examples include local La Leche League groups, peer counselors, and support groups offered through practices. Physicians can expand the network of support for breastfeeding by providing in-kind and financial support for local breastfeeding support groups.

Printed Materials

Any material offered to women should be checked for accuracy and content, and should be provided to families during their first contact with a health care system. Excellent alternatives for literature from manufacturers include resources from the American Academy of Pediatrics, American Congress of Obstetricians and Gynecologists, American Academy of Family Physicians, Academy of Breastfeeding Medicine, La Leche League International, Wellstart International, and childbirth organizations.

Potential Barriers to Effective Breastfeeding

Barriers to breastfeeding should be anticipated and discouraged, especially those that may be encountered early in the postpartum period. New mothers often have questions about returning to work and using electric breast pumps. In one study, 1 of the top 3 reasons women gave for not breastfeeding was "could not breastfeed because had to return to work." Anticipating this concern and providing instruction about expression and storage assistance and support could improve breastfeeding duration. See Chapters 10 and 11 for a discussion on employment and the use of breast pumps. Physicians can encourage employers in their community to adopt workplace practices that support breastfeeding.

The Business Aspect of Breastfeeding

The lactation aspects of a pediatric practice could be viewed in a business model for the improvement of the practice. In any service industry, if 75% of the clients want or need your product, you have made a good decision to apply your services to that group. Thus, the national average of 75% of women initiating breastfeeding gives substantial reason for focusing a practice toward assisting these mothers. Physicians can be key leaders in promoting and supporting breastfeeding. They need to appreciate breastfeeding from a larger business context.

Breastfeeding Support Services

Many practices may be able to provide delivery of outpatient breastfeeding medicine services. These services may incorporate many of the personnel mentioned earlier including lactation specialists, nursing staff, doulas, and peer counselors. Depending on the model, breastfeeding support services can be profitable, neutral, or operate with net losses. If operated efficiently and effectively, breastfeeding support services can be sustainable and a significant asset for a primary care practice and its patients.

Coding, Billing, and Reimbursement

Resources are available to assist physicians with reimbursement for outpatient breastfeeding services. The AAP has created one such document, "Supporting Breastfeeding and Lactation: The Primary Care Pediatrician's Guide to Getting Paid." This resource was updated in November 2010 and is available online (http://www2.aap.org/breastfeeding/files/pdf/coding.pdf).

Breast Pumps and Other Breastfeeding Accessories

In some practices, renting and/or selling breast pumps and other breastfeed-ing accessories can be a value-added service that is profitable. However, ordering, stocking, insuring, maintaining inventory, dealing with defective or damaged equipment, and other issues do require time and effort.

National Initiatives

AAP Breastfeeding Residency Curriculum

Providing pediatricians with the latest scientific information, educational materials, and strategies for increasing breastfeeding rates toward Healthy People 2020 national goals, the AAP Breastfeeding Residency Curriculum has expanded the educational outreach to include obstetricians, family physicians, public health representatives, and physicians' training programs with an emphasis on culturally effective breastfeeding promotion and support to families with racially and ethnically diverse backgrounds. Implementation of the curriculum improves breastfeeding management and success.

Business Case for Breastfeeding

A comprehensive resource for those helping breastfeeding women as they return to the workforce, The Business Case for Breastfeeding is a program designed to educate employers about the value of supporting breastfeeding employees in the workplace. The program highlights how such support contributes to the success of the entire business and offers tools to help employers provide worksite lactation support and privacy for breastfeeding mothers to express milk. The program also offers guidance to employees on breastfeeding and working.

Patient Protection and Affordable Care Act Breastfeeding Provisions

Section 4207 of the Patient Protection and Affordable Care Act states that employers shall provide breastfeeding employees with "reasonable break time" and a private, nonbathroom place to express breast milk during the workday, up until the child's first birthday.

Internal Revenue Service Tax Incentives

The Internal Revenue Service allows mothers to use pretax money from their flexible spending accounts to cover the cost of breast pumps and other breastfeeding-related supplies. Those mothers who do not have flexible spending accounts may deduct breastfeeding supply costs if their total unreimbursed medical expenses exceed 7.5% of their adjusted gross income and they itemize their tax returns.

Strategies for Implementation

Providing support, time, and effort up front is valuable and cost-effective. The following examples are included to stimulate thinking about possibilities in the hospital and the office practice.

- *Hospital strategies* to promote breastfeeding at various hospitals have been successful (see Table 6-1 and Box 6-3).
- *The day 3 to 5 follow-up visit* should be scheduled before hospital discharge so the infant can be evaluated in the office or clinic. At that time, history, weight, and physical examination can be completed and breastfeeding observed. If after the routine visit between 3 and 5 days the physician has concerns about breastfeeding, a problem-focused visit can be scheduled before the next routine checkup or referral can be made to a qualified lactation specialist (see Box 8-3).
- *Office Visits.* Developing partnerships and a collaborative breastfeeding agenda with others in the community is an effective way to strengthen breastfeeding management (Box 17-1).
- *Growth Curves.* Because breastfeeding is the normative way of feeding an infant, and to avoid labeling breastfed infants as growing poorly, the World Health Organization growth curves should be used to monitor the growth of all infants (see Chapter 8).
- *Subsequent Visits.* Anticipatory guidance is outlined in checklists pertinent to each health supervision visit (see Chapter 8).

Box 17-1. Selected Strategies Used to Encourage Breastfeeding in the Office

- Work with family life educators and home health nurses to ensure that the same breastfeeding messages are given.
- Offer prenatal classes beneficial for patients.
- Employ lactation specialists in the practice under the team leadership of the physician.
- Provide positive feedback to mothers (present a Certificate of Achievement for breastfeeding at each visit).
- Develop and support office and community-based breastfeeding activities.
- Encourage breastfeeding education in schools.
- Introduce breastfeeding benefits during an adolescent's office visit.

Selected References

1. ABM clinical protocol #14: Breastfeeding-friendly physician's office, part 1: optimizing care for infants and children. *Breastfeed Med.* 2006;1:115–119

2. American Academy of Pediatrics. *Supporting Breastfeeding and Lactation: The Primary Care Pediatrician's Guide to Getting Paid.* http://www2.aap.org/breastfeeding/files/pdf/coding.pdf. Accessed September 3, 2013

3. American Academy of Pediatrics Medical Home Initiatives for Children With Special Needs Project Advisory Committee. The medical home. *Pediatrics.* 2002;110:184–186

4. Arora S, McJunkin C, Wehrer J, Kuhn P. Major factors influencing breastfeeding rates: mother's perception of father's attitude and milk supply. *Pediatrics.* 2000;106:e67

5. Bartick M, Reinhold A. The burden of suboptimal breastfeeding in the United States: a pediatric cost analysis. *Pediatrics.* 2010;125:e1048–e1056

6. Bunik M. *Breastfeeding Telephone Triage and Advice.* Elk Grove Village, IL: American Academy of Pediatrics; 2013

7. Feldman-Winter LB, Barone L, Milcarek B, et al. Residency curriculum improves breastfeeding care. *Pediatrics.* 2010;126:289–297

8. Feldman-Winter LB, Schanler RJ, O'Connor KG, Lawrence RA. Pediatricians and the promotion and support of breastfeeding. *Arch Pediatr Adolesc Med.* 2008;162:1142–1149

9. Freed GL, Clark SJ, Lohr JA, Sorenson JR. Pediatrician involvement in breast-feeding promotion: a national study of residents and practitioners. *Pediatrics.* 1995;96:490–494

10. Grummer-Strawn LM, Reinold C, Krebs NF. Use of World Health Organization and CDC growth charts for children aged 0–59 months in the United States. *MMWR Recomm Rep.* 2010;59(RR-9):1–15

11. Howard C, Howard F, Lawrence R, Andresen E, DeBlieck E, Weitzman M. Office prenatal formula advertising and its effect on breastfeeding patterns. *Obstet Gynecol.* 2000;95:296–303

12. Howard FM, Howard CR, Weitzman M. The physician as advertiser: the unintentional discouragement of breast-feeding. *Obstet Gynecol.* 1993;81:1048–1051

13. Lu MC, Lange L, Slusser W, Hamilton J, Halfon N. Provider encouragement of breast-feeding: evidence from a national survey. *Obstet Gynecol.* 2001;97:290–295

14. Merewood A, Philipp BL. Becoming Baby-Friendly: overcoming the issue of accepting free formula. *J Hum Lact.* 2000;16:279–282

15. Perez-Escamilla R, Pollitt E, Lonnerdal B, Dewey KG. Infant feeding policies in maternity wards and their effect on breastfeeding success: an analytical overview. *Am J Public Health.* 1994;84:89–97

16. Perrine CG, Scanlon KS, Odom E, Grummer-Strawn LM. Baby-Friendly hospital practices and meeting exclusive breastfeeding intention. *Pediatrics.* 2012;130:54–60

17. Philipp BL. Every call is an opportunity. Supporting breastfeeding mothers over the telephone. *Pediatr Clin North Am.* 2001;48:525–532

18. Philipp BL, Cadwell K. Fielding questions about breastfeeding. *Contemp Pediatr.* 1999;16:149–164

19. Philipp BL, Merewood A, O'Brien S. Physicians and breastfeeding promotion in the United States: a call for action. *Pediatrics.* 2001;107:584–587

20. Pugin E, Valdes V, Labbok MH, Perez A, Aravena R. Does prenatal breastfeeding skills group education increase the effectiveness of a comprehensive breastfeeding promotion program? *J Hum Lact.* 1996;12:15–19

21. Schanler RJ, O'Connor KG, Lawrence RA. Pediatricians' practices and attitudes regarding breastfeeding promotion. *Pediatrics.* 1999;103:e35

22. Snell BJ, Krantz M, Keeton R, Delgado K, Peckham C. The association of formula samples given at hospital discharge with the early duration of breastfeeding. *J Hum Lact.* 1992;8:67–72

23. Taveras EM, Capra AM, Braveman PA, Jensvold NG, Escobar GJ, Lieu TA. Clinician support and psychosocial risk factors associated with breastfeeding discontinuation. *Pediatrics.* 2003;112:108–115

24. US Department of Health and Human Services. *The Surgeon General's Call to Action to Support Breastfeeding.* Washington, DC: US Department of Health and Human Services, Office of the Surgeon General; 2011

25. Wolynn T. Breastfeeding—so easy even a doctor can support it. *Breastfeed Med.* 2011;6:345–347

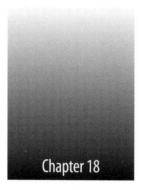

Chapter 18

Breastfeeding Issues During Disasters

A disaster, whether natural or human-made, often deprives people of food, clean water, heat, shelter, clothing, medicine, and other necessary resources needed to survive. Infants are at highest risk; therefore, rescue organizations rush to send infant formula to the affected area. However, because access to potable water and sterile feeding utensils is usually limited, the formula is often not usable. Breastfeeding provides the cleanest and safest infant and young child nutrition in any situation. Breastfeeding is sanitary, and it requires no electricity or refrigeration for preparation or storage. Human milk is the most appropriate nutrition, readily available without dependence on supplies, and is at the right temperature without the need for warming or cooling. In addition, it keeps the baby in contact with the mother, which prevents hypothermia from exposure. It is protective against infectious diseases, especially diarrhea and respiratory illnesses, which are at increased risks during a disaster. The security and warmth provided by breastfeeding is crucial for both mothers and children in the chaotic circumstances of an emergency. In addition, breastfeeding allows the mother to independently provide for her child despite the helplessness that occurs during a disaster.

Infant formula has many disadvantages during a disaster. It may not be available initially, or supplies may run out before the situation is resolved. It may become contaminated. Errors in formula preparation can occur at any time, especially during the chaos of a disaster. Water that is mixed with powdered or concentrated formula may be contaminated, and there may be no method to sterilize the formula, bottles, or nipples. In addition, if there is no electricity, opened prepared formula cannot be preserved by refrigeration. Therefore, the goal of infant disaster relief and the best way to save vulnerable infants must be to protect the breastfeeding relationship and to help women who have stopped lactating return to breastfeeding (relactation). Food supplies should be used to feed the mother, not the infant. By feeding her, you are helping both the mother and infant, and harming neither.

Disaster Preparation

To be effective, disaster preparation must begin before a disaster. Educated health care professionals should provide breastfeeding education to emergency relief agencies (all supervisory, technical, and nontechnical staff and volunteer workers) for these agencies to appropriately support and protect breastfeeding in emergencies. In addition to the practicalities of breastfeeding support, this education should also address the cultural expectations and personal experiences of staff and volunteers that may present barriers to understanding and implementing breastfeeding support. Key information about infant and young child feeding needs to be integrated into routine rapid assessment procedures and emergency preparedness plans. Emergency preparedness must include strategies to prevent separation of mothers and infants during evacuation, transport, and sheltering, as well as a unification plan for those who do become separated during an emergency. For those infants who despite best efforts will need formula, standards need to be established to ensure the safe storage and feeding of purchased and donated infant formula. For example, ready to feed is much more appropriate than formula that needs a sterile water supply to mix before feeding.

Breastfeeding Support During the Disaster

During the disaster, the role of health care professionals becomes even more crucial. In the immediate postdisaster period, an important role for health care professionals is to advocate to keep families together by creating safe havens for pregnant and breastfeeding mothers. These havens should provide security, counseling, clean water, and food. They should provide a safe environment for breastfeeding or expressing milk, including providing a private area or a way to breastfeed discreetly if the mother desires it. Health care professionals can contribute to the creation of havens by using offices, hospitals, or forming them within other shelters. They should identify breastfeeding mothers on arrival at the shelter and provide them with education, assurance, and support to sustain and increase their milk supply. Mothers who birth during a disaster period should be advised of the life-saving importance of breastfeeding and should be supported to initiate and continue breastfeeding.

Mothers should be assured that stress does not cause milk to dry up and that even malnourished women can breastfeed successfully. They should be encouraged to exclusively breastfeed as much as is feasible and taught that optimal human milk supply is maintained by infant demand. Mothers of recently weaned infants and young children should be informed that relactation is a realistic possibility. Lactating women must be included in the priority list for clean water and food. Mothers should be shown how to express milk by hand, if milk expression is needed. If there is a shortage of safe, complementary foods for infants older than 6 months, health care professionals can assure mothers that their milk can contribute significant nutrition in the absence of other foods for the first year of life and beyond. It is the perfect emergency food source.

During a disaster, assessment of the lactating infant needs to include hydration and nutritional status. Lactating women may be immunized as recommended for adults and adolescents to protect against measles, mumps, rubella, tetanus, diphtheria, pertussis, influenza, *Streptococcus pneumoniae*, *Neisseria meningitis*, hepatitis A, hepatitis B, varicella, and inactivated polio. Antibiotics and other medications can also be given to lactating women during a disaster, because they are usually compatible with breastfeeding. Although little DEET gets into human milk, if it is recommended as an insect repellant, it is best to limit the amount to which the lactating mother is exposed. It should be applied only to clothing and exposed skin, such as hands and face, and never to the breast area.

Health care professionals should advocate for optimal feeding options for orphaned infants and infants separated from their mothers, or when the mother cannot lactate. When a mother's own milk is not available, the next best option is donor human milk. Although pasteurized donor milk from a regulated milk bank is preferred, it has to be transported into the disaster area frozen and maintained frozen or refrigerated until fed to babies. The nature of a disaster is that this infrastructure is often not present in the early days, so pasteurized donor human milk is not a viable option until it is in place. Another option is termed "informal" human milk donation— that is, wet nursing or expressed human milk from volunteers. If informal human milk donation is used, the parent or person responsible for the baby must understand the risks and benefits of feeding unpasteurized human milk (see Chapter 11). If formula is given, health care professionals should recommend ready-to-feed formula. Concentrated or powdered formula should be used only if bottled or boiled water is available. Water that has been treated with iodine or chlorine tablets should not be used, except as a last resort. Infant feeding practices and resources should be assessed, coordinated, and monitored throughout the disaster. Mothers who are separated from their infants should be encouraged and assisted to express their milk to maintain their milk production and, possibly, serve as a human milk donor to other babies until reunited with her own.

As the shelter environment stabilizes over time, priority should be given to providing refrigeration and transportation support for pasteurized donor human milk, providing appropriate complementary foods for children older than 6 months, and including skilled lactation care providers in the team of trained emergency workers.

Relactation

For some mothers and babies, relactation, which is a resumption of lactation once breastfeeding has stopped, is possible (see Chapter 15). Steps to induce relactation include encouraging the mother to start skin-to-skin contact and frequent suckling by the infant, as often as continuously to every 2 hours. Supplements should be preferentially given as the infant suckles at the breast with a Supplemental Nursing System (SNS) if the means to clean the equipment in a sanitary manner exist. The mother's milk supply often increases gradually over days to weeks and supplementation should decrease accordingly. Signs of milk production include an increase in breast size or fullness, less consumption of supplement, infant satisfaction after feeding at the breast, and stool changes to softer, more yellow consistency. Careful assessment of the infant's nutritional and hydration status by the mother and health care professionals is critical during this process. Relactation is more successful if the infant was recently weaned, if the mother is still occasionally nursing, or if the infant is younger than 6 months. It is, however, possible in older infants and in mothers who never nursed (induced lactation). Necessary conditions are a highly motivated mother, stimulation of the breasts, and ongoing support.

Radiation

When a leak or explosion occurs at a nuclear reactor site, ionizing radiation is released, most often as radioactive iodine. Once out of the closest zone where radiation burns and immediate life-threatening effects occur (external radiation exposure), the concern becomes the ingestion of contaminated food, milk, and water, or the inhalation of radiation gas (internal radiation exposure). Children are particularly vulnerable because the "heavy" particles rapidly fall to the ground, settling in the area where babies and small children "live." Because children also have higher minute ventilation than adults, they are at greater risk for breathing in more of the aerosolized particles. Radioactive iodine is actively transferred into mammalian milk, both human and bovine, making these sources of nutrition potential risks for this vulnerable population. If contaminated water is used to mix formula for babies, it serves as another source for internal radiation exposure. Radioactive iodine is rapidly taken up into the thyroid gland and can ultimately cause thyroid cancer. The rate of thyroid cancer in children who were 0 to 4 years of age at the time of the Chernobyl reactor accident has been as much as 100-fold compared with pre-Chernobyl rates. These cancers occurred in children exposed to very low levels of radioiodine exposure; marked increases were seen in children exposed to 5 cGy radiation to the thyroid, whereas a few cases have even occurred in children exposed to 1 cGy.

Potassium iodide (KI) is recommended for children, infants, and pregnant or lactating women at a predicted thyroid exposure of 1 cGy or more according to the World Health Organization and 5 cGy or more according to the Centers for Disease Control and Prevention. Treatment with KI protects individuals from radioactive iodine because it competitively blocks radioactive iodine from being absorbed by the thyroid gland. After saturation with KI, no further radioactive iodine or KI can be absorbed for the next 24 hours. There is, however, a critical time period for taking KI, optimally being pre-exposure followed by immediate post-exposure.. By 12 hours after exposure, there is little protective effect. Once radioactive iodine has entered the thyroid, KI cannot remove it or reverse the health effects it causes. Because the protective effect of KI lasts approximately 24 hours, KI should be dosed daily for the mother. However, repeat dosing of KI should be avoided in the newborn to minimize the risk for hypothyroidism.

Although there is great concern with potentially contaminated human milk, we recommend that in times of disaster, mothers exposed to nonlethal levels of radiation can and should breastfeed. Breastfeeding decisions should be based on levels of exposure and availability of human milk substitutes. Formula may be unsafe depending on local water levels; cow milk also may be unsafe. Ready-to-feed formula is an option if available. The breastfeeding mother should take daily doses of 130 mg KI until a risk for significant exposure to radioiodine, either by inhalation or ingestion, no longer exists, as it will protect the mother and baby, and may reduce radiation levels in her milk.

The infant should receive 1 dose of 16 mg if 1 month or younger and 32 mg if older than 1 month, because a larger dose increases the baby's risk for hypothyroidism. The thyroid function of the infant should be monitored and thyroid hormone therapy prescribed if hypothyroidism develops. Because infants are particularly vulnerable to radiation, they should get priority, along with their mothers, for evacuation and control of the food supply. If KI is not available and safe formula is available, formula supplementation should be provided as a temporary solution until KI becomes available or the public health authorities declare breastfeeding safe again. If this decision is made, mothers must be supported to express their milk to maintain their milk supply until the baby can resume breastfeeding.

Selected References

1. American Academy of Pediatrics. Infant nutrition during a disaster: breastfeeding and other options. 2007. http://www.aap.org/breastfeeding/files/pdf/InfantNutritionDisaster.pdf. Accessed September 3, 2013
2. American Academy of Pediatrics Committee on Environmental Health. Radiation disasters and children. *Pediatrics.* 2003;111:1455–1466
3. American College of Obstetricians and Gynecologists Committee on Obstetric Practice. Committee opinion no. 555: hospital disaster preparedness for obstetricians and facilities providing maternity care. *Obstet Gynecol.* 2013;121(3):696–699
4. Infant and Young Child Feeding in Emergencies Core Group. *Infant and Young Child Feeding in Emergencies: Operational Guidance for Emergency Relief Staff and Programme Managers.* v 2.1. Oxford, United Kingdom: Infant and Young Child Feeding in Emergencies Core Group, Emergency Nutrition Network; 2007
5. Ip S, Chung M, Raman G, et al. *Breastfeeding and Maternal and Infant Health Outcomes in Developed Countries.* Rockville, MD: Agency for Healthcare Research and Quality; 2007. Evidence Report/Technology Assessment No. 153
6. Lawrence R. Disasters at home and abroad. *Breastfeed Med.* 2011;6:53–54
7. National Commission on Children and Disasters. Appendix D: children and disasters: the role of state and local governments in protecting this vulnerable population. In: *2010 Report to the President and Congress.* Rockville, MD: Agency for Healthcare Research and Quality; 2010. AHRQ Publication No. 10-M037
8. US Breastfeeding Committee. Breastfeeding: a vital emergency response. Are you ready? 2009. http://www.usbreastfeeding.org/LinkClick.aspx?link= Publications%2fBF-Emergency-Response-2009-USBC.pdf&tabid=70&mid=388. Accessed September 3, 2013
9. US Department of Health and Human Services, Food and Drug Administration Center for Drug Evaluation and Research (CDER). *Potassium Iodide as a Thyroid Blocking Agent in Radiation Emergencies.* December 2001. http://www.fda.gov/downloads/Drugs/Guidance ComplianceRegulatoryInformation/Guidances/ucm080542.pdf. Accessed September 3, 2013
10. Wellstart International. Infant and young child feeding in emergency situations. http://wellstart.org/Infant_feeding_emergency.pdf. Updated September 2005. Accessed September 3, 2013
11. World Health Organization. *Guiding Principles for Feeding Infants and Young Children During Emergencies.* Geneva, Switzerland: World Health Organization; 2004
12. World Health Organization/United Nations Children's Fund. *Global Strategy for Infant and Young Child Feeding.* Geneva, Switzerland: World Health Organization; 2003

Breastfeeding Resources

Publications

Breastfeeding: A Guide for the Medical Profession
Lawrence, RA, and Lawrence, RM
7th edition, 2011
Elsevier Mosby, Inc
www.us.elsevierhealth.com

Breastfeeding Answers Made Simple: A Guide for Helping Mothers
Mohrbacher, N
1st edition, 2010
Hale Publishing
800/378-1317
www.ibreastfeeding.com

Breastfeeding and Diseases
Buescher, S, and Hatcher, SW
1st edition, 2009
Hale Publishing
800/378-1317
www.ibreastfeeding.com

Breastfeeding and Human Lactation
Riordan, J, and Wambach, K
4th edition, 2010
Jones and Bartlett Publishers
800/832-0034
www.jblearning.com

Breastfeeding in the United States: A National Agenda
United States Breastfeeding Committee
2001
US Department of Health and Human Services, Health Resources and Services Administration, Maternal and Child Health Bureau
www.usbreastfeeding.org

Breastfeeding Medicine
Journal of the Academy of Breastfeeding Medicine
Mary Ann Liebert, Inc
www.liebertpub.com

Breastfeeding Telephone Triage and Advice
Bunik, M
1st edition, 2013
American Academy of Pediatrics
888/227-1770
www.aap.org

Publications *(continued)*

Bright Futures Guidelines for Health Supervision of Infants, Children, and Adolescents
Hagan, J, Duncan, P, and Shaw, J, eds
3rd edition, 2008
American Academy of Pediatrics
888/227-1770
www.aap.org

Checklists for Breastfeeding Health Supervision
American Academy of Pediatrics
    Section on Breastfeeding
2nd edition, 2013
American Academy of Pediatrics
888/227-1770
www.aap.org

Clinical Therapy in Breastfeeding Patients
Hale, TW, and Berens, P
3rd edition, 2010
Hale Publishing
800/378-1317
www.ibreastfeeding.com

Drugs in Pregnancy and Lactation: A Reference Guide to Fetal and Neonatal Risk
Briggs, GG, Freeman, RK, and Yaffe, SJ
9th edition, 2011
Lippincott Williams & Wilkins
800/683-3030
www.lww.com

Encounters With Children: Pediatric Behavior and Development
Dixon, SD, and Stein, MT
4th edition, 2005
Elsevier Mosby, Inc
www.us.elsevierhealth.com

Family Physicians Supporting Breastfeeding (*Position Paper*)
American Academy of Family
    Physicians, Breastfeeding
    Advisory Committee
Fall 2008
American Academy of Family
    Physicians
www.aafp.org/online/en/
home/policy/policies/b/
breastfeedingpositionpaper.html

Guidelines for Perinatal Care
American Academy of Pediatrics,
    American College of Obstetricians
    and Gynecologists
7th edition, 2012
American Academy of Pediatrics,
    American College of Obstetricians
    and Gynecologists
888/227-1770
www.aap.org

Journal of Human Lactation
International Lactation Consultants
    Association
Sage Publications
http://jhl.sagepub.com/

Little Green Book of Breastfeeding Management
Hertz, G
5th edition, 2011
Hale Publishing
800/378-1317
www.ibreastfeeding.com

Medications and Mothers' Milk
Hale, TW
15th edition, 2012
Hale Publishing
800/378-1317
www.ibreastfeeding.com

Nonprescription Drugs for the Breastfeeding Mother
Nice, F
2nd edition, 2011
Hale Publishing
800/378-1317
www.ibreastfeeding.com

Pediatric Nutrition Handbook
American Academy of Pediatrics
 Committee on Nutrition
6th edition, 2009
American Academy of Pediatrics
888/227-1770
www.aap.org

Supporting Breastfeeding and Lactation: The Primary Care Pediatrician's Guide to Getting Paid
2010
American Academy of Pediatrics
http://www2.aap.org/breastfeeding/
files/pdf/coding.pdf

Ten Steps to Support Parents' Choice to Breastfeed Their Baby
Breastfeeding Promotion in
 Physicians' Office Practices
2003
American Academy of Pediatrics
www.aap.org/breastfeeding

Textbook of Human Lactation
Hale, TW, and Hartmann, PE
1st edition, 2007
Hale Publishing
800/378-1317
www.ibreastfeeding.com

The Surgeon General's Call to Action to Support Breastfeeding
Department of Health and Human
 Services Office of the Surgeon
 General
2011
Department of Health and Human
 Services Office of the Surgeon
 General
800/994-9662
www.surgeongeneral.gov

Breastfeeding Education and Training

Breastfeeding Basics
O'Connor, M, Lewin, L, and CWRU
University Hospitals of Cleveland,
1998
www.breastfeedingbasics.org

Breastfeeding Residency Curriculum
American Academy of Pediatrics
Breastfeeding Promotion in
Physicians' Office Practices,
Phase III, 2008
www.aap.org/breastfeeding/
curriculum

Breastfeeding Training Course
University of Virginia School
of Medicine and Virginia,
Department of Health, 2013
http://bfconsortium.org/

Lactation Management Self-Study Modules
Wellstart International
3rd Edition, 2009
www.wellstart.org

Books for Parents

Breastfeeding Your Baby: Answers to Common Questions
American Academy of Pediatrics
2012
American Academy of Pediatrics
888/227-1770
www.aap.org

Breastfeeding, A Guide to Getting Started (video and companion booklet)
Morton, J
2nd version, 2009
Breastmilk Solutions
831/219-5021
www.breastmilksolutions.com

Great Expectations: The Essential Guide to Breastfeeding
Neifert, M
2009
Sterling Publishing
www.sterlingpublishing.com

New Mother's Guide to Breastfeeding
Meek, JY, ed
American Academy of Pediatrics
2nd edition, 2011
Bantam
888/227-1770
www.aap.org

The Nursing Mother's Companion
Huggins, K
6th edition, 2010
Harvard Common Press
www.harvardcommonpress.com

The Womanly Art of Breastfeeding
Wiessinger, D, West, D, and Pitman, T
8th edition, 2010
La Leche League International
847/519-7730
www.llli.org

Internet Resources

Academy of Breastfeeding Medicine
www.bfmed.org

American Academy of Family Physicians
www.aafp.org
familydoctor.org

American Academy of Pediatrics
www.aap.org/breastfeeding
www.healthychildren.org

American College of Obstetricians and Gynecologists
www.acog.org

Baby-Friendly USA
www.babyfriendlyusa.org

Baby Milk Action
www.babymilkaction.org

Breastfeeding Federal Legislative Updates
www.maloney.house.gov/issue/
breastfeeding

Breastfeeding Task Force of Greater Los Angeles
www.breastfeedingtaskforla.org

Business Case for Breastfeeding
(Office on Women's Health)
www.womenshealth.gov/
breastfeeding/government-in-action/
business-case.html

Centers for Disease Control and Prevention
www.cdc.gov

Children's Defense Fund
www.childrensdefense.org

Coalition for Improving Maternity Services
www.motherfriendly.org

DHHS–Healthcare.gov
(Information about Affordable Care Act)
www.healthcare.gov

Food and Drug Administration
www.fda.gov

Healthy People 2020 (National Objectives)
www.HealthyPeople.gov

Human Lactation Center (University of Rochester Medical Center)
www.urmc.rochester.edu/
childrens-hospital/neonatology/
lactation.aspx

Human Milk Banking Association of North America
www.hmbana.org

INFACT Canada: Infant Feeding Action Coalition
www.infactcanada.ca

International Baby Food Action Network
www.ibfan.org

International Board of Lactation Consultant Examiners
www.iblce.org

Internet Resources (continued)

International Childbirth Education Association
www.icea.org

International Code of Marketing of Breast-milk Substitutes
www.who.int/nutrition/publications/infantfeeding/9241541601/en/

International Lactation Consultant Association
www.ilca.org

International Society for Research in Human Milk and Lactation
www.isrhml.org

La Leche League International
www.lalecheleague.org

LactMed–Drugs and Lactation Database
www.toxnet.nlm.nih.gov/cgi-bin/sis/htmlgen?LACT

Linkages
www.linkagesproject.org

National Healthy Mothers, Healthy Babies Coalition
www.hmhb.org

National Institutes of Health
www.nih.gov

National WIC Association
www.nwica.org

The InfantRisk Center
www.infantrisk.com

United Nation Children's Fund
www.unicef.org

United States Surgeon General's Call to Action (Breastfeeding Support)
www.surgeongeneral.gov/initiatives/index.html

US Breastfeeding Committee
www.usbreastfeeding.org

US Department of Health and Human Services
www.dhhs.gov

US Food and Drug Administration
www.fda.gov/medwatch

USDA Food and Nutrition Service
www.fns.usda.gov/wic

World Alliance for Breastfeeding Action
www.waba.org.my

Please note: Inclusion in this publication does not imply an endorsement by the AAP or ACOG. The AAP and ACOG are not responsible for the content of the resources mentioned. Addresses, phone numbers, and Web site addresses are as current as possible, but may change at any time.

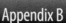

Appendix B

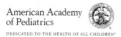

American Academy
of Pediatrics

DEDICATED TO THE HEALTH OF ALL CHILDREN®

POLICY STATEMENT

Breastfeeding and the Use of Human Milk

SECTION ON BREASTFEEDING

KEY WORDS
breastfeeding, complementary foods, infant nutrition, lactation,
human milk, nursing

ABBREVIATIONS
AAP—American Academy of Pediatrics
AHRQ—Agency for Healthcare Research and Quality
CDC—Centers for Disease Control and Prevention
CI—confidence interval
CMV—cytomegalovirus
DHA—docosahexaenoic acid
NEC—necrotizing enterocolitis
OR—odds ratio
SIDS—sudden infant death syndrome
WHO—World Health Organization

www.pediatrics.org/cgi/doi/10.1542/peds.2011-3552

doi:10.1542/peds.2011-3552

PEDIATRICS (ISSN Numbers: Print, 0031-4005; Online, 1098-4275).

Copyright © 2012 by the American Academy of Pediatrics

abstract

Breastfeeding and human milk are the normative standards for infant
feeding and nutrition. Given the documented short- and long-term medical and neurodevelopmental advantages of breastfeeding, infant nutrition should be considered a public health issue and not only
a lifestyle choice. The American Academy of Pediatrics reaffirms its
recommendation of exclusive breastfeeding for about 6 months, followed by continued breastfeeding as complementary foods are introduced, with continuation of breastfeeding for 1 year or longer as
mutually desired by mother and infant. Medical contraindications to
breastfeeding are rare. Infant growth should be monitored with the
World Health Organization (WHO) Growth Curve Standards to avoid mislabeling infants as underweight or failing to thrive. Hospital routines
to encourage and support the initiation and sustaining of exclusive breastfeeding should be based on the American Academy of
Pediatrics-endorsed WHO/UNICEF "Ten Steps to Successful Breastfeeding." National strategies supported by the US Surgeon General's Call
to Action, the Centers for Disease Control and Prevention, and The
Joint Commission are involved to facilitate breastfeeding practices in
US hospitals and communities. Pediatricians play a critical role in
their practices and communities as advocates of breastfeeding and
thus should be knowledgeable about the health risks of not breastfeeding, the economic benefits to society of breastfeeding, and the
techniques for managing and supporting the breastfeeding dyad. The
"Business Case for Breastfeeding" details how mothers can maintain
lactation in the workplace and the benefits to employers who facilitate this practice. *Pediatrics* 2012;129:e827–e841

INTRODUCTION

Six years have transpired since publication of the last policy statement
of the American Academy of Pediatrics (AAP) regarding breastfeeding.[1]
Recently published research and systematic reviews have reinforced
the conclusion that breastfeeding and human milk are the reference
normative standards for infant feeding and nutrition. The current
statement updates the evidence for this conclusion and serves as
a basis for AAP publications that detail breastfeeding management
and infant nutrition, including the *AAP Breastfeeding Handbook for
Physicians*,[2] *AAP Sample Hospital Breastfeeding Policy for Newborns*,[3]
AAP Breastfeeding Residency Curriculum,[4] and the *AAP Safe and
Healthy Beginnings Toolkit*.[5] The AAP reaffirms its recommendation
of exclusive breastfeeding for about 6 months, followed by continued
breastfeeding as complementary foods are introduced, with continuation

of breastfeeding for 1 year or longer as mutually desired by mother and infant.

EPIDEMIOLOGY

Information regarding breastfeeding rates and practices in the United States is available from a variety of government data sets, including the Centers for Disease Control and Prevention (CDC) National Immunization Survey,[6] the NHANES,[7] and Maternity Practices and Infant Nutrition and Care.[8] Drawing on these data and others, the CDC has published the "Breastfeeding Report Card," which highlights the degree of progress in achieving the breastfeeding goals of the Healthy People 2010 targets as well as the 2020 targets (Table 1).[9–11]

The rate of initiation of breastfeeding for the total US population based on the latest National Immunization Survey data are 75%.[11] This overall rate, however, obscures clinically significant sociodemographic and cultural differences. For example, the breastfeeding initiation rate for the Hispanic or Latino population was 80.6%, but for the non-Hispanic black or African American population, it was 58.1%. Among low-income mothers (participants in the Special Supplemental Nutrition Program for Women, Infants, and Children [WIC]), the breastfeeding initiation rate was 67.5%, but in those

with a higher income ineligible for WIC, it was 84.6%.[12] Breastfeeding initiation rate was 37% for low-income non-Hispanic black mothers.[7] Similar disparities are age-related; mothers younger than 20 years initiated breastfeeding at a rate of 59.7% compared with the rate of 79.3% in mothers older than 30 years. The lowest rates of initiation were seen among non-Hispanic black mothers younger than 20 years, in whom the breastfeeding initiation rate was 30%.[7]

Although over the past decade, there has been a modest increase in the rate of "any breastfeeding" at 3 and 6 months, in none of the subgroups have the Healthy People 2010 targets been reached. For example, the 6-month "any breastfeeding" rate for the total US population was 43%, the rate for the Hispanic or Latino subgroup was 46%, and the rate for the non-Hispanic black or African American subgroup was only 27.5%. Rates of exclusive breastfeeding are further from Healthy People 2010 targets, with only 13% of the US population meeting the recommendation to breastfeed exclusively for 6 months. Thus, it appears that although the breastfeeding initiation rates have approached the 2010 Healthy People targets, the targets for duration of any breastfeeding and exclusive breastfeeding have not been met.

Furthermore, 24% of maternity services provide supplements of commercial infant formula as a general practice in the first 48 hours after birth. These observations have led to the conclusion that the disparities in breastfeeding rates are also associated with variations in hospital routines, independent of the populations served. As such, it is clear that greater emphasis needs to be placed on improving and standardizing hospital-based practices to realize the newer 2020 targets (Table 1).

INFANT OUTCOMES

Methodologic Issues

Breastfeeding results in improved infant and maternal health outcomes in both the industrialized and developing world. Major methodologic issues have been raised as to the quality of some of these studies, especially as to the size of the study populations, quality of the data set, inadequate adjustment for confounders, absence of distinguishing between "any" or "exclusive" breastfeeding, and lack of a defined causal relationship between breastfeeding and the specific outcome. In addition, there are inherent practical and ethical issues that have precluded prospective randomized interventional trials of different feeding regimens. As such, the majority of published reports are observational cohort studies and systematic reviews/meta-analyses.

To date, the most comprehensive publication that reviews and analyzes the published scientific literature that compares breastfeeding and commercial infant formula feeding as to health outcomes is the report prepared by the Evidence-based Practice Centers of the Agency for Healthcare Research and Quality (AHRQ) of the US Department of Health Human Services titled *Breastfeeding and Maternal and Infant Health Outcomes in Developed Countries.*[13] The following sections summarize and update the AHRQ meta-analyses and provide an expanded analysis regarding health outcomes. Table 2 summarizes the dose-response relationship between the duration of breastfeeding and its protective effect.

Respiratory Tract Infections and Otitis Media

The risk of hospitalization for lower respiratory tract infections in the first year is reduced 72% if infants breastfed exclusively for more than 4 months.[13,14] Infants who exclusively breastfed for 4

TABLE 1 Healthy People Targets 2010 and 2020(%)

	2007[a]	2010 Target	2020 Target
Any breastfeeding			
Ever	75.0	75	81.9
6 mo	43.8	50	60.5
1 y	22.4	25	34.1
Exclusive breastfeeding			
To 3 mo	33.5	40	44.3
To 6 mo	13.8	17	23.7
Worksite lactation support	25	—	38.0
Formula use in first 2 d	25.6	—	15.6

[a] 2007 data reported in 2011.[10]

Appendix B: American Academy of Pediatrics Policy Statement: Breastfeeding and the Use of Human Milk

TABLE 2 Dose-Response Benefits of Breastfeeding[a]

Condition	% Lower Risk[b]	Breastfeeding	Comments	OR[c]	95% CI
Otitis media[13]	23	Any	—	0.77	0.64–0.91
Otitis media[13]	50	≥3 or 6 mo	Exclusive BF	0.50	0.36–0.70
Recurrent otitis media[15]	77	Exclusive BF	Compared with BF 4 to <6 mo[d]	1.95	1.06–3.59
Upper respiratory tract infection[17]	63	>6 mo	Exclusive BF	0.30	0.18–0.74
Lower respiratory tract infection[13]	72	≥4 mo	Exclusive BF	0.28	0.14–0.54
Lower respiratory tract infection[15]	77	Exclusive BF	Compared with BF 4 to <6 mo[d]	4.27	1.27–14.35
Asthma[13]	40	≥3 mo	Atopic family history	0.60	0.43–0.82
Asthma[13]	26	≥3 mo	No atopic family history	0.74	0.6–0.92
RSV bronchiolitis[16]	74	>4 mo	—	0.26	0.074–0.9
NEC[19]	77	NICU stay	Preterm infants Exclusive HM	0.23	0.51–0.94
Atopic dermatitis[27]	27	>3 mo	Exclusive BF negative family history	0.84	0.59–1.19
Atopic dermatitis[27]	42	>3 mo	Exclusive BF positive family history	0.58	0.41–0.92
Gastroenteritis[13,14]	64	Any	—	0.36	0.32–0.40
Inflammatory bowel disease[32]	31	Any	—	0.69	0.51–0.94
Obesity[13]	24	Any	—	0.76	0.67–0.86
Celiac disease[31]	52	>2 mo	Gluten exposure when BF	0.48	0.40–0.89
Type 1 diabetes[13,42]	30	>3 mo	Exclusive BF	0.71	0.54–0.93
Type 2 diabetes[13,43]	40	Any	—	0.61	0.44–0.85
Leukemia (ALL)[13,46]	20	>6 mo	—	0.80	0.71–0.91
Leukemia (AML)[13,45]	15	>6 mo	—	0.85	0.73–0.98
SIDS[13]	36	Any >1 mo	—	0.64	0.57–0.81

ALL, acute lymphocytic leukemia; AML, acute myelogenous leukemia; BF, breastfeeding; HM, human milk; RSV, respiratory syncytial virus.
[a] Pooled data.
[b] % lower risk refers to lower risk while BF compared with feeding commercial infant formula or referent group specified.
[c] OR expressed as increase risk for commercial formula feeding.
[d] Referent group is exclusive BF ≥6 months.

to 6 months had a fourfold increase in the risk of pneumonia compared with infants who exclusively breastfed for more than 6 months.[15] The severity (duration of hospitalization and oxygen requirements) of respiratory syncytial virus bronchiolitis is reduced by 74% in infants who breastfed exclusively for 4 months compared with infants who never or only partially breastfed.[16]

Any breastfeeding compared with exclusive commercial infant formula feeding will reduce the incidence of otitis media (OM) by 23%.[13] Exclusive breastfeeding for more than 3 months reduces the risk of otitis media by 50%. Serious colds and ear and throat infections were reduced by 63% in infants who exclusively breastfed for 6 months.[17]

Gastrointestinal Tract Infections

Any breastfeeding is associated with a 64% reduction in the incidence of nonspecific gastrointestinal tract infections, and this effect lasts for 2 months after cessation of breastfeeding.[13,14,17,18]

Necrotizing Enterocolitis

Meta-analyses of 4 randomized clinical trials performed over the period 1983 to 2005 support the conclusion that feeding preterm infants human milk is associated with a significant reduction (58%) in the incidence of necrotizing enterocolitis (NEC).[13] A more recent

study of preterm infants fed an exclusive human milk diet compared with those fed human milk supplemented with cow-milk-based infant formula products noted a 77% reduction in NEC.[19] One case of NEC could be prevented if 10 infants received an exclusive human milk diet, and 1 case of NEC requiring surgery or resulting in death could be prevented if 8 infants received an exclusive human milk diet.[19]

Sudden Infant Death Syndrome and Infant Mortality

Meta-analyses with a clear definition of degree of breastfeeding and adjusted for confounders and other known risks for sudden infant death syndrome (SIDS) note that breastfeeding is associated with a 36% reduced risk of SIDS.[13] Latest data comparing any versus exclusive breastfeeding reveal that for any breastfeeding, the multivariate odds ratio (OR) is 0.55 (95% confidence interval [CI], 0.44–0.69). When computed for exclusive breastfeeding, the OR is 0.27 (95% CI, 0.27–0.31).[20] A proportion (21%) of the US infant mortality has been attributed, in part, to the increased rate of SIDS in infants who were never breastfed.[21] That the positive effect of breastfeeding on SIDS rates is independent of sleep position was confirmed in a large case-control study of supine-sleeping infants.[22,23]

It has been calculated that more than 900 infant lives per year may be saved in the United States if 90% of mothers exclusively breastfed for 6 months.[24] In the 42 developing countries in which 90% of the world's childhood deaths occur, exclusive breastfeeding for 6 months and weaning after 1 year is the most effective intervention, with the potential of preventing more than 1 million infant deaths per year, equal to preventing 13% of the world's childhood mortality.[25]

Allergic Disease

There is a protective effect of exclusive breastfeeding for 3 to 4 months in reducing the incidence of clinical asthma, atopic dermatitis, and eczema by 27% in a low-risk population and up to 42% in infants with positive family history.[13,26] There are conflicting studies that examine the timing of adding complementary foods after 4 months and the risk of allergy, including food allergies, atopic dermatitis, and asthma, in either the allergy-prone or nonatopic individual.[26] Similarly, there are no convincing data that delaying introduction of potentially allergenic foods after 6 months has any protective effect.[27–30] One problem in analyzing this research is the low prevalence of exclusive breastfeeding at 6 months in the study populations. Thus, research outcomes in studies that examine the development of atopy and the timing of introducing solid foods in partially breastfed infants may not be applicable to exclusively breastfed infants.

Celiac Disease

There is a reduction of 52% in the risk of developing celiac disease in infants who were breastfed at the time of gluten exposure.[31] Overall, there is an association between increased duration of breastfeeding and reduced risk of celiac disease when measured as the presence of celiac antibodies. The critical protective factor appears to be not the timing of the gluten exposure but the overlap of breastfeeding at the time of the initial gluten ingestion. Thus, gluten-containing foods should be introduced while the infant is receiving only breast milk and not infant formula or other bovine milk products.

Inflammatory Bowel Disease

Breastfeeding is associated with a 31% reduction in the risk of childhood inflammatory bowel disease.[32] The protective effect is hypothesized to result from the interaction of the immunomodulating effect of human milk and the underlying genetic susceptibility of the infant. Different patterns of intestinal colonization in breastfed versus commercial infant formula–fed infants may add to the preventive effect of human milk.[33]

Obesity

Because rates of obesity are significantly lower in breastfed infants, national campaigns to prevent obesity begin with breastfeeding support.[34,35] Although complex factors confound studies of obesity, there is a 15% to 30% reduction in adolescent and adult obesity rates if any breastfeeding occurred in infancy compared with no breastfeeding.[13,36] The Framingham Offspring study noted a relationship of breastfeeding and a lower BMI and higher high-density lipoprotein concentration in adults.[37] A sibling difference model study noted that the breastfed sibling weighed 14 pounds less than the sibling fed commercial infant formula and was less likely to reach BMI obesity threshold.[38] The duration of breastfeeding also is inversely related to the risk of overweight; each month of breastfeeding being associated with a 4% reduction in risk.[14]

The interpretation of these data is confounded by the lack of a definition in many studies of whether human milk was given by breastfeeding or by bottle. This is of particular importance, because breastfed infants self-regulate intake volume irrespective of maneuvers that increase available milk volume, and the early programming of self-regulation, in turn, affects adult weight gain.[39] This concept is further supported by the observations that infants who are fed by bottle, formula, or expressed breast milk will have increased bottle emptying, poorer self-regulation, and excessive weight gain in late infancy (older than 6 months) compared with infants who only nurse from the breast.[40,41]

Diabetes

Up to a 30% reduction in the incidence of type 1 diabetes mellitus is reported for infants who exclusively breastfed for at least 3 months, thus avoiding exposure to cow milk protein.[13,42] It has been postulated that the putative mechanism in the development of type 1 diabetes mellitus is the infant's exposure to cow milk β-lactoglobulin, which stimulates an immune-mediated process cross-reacting with pancreatic β cells. A reduction of 40% in the incidence of type 2 diabetes mellitus is reported, possibly reflecting the long-term positive effect of breastfeeding on weight control and feeding self-regulation.[43]

Childhood Leukemia and Lymphoma

There is a reduction in leukemia that is correlated with the duration of breastfeeding.[14,44] A reduction of 20% in the risk of acute lymphocytic leukemia and 15% in the risk of acute myeloid leukemia in infants breastfed for 6 months or longer.[45,46] Breastfeeding for less than 6 months is protective but of less magnitude (approximately 12% and 10%, respectively). The question of whether the protective effect of breastfeeding is a direct mechanism of human milk on malignancies or secondarily mediated by its reduction of early childhood infections has yet to be answered.

Neurodevelopmental Outcomes

Consistent differences in neurodevelopmental outcome between breastfed and commercial infant formula–fed infants have been reported, but the outcomes are confounded by differences in parental education, intelligence, home environment, and socioeconomic status.[13,47] The large, randomized Promotion of Breastfeeding Intervention Trial provided evidence that adjusted outcomes of intelligence scores and teacher's ratings are significantly greater in breastfed infants.[48–50] In

Appendix B: American Academy of Pediatrics Policy Statement: Breastfeeding and the Use of Human Milk

addition, higher intelligence scores are noted in infants who exclusively breastfed for 3 months or longer, and higher teacher ratings were observed if exclusive breastfeeding was practiced for 3 months or longer. Significantly positive effects of human milk feeding on long-term neurodevelopment are observed in preterm infants, the population more at risk for these adverse neurodevelopmental outcomes.[51–54]

PRETERM INFANTS

There are several significant short- and long-term beneficial effects of feeding preterm infants human milk. Lower rates of sepsis and NEC indicate that human milk contributes to the development of the preterm infant's immature host defense.[19,55–59] The benefits of feeding human milk to preterm infants are realized not only in the NICU but also in the fewer hospital readmissions for illness in the year after NICU discharge.[51,52] Furthermore, the implications for a reduction in incidence of NEC include not only lower mortality rates but also lower long-term growth failure and neurodevelopmental disabilities.[60,61] Clinical feeding tolerance is improved, and the attainment of full enteral feeding is hastened by a diet of human milk.[51,52,59]

Neurodevelopmental outcomes are improved by the feeding of human milk. Long-term studies at 8 years of age through adolescence suggest that intelligence test results and white matter and total brain volumes are greater in subjects who had received human milk as infants in the NICU.[53,54] Extremely preterm infants receiving the greatest proportion of human milk in the NICU had significantly greater scores on mental, motor, and behavior ratings at ages 18 months and 30 months.[51,52] These data remain significant after adjustment for confounding factors, such as maternal age, education, marital status, race, and infant morbidities.

These neurodevelopmental outcomes are associated with predominant and not necessarily exclusive human milk feeding. Human milk feeding in the NICU also is associated with lower rates of severe retinopathy of prematurity.[62,63] Long-term studies of preterm infants also suggest that human milk feeding is associated with lower rates of metabolic syndrome, and in adolescents, it is associated with lower blood pressures and low-density lipoprotein concentrations and improved leptin and insulin metabolism.[64,65]

The potent benefits of human milk are such that all preterm infants should receive human milk (Table 3). Mother's own milk, fresh or frozen, should be the primary diet, and it should be fortified appropriately for the infant born weighing less than 1.5 kg. If mother's own milk is unavailable despite significant lactation support, pasteurized donor milk should be used.[19,66] Quality control of pasteurized donor milk is important and should be monitored. New data suggest that mother's own milk can be stored at refrigerator temperature (4°C) in the NICU for as long as 96 hours.[67] Data on thawing, warming, and prolonged storage need updating. Practices should involve protocols that prevent misadministration of milk.

MATERNAL OUTCOMES

Both short- and long-term health benefits accrue to mothers who breastfeed. Such mothers have decreased postpartum blood loss and more rapid involution of the uterus. Continued breastfeeding leads to increased child spacing secondary to lactational amenorrhea. Prospective cohort studies have noted an increase in postpartum depression in mothers who do not breastfeed or who wean early.[68] A large prospective study on child abuse and neglect perpetuated by mothers found, after correcting for potential

TABLE 3 Recommendations on Breastfeeding Management for Preterm Infants

1. All preterm infants should receive human milk.
   - Human milk should be fortified, with protein, minerals, and vitamins to ensure optimal nutrient intake for infants weighing <1500 g at birth.
   - Pasteurized donor human milk, appropriately fortified, should be used if mother's own milk is unavailable or its use is contraindicated.
2. Methods and training protocols for manual and mechanical milk expression must be available to mothers.
3. Neonatal intensive care units should possess evidence-based protocols for collection, storage, and labeling of human milk.[150]
4. Neonatal intensive care units should ensure that practices do not prevent the misadministration of human milk (http://www.cdc.gov/breastfeeding/recommendations/other_mothers_milk.htm).
5. There are no data to support routinely culturing human milk for bacterial or other organisms.[151]

confounders, that the rate of abuse/neglect was significantly increased for mothers who did not breastfeed as opposed to those who did (OR: 2.6; 95% CI: 1.7–3.9).[69]

Studies of the overall effect of breastfeeding on the return of the mothers to their pre-pregnancy weight are inconclusive, given the large numbers of confounding factors on weight loss (diet, activity, baseline BMI, ethnicity).[13] In a covariate-adjusted study of more than 14 000 women postpartum, mothers who exclusively breastfed for longer than 6 months weighed 1.38 kg less than those who did not breastfeed.[70] In mothers without a history of gestational diabetes, breastfeeding duration was associated with a decreased risk of type 2 diabetes mellitus; for each year of breastfeeding, there was a decreased risk of 4% to 12%.[71,72] No beneficial effect for breastfeeding was noted in mothers who were diagnosed with gestational diabetes.

The longitudinal Nurses Health Study noted an inverse relationship between the cumulative lifetime duration of breastfeeding and the development of rheumatoid arthritis.[73] If cumulative duration of breastfeeding exceeded 12 months, the relative risk of rheumatoid arthritis was 0.8 (95% CI: 0.8–1.0), and if the cumulative duration of breastfeeding was longer than 24 months, the relative risk of rheumatoid arthritis was 0.5 (95% CI: 0.3–0.8).[73] An association between cumulative lactation experience and the incidence of adult cardiovascular disease was reported by the Women's Health Initiative in a longitudinal study of more than 139 000 postmenopausal women.[74] Women with a cumulative lactation history of 12 to 23 months had a significant reduction in hypertension (OR: 0.89; 95% CI: 0.84–0.93), hyperlipidemia (OR: 0.81; 95% CI: 0.76–0.87), cardiovascular disease (OR: 0.90; 95% CI: 0.85–0.96), and diabetes (OR: 0.74; 95% CI: 0.65–0.84).

Cumulative lactation experience also correlates with a reduction in both breast (primarily premenopausal) and ovarian cancer.[13,14,75] Cumulative duration of breastfeeding of longer than 12 months is associated with a 28% decrease in breast cancer (OR: 0.72; 95% CI: 0.65–0.8) and ovarian cancer (OR: 0.72; 95% CI: 0.54–0.97).[76] Each year of breastfeeding has been calculated to result in a 4.3% reduction in breast cancer.[76,77]

ECONOMIC BENEFITS

A detailed pediatric cost analysis based on the AHRQ report concluded that if 90% of US mothers would comply with the recommendation to breastfeed exclusively for 6 months, there would be a savings of $13 billion per year.[24] The savings do not include those related to a reduction in parental absenteeism from work or adult deaths from diseases acquired in childhood, such as asthma, type 1 diabetes mellitus, or obesity-related conditions. Strategies that increase the number of mothers who breastfeed exclusively for about 6 months would be of great economic benefit on a national level.

DURATION OF EXCLUSIVE BREASTFEEDING

The AAP recommends exclusive breastfeeding for about 6 months, with continuation of breastfeeding for 1 year or longer as mutually desired by mother and infant, a recommendation concurred to by the WHO[78] and the Institute of Medicine.[79]

Support for this recommendation of exclusive breastfeeding is found in the differences in health outcomes of infants breastfed exclusively for 4 vs 6 months, for gastrointestinal disease, otitis media, respiratory illnesses, and atopic disease, as well as differences in maternal outcomes of delayed menses and postpartum weight loss.[15,18,80]

Compared with infants who never breastfed, infants who were exclusively breastfed for 4 months had significantly greater incidence of lower respiratory tract illnesses, otitis media, and diarrheal disease than infants exclusively breastfed for 6 months or longer.[15,18] When compared with infants who exclusively breastfed for longer than 6 months, those exclusively breastfed for 4 to 6 months had a fourfold increase in the risk of pneumonia.[15] Furthermore, exclusively breastfeeding for 6 months extends the period of lactational amenorrhea and thus improves child spacing, which reduces the risk of birth of a preterm infant.[81]

The AAP is cognizant that for some infants, because of family and medical history, individual developmental status, and/or social and cultural dynamics, complementary feeding, including gluten-containing grains, begins earlier than 6 months of age.[82,83] Because breastfeeding is immunoprotective, when such complementary foods are introduced, it is advised that this be done while the infant is feeding only breastmilk.[82] Mothers should be encouraged to continue breastfeeding through the first

year and beyond as more and varied complementary foods are introduced.

CONTRAINDICATIONS TO BREASTFEEDING

There are a limited number of medical conditions in which breastfeeding is contraindicated, including an infant with the metabolic disorder of classic galactosemia. Alternating breastfeeding with special protein-free or modified formulas can be used in feeding infants with other metabolic diseases (such as phenylketonuria), provided that appropriate blood monitoring is available. Mothers who are positive for human T-cell lymphotrophic virus type I or II[84] or untreated brucellosis[85] should not breastfeed nor provide expressed milk to their infants Breastfeeding should not occur if the mother has active (infectious) untreated tuberculosis or has active herpes simplex lesions on her breast; however, expressed milk can be used because there is no concern about these infectious organisms passing through the milk. Breastfeeding can be resumed when a mother with tuberculosis is treated for a minimum of 2 weeks and is documented that she is no longer infectious.[86] Mothers who develop varicella 5 days before through 2 days after delivery should be separated from their infants, but their expressed milk can be used for feeding.[87] In 2009, the CDC recommended that mothers acutely infected with H1N1 influenza should temporarily be isolated from their infants until they are afebrile, but they can provide expressed milk for feeding.[88]

In the industrialized world, it is not recommended that HIV-positive mothers breastfeed. However, in the developing world, where mortality is increased in non-breastfeeding infants from a combination of malnutrition and infectious diseases, breastfeeding may outweigh the risk of the acquiring HIV infection

FROM THE AMERICAN ACADEMY OF PEDIATRICS

from human milk. Infants in areas with endemic HIV who are exclusively breastfed for the first 3 months are at a lower risk of acquiring HIV infection than are those who received a mixed diet of human milk and other foods and/or commercial infant formula.[89] Recent studies document that combining exclusive breastfeeding for 6 months with 6 months of antiretroviral therapy significantly decreases the postnatal acquisition of HIV-1.[90,91]

There is no contraindication to breastfeeding for a full-term infant whose mother is seropositive for cytomegalovirus (CMV). There is a possibility that CMV acquired from mother's milk may be associated with a late-onset sepsis-like syndrome in the extremely low birth weight (birth weight <1500 g) preterm infant. Although not associated with long-term abnormalities, such a syndrome may warrant antiviral therapy.[92] The value of routinely feeding human milk from seropositive mothers to preterm infants outweighs the risks of clinical disease, especially because no long-term neurodevelopmental abnormalities have been reported.[93] Freezing of milk reduces but does not eliminate CMV.[94] Heating, either as Holder pasteurization (heating at 62.5°C for 30 minutes) or high-temperature short pasteurization (72°C for 5–10 seconds) eliminates the viral load from the milk but also affects bioactive factors and nutrients.[95] Thus, fresh mother's own milk is preferable for routinely feeding all preterm infants.

Maternal substance abuse is not a categorical contraindication to breastfeeding. Adequately nourished narcotic-dependent mothers can be encouraged to breastfeed if they are enrolled in a supervised methadone maintenance program and have negative screening for HIV and illicit drugs.[96] Street drugs such as PCP (phencyclidine), cocaine, and cannabis can be detected in human milk, and their use by breastfeeding mothers is of concern, particularly with regard to the infant's long-term neurobehavioral development and thus are contraindicated.[97] Alcohol is not a galactogogue; it may blunt prolactin response to suckling and negatively affects infant motor development.[98,99] Thus, ingestion of alcoholic beverages should be minimized and limited to an occasional intake but no more than 0.5 g alcohol per kg body weight, which for a 60 kg mother is approximately 2 oz liquor, 8 oz wine, or 2 beers.[100] Nursing should take place 2 hours or longer after the alcohol intake to minimize its concentration in the ingested milk.[101] Maternal smoking is not an absolute contraindication to breastfeeding but should be strongly discouraged, because it is associated with an increased incidence in infant respiratory allergy[102] and SIDS.[103] Smoking should not occur in the presence of the infant so as to minimize the negative effect of secondary passive smoke inhalation.[104] Smoking is also a risk factor for low milk supply and poor weight gain.[105,106]

MATERNAL DIET

Well-nourished lactating mothers have an increased daily energy need of 450 to 500 kcal/day that can be met by a modest increase in a normally balanced varied diet.[107–109] Although dietary reference intakes for breastfeeding mothers are similar to or greater than those during pregnancy, there is no routine recommendation for maternal supplements during lactation.[108,109,110] Many clinicians recommend the continued use of prenatal vitamin supplements during lactation.[109]

The mother's diet should include an average daily intake of 200 to 300 mg of the ω-3 long-chain polyunsaturated fatty acids (docosahexaenoic acid [DHA]) to guarantee a sufficient concentration of preformed DHA in the milk.[111,112] Consumption of 1 to 2 portions of fish (eg, herring, canned light tuna, salmon) per week will meet this need. The concern regarding the possible risk from intake of excessive mercury or other contaminants is offset by the neurobehavioral benefits of an adequate DHA intake and can be minimized by avoiding the intake of predatory fish (eg, pike, marlin, mackerel, tile fish, swordfish).[113] Poorly nourished mothers or those on selective vegan diets may require a supplement of DHA as well as multivitamins.

MATERNAL MEDICATIONS

Recommendations regarding breastfeeding in situations in which the mother is undergoing either diagnostic procedures or pharmacologic therapy must balance the benefits to the infant and the mother against the potential risk of drug exposure to the infant. There are only a limited number of agents that are contraindicated, and an appropriate substitute usually can be found. The most comprehensive, up-to-date source of information regarding the safety of maternal medications when the mother is breastfeeding is LactMed, an Internet-accessed source published by the National Library of Medicine/National Institutes of Health.[114] A forthcoming AAP policy statement on the transfer of drugs and other chemicals into human milk will provide additional recommendations, with particular focus on psychotropic drugs, herbal products, galactogogues, narcotics, and pain medications.[115] In general, breastfeeding is not recommended when mothers are receiving medication from the following classes of drugs: amphetamines, chemotherapy agents, ergotamines, and statins.

There are a wide variety of maternally administered psychotropic agents for which there are inadequate pharmacologic data with regard to human milk and/or nursing infant's blood concentrations. In addition, data regarding the long-term neurobehavioral effects from exposure to these agents during the critical developmental period of early infancy are lacking. A recent comprehensive review noted that of the 96 psychotropic drugs available, pharmacologic and clinical information was only available for 62 (65%) of the drugs.[116] In only 19 was there adequate information to allow for defining a safety protocol and thus qualifying to be compatible for use by lactating mothers. Among the agents considered to be least problematic were the tricyclic antidepressants amitriptyline and clomipramine and the selective serotonin-reuptake inhibitors paroxetine and sertraline.

Detailed guidelines regarding the necessity for and duration of temporary cessation of breastfeeding after maternal exposure to diagnostic radioactive compounds are provided by the US Nuclear Regulatory Commission and in medical reviews.[117–119] Special precaution should be followed in the situation of breastfeeding infants with glucose-6-phosphate-dehydrogenase deficiency. Fava beans, nitrofurantoin, primaquine, and phenazopyridine should be avoided by the mother to minimize the risk of hemolysis in the infant.[120]

HOSPITAL ROUTINES

The Sections on Breastfeeding and Perinatal Pediatrics have published the Sample Hospital Breastfeeding Policy that is available from the AAP Safe and Healthy Beginnings Web site.[3,5] This sample hospital policy is based on the detailed recommendations of the previous AAP policy statement "Breastfeeding and the Use of Human Milk"[1] as well as the principles of the 1991 WHO/UNICEF publication "Tens Steps to Successful Breastfeeding" (Table 4)[121] and provides a template for developing a uniform hospital policy for support of breastfeeding.[122] In particular,

emphasis is placed on the need to revise or discontinue disruptive hospital policies that interfere with early skin-to-skin contact, that provide water, glucose water, or commercial infant formula without a medical indication, that restrict the amount of time the infant can be with the mother, that limit feeding duration, or that provide unlimited pacifier use.

In 2009, the AAP endorsed the Ten Steps program (see Table 4). Adherence to these 10 steps has been demonstrated to increase rates of breastfeeding initiation, duration, and exclusivity.[122,123] Implementation of the following 5 postpartum hospital practices has been demonstrated to increase breastfeeding duration, irrespective of socioeconomic status: breastfeeding in the first hour after birth, exclusive breastfeeding, rooming-in, avoidance of pacifiers, and receipt of telephone number for support after discharge from the hospital.[124]

The CDC National Survey of Maternity Practices in Infant Nutrition and Care has assessed the lactation practices in more than 80% of US hospitals and noted that the mean score for implementation of the Ten Steps was only 65%.[34,125] Fifty-eight percent of hospitals erroneously advised mothers to limit suckling at the breast to a specified length of time, and 41% of the hospitals gave pacifiers to more than some of their newborns—both practices that have been documented to lower breastfeeding rates and duration.[126] The survey noted that in 30% of all birth centers, more than half of all newborns received supplementation commercial infant formula, a practice associated with shorter duration of breastfeeding and less exclusivity.[34,125] As indicated in the benefits section, this early supplementation may affect morbidity outcomes in this population. The survey also reported that 66% of hospitals

reported that they distributed to breastfeeding mothers discharge packs that contained commercial infant formula, a practice that has been documented to negatively affect exclusivity and duration of breastfeeding.[127] Few birth centers have model hospital policies (14%) and support breastfeeding mothers after hospital discharge (27%). Only 37% of centers practice more than 5 of the 10 Steps and only 3.5% practice 9 to 10 Steps.[34]

There is, thus, a need for a major conceptual change in the organization of the hospital services for the mother and infant dyad (Table 5). This requires that medical and nursing routines and practices adjust to the principle that breastfeeding should begin within the first hour after birth (even for Cesarean deliveries) and that infants must be continuously accessible to the mother by rooming-in

TABLE 4 WHO/UNICEF Ten Steps to Successful Breastfeeding

1. Have a written breastfeeding policy that is routinely communicated to all health care staff.
2. Train all health care staff in the skills necessary to implement this policy.
3. Inform all pregnant women about the benefits and management of breastfeeding.
4. Help mothers initiate breastfeeding within the first hour of birth.
5. Show mothers how to breastfeed and how to maintain lactation even if they are separated from their infants.
6. Give newborn infants no food or drink other than breast milk, unless medically indicated.
7. Practice rooming-in (allow mothers and infants to remain together) 24 h a day.
8. Encourage breastfeeding on demand.
9. Give no artificial nipples or pacifiers to breastfeeding infants.[a]
10. Foster the establishment of breastfeeding support groups and refer mothers to them on discharge from hospital.

[a] The AAP does not support a categorical ban on pacifiers because of their role in SIDS risk reduction and their analgesic benefit during painful procedures when breastfeeding cannot provide the analgesia. Pacifier use in the hospital in the neonatal period should be limited to specific medical indications such as pain reduction and calming in a drug-exposed infant, for example. Mothers of healthy term breastfed infants should be instructed to delay pacifier use until breastfeeding is well-established, usually about 3 to 4 wk after birth.

arrangements that facilitate around-the-clock, on-demand feeding for the healthy infant. Formal staff training should not only focus on updating knowledge and techniques for breast-feeding support but also should acknowledge the need to change attitudes and eradicate unsubstantiated beliefs about the supposed equivalency of breastfeeding and commercial infant formula feeding. Emphasis should be placed on the numerous benefits of exclusive breastfeeding. The importance of addressing the issue of the impact of hospital practices and policies on breastfeeding outcomes is highlighted by the decision of The Joint Commission to adopt the rate of exclusive breast milk feeding as a Perinatal Care Core Measure.[127] As such, the rate of exclusive breastfeeding during the hospital stay has been confirmed as a critical variable when measuring the quality of care provided by a medical facility.

Pacifier Use

Given the documentation that early use of pacifiers may be associated with less successful breastfeeding, pacifier use in the neonatal period should be limited to specific medical situations.[128] These include uses for pain relief, as a calming agent, or as part of structured program for enhancing oral motor function. Because pacifier use has been associated with a reduction in SIDS incidence, mothers of healthy term infants should be instructed to use pacifiers at infant nap or sleep time after breastfeeding is well established, at approximately 3 to 4 weeks of age.[129–131]

Vitamins and Mineral Supplements

Intramuscular vitamin K_1 (phytonadione) at a dose of 0.5 to 1.0 mg should routinely be administered to all infants on the first day to reduce the risk of hemorrhagic disease of the newborn.[132] A delay of administration until after the first feeding at the breast but not later than 6 hours of age is recommended. A single oral dose of vitamin K should not be used, because the oral dose is variably absorbed and does not provide adequate concentrations or stores for the breastfed infant.[132]

Vitamin D deficiency/insufficiency and rickets has increased in all infants as a result of decreased sunlight exposure secondary to changes in lifestyle, dress habits, and use of topical sunscreen preparations. To maintain an adequate serum vitamin D concentration, all breastfed infants routinely should receive an oral supplement of vitamin D, 400 U per day, beginning at hospital discharge.[133]

Supplementary fluoride should not be provided during the first 6 months. From age 6 months to 3 years, fluoride supplementation should be limited to infants residing in communities where the fluoride concentration in the water is <0.3 ppm.[134] Complementary food rich in iron and zinc should be introduced at about 6 months of age. Supplementation of oral iron drops before 6 months may be needed to support iron stores.

Premature infants should receive both a multivitamin preparation and an oral iron supplement until they are ingesting a completely mixed diet and their growth and hematologic status are normalized.

GROWTH

The growth pattern of healthy term breastfed infants differs from the existing CDC "reference" growth curves, which are primarily based on data from few breastfeeding infants. The WHO multicenter curves are based on combined longitudinal data from healthy breastfed infants from birth to 24 months and cross-sectional data from 2 to 5 years of the same children from 6 diverse geographical areas

TABLE 5 Recommendations on Breastfeeding Management for Healthy Term Infants

1. Exclusive breastfeeding for about 6 mo
   • Breastfeeding preferred; alternatively expressed mother's milk, or donor milk
   • To continue for at least the first year and beyond for as long as mutually desired by mother and child
   • Complementary foods rich in iron and other micronutrients should be introduced at about 6 mo of age
2. Peripartum policies and practices that optimize breastfeeding initiation and maintenance should be compatible with the AAP and Academy of Breastfeeding Medicine Model Hospital Policy and include the following:
   • Direct skin-to-skin contact with mothers immediately after delivery until the first feeding is accomplished and encouraged throughout the postpartum period
   • Delay in routine procedures (weighing, measuring, bathing, blood tests, vaccines, and eye prophylaxis) until after the first feeding is completed
   • Delay in administration of intramuscular vitamin K until after the first feeding is completed but within 6 h of birth
   • Ensure 8 to 12 feedings at the breast every 24 h
   • Ensure formal evaluation and documentation of breastfeeding by trained caregivers (including position, latch, milk transfer, examination) at least for each nursing shift
   • Give no supplements (water, glucose water, commercial infant formula, or other fluids) to breastfeeding newborn infants unless medically indicated using standard evidence-based guidelines for the management of hyperbilirubinemia and hypoglycemia
   • Avoid routine pacifier use in the postpartum period
   • Begin daily oral vitamin D drops (400 IU) at hospital discharge
3. All breastfeeding newborn infants should be seen by a pediatrician at 3 to 5 d of age, which is within 48 to 72 h after discharge from the hospital
   • Evaluate hydration (elimination patterns)
   • Evaluate body wt gain (body wt loss no more than 7% from birth and no further wt loss by day 5: assess feeding and consider more frequent follow-up)
   • Discuss maternal/infant issues
   • Observe feeding
4. Mother and infant should sleep in proximity to each other to facilitate breastfeeding
5. Pacifier should be offered, while placing infant in back-to-sleep-position, no earlier than 3 to 4 wk of age and after breastfeeding has been established

e835

(Brazil, Ghana, India, Norway, Oman, and the United States).[135] As such, the WHO curves are "standards" and are the normative model for growth and development irrespective of infant ethnicity or geography reflecting the optimal growth of the breastfed infant.[136] Use of the WHO curves for the first 2 years allows for more accurate monitoring of weight and height for age and, in comparison with use of the CDC reference curves, results in more accurate (lower) rates of undernutrition and short stature and (higher) rates of overweight. Furthermore, birth to 6-month growth charts are available where the curves are magnified to permit monitoring of weight trajectories. As such, the WHO curves serve as the best guide for assessing lactation performance because they minimize mislabeling clinical situations as inadequate breastfeeding and identify more accurately and promptly overweight and obese infants. As of September 2010, the CDC, with the concurrence of the AAP, recommended the use of the WHO curves for all children younger than 24 months.[137,138]

ROLE OF THE PEDIATRICIAN

Pediatricians have a critical role in their individual practices, communities, and society at large to serve as advocates and supporters of successful breastfeeding (Table 6).[139] Despite this critical role, studies have demonstrated lack of preparation and knowledge and declining attitudes regarding the feasibility of breastfeeding.[140] The AAP Web site[141] provides a wealth of breastfeeding-related material and resources to assist and support pediatricians in their critical role as advocates of infant well-being. This includes the Safe and Healthy Beginnings toolkit,[5] which includes resources for physician's office for promotion of breastfeeding in a busy pediatric practice setting, a pocket

TABLE 6 Role of the Pediatrician

1. Promote breastfeeding as the norm for infant feeding.
2. Become knowledgeable in the principles and management of lactation and breastfeeding.
3. Develop skills necessary for assessing the adequacy of breastfeeding.
4. Support training and education for medical students, residents and postgraduate physicians in breastfeeding and lactation.
5. Promote hospital policies that are compatible with the AAP and Academy of Breastfeeding Medicine Model Hospital Policy and the WHO/UNICEF "Ten Steps to Successful Breastfeeding."
6. Collaborate with the obstetric community to develop optimal breastfeeding support programs.
7. Coordinate with community-based health care professionals and certified breastfeeding counselors to ensure uniform and comprehensive breastfeeding support.

guide for coding to facilitate appropriate payment, suggested guidelines for telephone triage of maternal breastfeeding concerns, and information regarding employer support for breastfeeding in the workplace. Evidence-based protocols from organizations such as the Academy of Breastfeeding Medicine provide detailed clinical guidance for management of specific issues, including the recommendations for frequent and unrestricted time for breastfeeding so as to minimize hyperbilirubinemia and hypoglycemia.[4,142,143] The critical role that pediatricians play is highlighted by the recommended health supervision visit at 3 to 5 days of age, which is within 48 to 72 hours after discharge from the hospital, as well as pediatricians support of practices that avoid non–medically indicated supplementation with commercial infant formula.[144]

Pediatricians also should serve as breastfeeding advocates and educators and not solely delegate this role to staff or nonmedical/lay volunteers. Communicating with families that breastfeeding is a medical priority that is enthusiastically recommended by their personal pediatrician will build

support for mothers in the early weeks postpartum. To assist in the education of future physicians, the AAP recommends using the evidence-based Breastfeeding Residency Curriculum,[4] which has been demonstrated to improve knowledge, confidence, practice patterns, and breastfeeding rates. The pediatrician's own office-based practice should serve as a model for how to support breastfeeding in the workplace. The pediatrician should also take the lead in encouraging the hospitals with which he or she is affiliated to provide proper support and facilities for their employees who choose to continue to breastfeed.

BUSINESS CASE FOR BREASTFEEDING

A mother/baby-friendly worksite provides benefits to employers, including a reduction in company health care costs, lower employee absenteeism, reduction in employee turnover, and increased employee morale and productivity.[145,146] The return on investment has been calculated that for every $1 invested in creating and supporting a lactation support program (including a designated pump site that guarantees privacy, availability of refrigeration and a hand-washing facility, and appropriate mother break time) there is a $2 to $3 dollar return.[147] The Maternal and Child Health Bureau of the US Department of Health and Human Services, with support from the Office of Women's Health, has created a program, "The Business Case for Breastfeeding," that provides details of economic benefits to the employer and toolkits for the creation of such programs.[148] The Patient Protection and Affordable Care Act passed by Congress in March 2010 mandates that employers provide "reasonable break time" for nursing mothers and private non-bathroom areas to express

FROM THE AMERICAN ACADEMY OF PEDIATRICS

breast milk during their workday.[149] The establishment of these initiatives as the standard workplace environment will support mothers in their goal of supplying only breast milk to their infants beyond the immediate postpartum period.

CONCLUSIONS

Research and practice in the 5 years since publication of the last AAP policy statement have reinforced the conclusion that breastfeeding and the use of human milk confer unique nutritional and nonnutritional benefits to the infant and the mother and, in turn, optimize infant, child, and adult health as well as child growth and development. Recently, published evidence-based studies have confirmed and quantitated the risks of not breastfeeding. Thus, infant feeding should not be considered as a lifestyle choice but rather as a basic health issue. As such, the pediatrician's role in advocating and supporting proper breastfeeding practices is essential and vital for the achievement of this preferred public health goal.[35]

LEAD AUTHORS

Arthur I. Eidelman, MD

Richard J. Schanler, MD

SECTION ON BREASTFEEDING EXECUTIVE COMMITTEE, 2011–2012
Margreete Johnston, MD
Susan Landers, MD
Larry Noble, MD
Kinga Szucs, MD
Laura Viehmann, MD

PAST CONTRIBUTING EXECUTIVE COMMITTEE MEMBERS
Lori Feldman-Winter, MD
Ruth Lawrence, MD

STAFF
Sunnah Kim, MS
Ngozi Onyema, MPH

REFERENCES

1. Gartner LM, Morton J, Lawrence RA, et al; American Academy of Pediatrics Section on Breastfeeding. Breastfeeding and the use of human milk. *Pediatrics*. 2005;115 (2):496–506

2. Schanler RJ, Dooley S, Gartner LM, Krebs NF, Mass SB. *Breastfeeding Handbook for Physicians*. Elk Grove Village, IL: American Academy of Pediatrics; Washington, DC: American College of Obstetricians and Gynecologists; 2006

3. American Academy of Pediatrics Section on Breastfeeding. Sample Hospital Breastfeeding Policy for Newborns. Elk Grove Village, IL: American Academy of Pediatrics; 2008

4. Feldman-Winter L, Barone L, Milcarek B, et al. Residency curriculum improves breastfeeding care. *Pediatrics*. 2010;126 (2):289–297

5. American Academy of Pediatrics. *Safe and Health Beginnings: A Resource Toolkit for Hospitals and Physicians' Offices*. Elk Grove Village, IL: American Academy of Pediatrics; 2008

6. Centers for Disease Control and Prevention. Breastfeeding Among U.S. Children Born 1999–2006, CDC National Immunization Survey. Atlanta, GA: Centers for Disease Control and Prevention; 2010

7. McDowell MM, Wang C-Y, Kennedy-Stephenson J. Breastfeeding in the United States: Findings from the National Health and Nutrition Examination Surveys, 1999–2006. NCHS Data Briefs, no. 5. Hyatsville, MD: National Center for Health Statistics; 2008

8. 2007 CDC National Survey of Maternity Practices in Infant Nutrition and Care.

Atlanta, GA: Centers for Disease Control and Prevention; 2009

9. Office of Disease Prevention and Health Promotion; US Department of Health and Human Services. Healthy People 2010. Available at: www.healthypeople.gov. Accessed June 3, 2011

10. Centers for Disease Control and Prevention. Breastfeeding report card—United States, 2010. Available at: www.cdc.gov/breastfeeding/data/reportcard.htm. Accessed June 3, 2011

11. U.S. Department of Health and Human Services. Maternal, infant, and child health. Healthy People 2020; 2010. Available at: http://healthypeople.gov/2020/topicsobjectives2020/overview.aspx? topicid=26. Accessed December 12, 2011

12. Centers for Disease Control and Prevention. Racial and ethnic differences in breastfeeding initiation and duration, by state National Immunization Survey, United States, 2004–2008. *MMWR Morb Mortal Wkly Rep*. 2010;59(11):327–334

13. Ip S, Chung M, Raman G, et al; Tufts-New England Medical Center Evidence-based Practice Center. Breastfeeding and maternal and infant health outcomes in developed countries. *Evid Rep Technol Assess (Full Rep)*. 2007;153(153):1–186

14. Ip S, Chung M, Raman G, Trikalinos TA, Lau J. A summary of the Agency for Healthcare Research and Quality's evidence report on breastfeeding in developed countries. *Breastfeed Med*. 2009;4(suppl 1):S17–S30

15. Chantry CJ, Howard CR, Auinger P. Full breastfeeding duration and associated decrease in respiratory tract infection in

US children. *Pediatrics*. 2006;117(2):425–432

16. Nishimura T, Suzue J, Kaji H. Breastfeeding reduces the severity of respiratory syncytial virus infection among young infants: a multi-center prospective study. *Pediatr Int*. 2009;51(6):812–816

17. Duijts L, Jaddoe VW, Hofman A, Moll HA. Prolonged and exclusive breastfeeding reduces the risk of infectious diseases in infancy. *Pediatrics*. 2010;126(1). Available at: www.pediatrics.org/cgi/content/full/126/1/e18

18. Quigley MA, Kelly YJ, Sacker A. Breastfeeding and hospitalization for diarrheal and respiratory infection in the United Kingdom Millennium Cohort Study. *Pediatrics*. 2007;119(4). Available at: www.pediatrics.org/cgi/content/full/119/4/e837

19. Sullivan S, Schanler RJ, Kim JH, et al. An exclusively human milk-based diet is associated with a lower rate of necrotizing enterocolitis than a diet of human milk and bovine milk-based products. *J Pediatr*. 2010;156(4):562–567, e1

20. Hauck FR, Thompson JMD, Tanabe KO, Moon RY, Vennemann MM. Breastfeeding and reduced risk of sudden infant death syndrome: a meta-analysis. *Pediatrics*. 2011;128(1):1–8

21. Chen A, Rogan WJ. Breastfeeding and the risk of postneonatal death in the United States. *Pediatrics*. 2004;113(5). Available at: www.pediatrics.org/cgi/content/full/113/5/e435

22. Task Force on Sudden Infant Death Syndrome. SIDS and other sleep-related infant deaths: expansion of recommendations for

a safe infant sleeping environment. *Pediatrics.* 2011;128(5):1030–1039

23. Vennemann MM, Bajanowski T, Brinkmann B, et al; GeSID Study Group. Does breastfeeding reduce the risk of sudden infant death syndrome? *Pediatrics.* 2009;123(3). Available at: www.pediatrics.org/cgi/content/full/123/3/e406

24. Bartick M, Reinhold A. The burden of suboptimal breastfeeding in the United States: a pediatric cost analysis. *Pediatrics.* 2010; 125(5). Available at: www.pediatrics.org/cgi/content/full/125/5/e1048

25. Jones G, Steketee RW, Black RE, Bhutta ZA, Morris SS; Bellagio Child Survival Study Group. How many child deaths can we prevent this year? *Lancet.* 2003;362(9377):65–71

26. Greer FR, Sicherer SH, Burks AW; American Academy of Pediatrics Committee on Nutrition. ; American Academy of Pediatrics Section on Allergy and Immunology. Effects of early nutritional interventions on the development of atopic disease in infants and children: the role of maternal dietary restriction, breastfeeding, timing of introduction of complementary foods, and hydrolyzed formulas. *Pediatrics.* 2008; 121(1):183–191

27. Zutavern A, Brockow I, Schaaf B, et al; LISA Study Group. Timing of solid food introduction in relation to atopic dermatitis and atopic sensitization: results from a prospective birth cohort study. *Pediatrics.* 2006;117(2):401–411

28. Poole JA, Barriga K, Leung DYM, et al. Timing of initial exposure to cereal grains and the risk of wheat allergy. *Pediatrics.* 2006;117(6):2175–2182

29. Zutavern A, Brockow I, Schaaf B, et al; LISA Study Group. Timing of solid food introduction in relation to eczema, asthma, allergic rhinitis, and food and inhalant sensitization at the age of 6 years: results from the prospective birth cohort study LISA. *Pediatrics.* 2008;121(1). Available at: www.pediatrics.org/cgi/content/full/121/1/e44

30. Nwaru BI, Erkkola M, Ahonen S, et al. Age at the introduction of solid foods during the first year and allergic sensitization at age 5 years. *Pediatrics.* 2010;125(1):50–59

31. Akobeng AK, Ramanan AV, Buchan I, Heller RF. Effect of breast feeding on risk of coeliac disease: a systematic review and meta-analysis of observational studies. *Arch Dis Child.* 2006;91(1):39–43

32. Barclay AR, Russell RK, Wilson ML, Gilmour WH, Satsangi J, Wilson DC. Systematic review: the role of breastfeeding in the development of pediatric inflammatory bowel disease. *J Pediatr.* 2009;155(3):421–426

33. Penders J, Thijs C, Vink C, et al. Factors influencing the composition of the intestinal microbiota in early infancy. *Pediatrics.* 2006;118(2):511–521

34. Perrine CG, Shealy KM, Scanlon KS, et al; Centers for Disease Control and Prevention (CDC). Vital signs: hospital practices to support breastfeeding—United States, 2007 and 2009. *MMWR Morb Mortal Wkly Rep.* 2011;60(30):1020–1025

35. U.S.Department of Health and Human Services, The Surgeon General's Call to Action to Support Breastfeeding. Available at: www.surgeongeneral.gov/topics/breastfeeding/ Accessed March 28, 2011

36. Owen CG, Martin RM, Whincup PH, Smith GD, Cook DG. Effect of infant feeding on the risk of obesity across the life course: a quantitative review of published evidence. *Pediatrics.* 2005;115(5):1367–1377

37. Parikh NI, Hwang SJ, Ingelsson E, et al. Breastfeeding in infancy and adult cardiovascular disease risk factors. *Am J Med.* 2009;122(7):656–663, e1

38. Metzger MW, McDade TW. Breastfeeding as obesity prevention in the United States: a sibling difference model. *Am J Hum Biol.* 2010;22(3):291–296

39. Dewey KG, Lönnerdal B. Infant self-regulation of breast milk intake. *Acta Paediatr Scand.* 1986;75(6):893–898

40. Li R, Fein SB, Grummer-Strawn LM. Association of breastfeeding intensity and bottle-emptying behaviors at early infancy with infants' risk for excess weight at late infancy. *Pediatrics.* 2008;122(suppl 2): S77–S84

41. Li R, Fein SB, Grummer-Strawn LM. Do infants fed from bottles lack self-regulation of milk intake compared with directly breastfed infants? *Pediatrics.* 2010;125(6). Available at: www.pediatrics.org/cgi/content/full/125/6/e1386

42. Rosenbauer J, Herzig P, Giani G. Early infant feeding and risk of type 1 diabetes mellitus—a nationwide population-based case-control study in pre-school children. *Diabetes Metab Res Rev.* 2008;24(3):211–222

43. Das UN. Breastfeeding prevents type 2 diabetes mellitus: but, how and why? *Am J Clin Nutr.* 2007;85(5):1436–1437

44. Bener A, Hoffmann GF, Afify Z, Rasul K, Tewfik I. Does prolonged breastfeeding reduce the risk for childhood leukemia and lymphomas? *Minerva Pediatr.* 2008;60 (2):155–161

45. Rudant J, Orsi L, Menegaux F, et al. Childhood acute leukemia, early common infections, and allergy: The ESCALE Study. *Am J Epidemiol.* 2010;172(9):1015–1027

46. Kwan ML, Buffler PA, Abrams B, Kiley VA. Breastfeeding and the risk of childhood leukemia: a meta-analysis. *Public Health Rep.* 2004;119(6):521–535

47. Der G, Batty GD, Deary IJ. Effect of breast feeding on intelligence in children: prospective study, sibling pairs analysis, and meta-analysis. *BMJ.* 2006;333(7575):945–950

48. Kramer MS, Fombonne E, Igumnov S, et al; Promotion of Breastfeeding Intervention Trial (PROBIT) Study Group. Effects of prolonged and exclusive breastfeeding on child behavior and maternal adjustment: evidence from a large, randomized trial. *Pediatrics.* 2008;121(3). Available at: www.pediatrics.org/cgi/content/full/121/3/e435

49. Kramer MS, Aboud F, Mironova E, et al; Promotion of Breastfeeding Intervention Trial (PROBIT) Study Group. Breastfeeding and child cognitive development: new evidence from a large randomized trial. *Arch Gen Psychiatry.* 2008;65(5):578–584

50. Kramer MS, Chalmers B, Hodnett ED, et al; PROBIT Study Group (Promotion of Breastfeeding Intervention Trial). Promotion of Breastfeeding Intervention Trial (PROBIT): a randomized trial in the Republic of Belarus. *JAMA.* 2001;285(4):413–420

51. Vohr BR, Poindexter BB, Dusick AM, et al; NICHD Neonatal Research Network. Beneficial effects of breast milk in the neonatal intensive care unit on the developmental outcome of extremely low birth weight infants at 18 months of age. *Pediatrics.* 2006;118(1). Available at: www.pediatrics.org/cgi/content/full/118/1/e115

52. Vohr BR, Poindexter BB, Dusick AM, et al; National Institute of Child Health and Human Development National Research Network. Persistent beneficial effects of breast milk ingested in the neonatal intensive care unit on outcomes of extremely low birth weight infants at 30 months of age. *Pediatrics.* 2007;120(4). Available at: www.pediatrics.org/cgi/content/full/120/4/e953

53. Lucas A, Morley R, Cole TJ. Randomised trial of early diet in preterm babies and later intelligence quotient. *BMJ.* 1998;317 (7171):1481–1487

54. Isaacs EB, Fischl BR, Quinn BT, Chong WK, Gadian DG, Lucas A. Impact of breast milk on intelligence quotient, brain size, and white matter development. *Pediatr Res.* 2010;67(4):357–362

55. Furman L, Taylor G, Minich N, Hack M. The effect of maternal milk on neonatal morbidity of very low-birth-weight infants. *Arch Pediatr Adolesc Med.* 2003;157(1):66–71

FROM THE AMERICAN ACADEMY OF PEDIATRICS

56. Lucas A, Cole TJ. Breast milk and neonatal necrotising enterocolitis. *Lancet.* 1990;336 (8730):1519–1523

57. Sisk PM, Lovelady CA, Dillard RG, Gruber KJ, O'Shea TM. Early human milk feeding is associated with a lower risk of necrotizing enterocolitis in very low birth weight infants. *J Perinatol.* 2007;27(7): 428–433

58. Meinzen-Derr J, Poindexter B, Wrage L, Morrow AL, Stoll B, Donovan EF. Role of human milk in extremely low birth weight infants' risk of necrotizing enterocolitis or death. *J Perinatol.* 2009;29(1):57–62

59. Schanler RJ, Shulman RJ, Lau C. Feeding strategies for premature infants: beneficial outcomes of feeding fortified human milk versus preterm formula. *Pediatrics.* 1999;103(6 pt 1):1150–1157

60. Hintz SR, Kendrick DE, Stoll BJ, et al; NICHD Neonatal Research Network. Neurodevelopmental and growth outcomes of extremely low birth weight infants after necrotizing enterocolitis. *Pediatrics.* 2005; 115(3):696–703

61. Shah DK, Doyle LW, Anderson PJ, et al. Adverse neurodevelopment in preterm infants with postnatal sepsis or necrotizing enterocolitis is mediated by white matter abnormalities on magnetic resonance imaging at term. *J Pediatr.* 2008; 153(2):170–175, e1

62. Hylander MA, Strobino DM, Dhanireddy R. Human milk feedings and infection among very low birth weight infants. *Pediatrics.* 1998;102(3). Available at: www.pediatrics. org/cgi/content/full/102/3/e38

63. Okamoto T, Shirai M, Kokubo M, et al. Human milk reduces the risk of retinal detachment in extremely low-birthweight infants. *Pediatr Int.* 2007;49(6):894–897

64. Lucas A. Long-term programming effects of early nutrition—implications for the preterm infant. *J Perinatol.* 2005;25(suppl 2):S2–S6

65. Singhal A, Cole TJ, Lucas A. Early nutrition in preterm infants and later blood pressure: two cohorts after randomised trials. *Lancet.* 2001;357(9254):413–419

66. Quigley MA, Henderson G, Anthony MY, McGuire W. Formula milk versus donor breast milk for feeding preterm or low birth weight infants. *Cochrane Database Syst Rev.* 2007;(4):CD002971

67. Slutzah M, Codipilly CN, Potak D, Clark RM, Schanler RJ. Refrigerator storage of expressed human milk in the neonatal intensive care unit. *J Pediatr.* 2010;156(1): 26–28

68. Henderson JJ, Evans SF, Straton JA, Priest SR, Hagan R. Impact of postnatal depression on breastfeeding duration. *Birth.* 2003;30 (3):175–180

69. Strathearn L, Mamun AA, Najman JM, O'Callaghan MJ. Does breastfeeding protect against substantiated child abuse and neglect? A 15-year cohort study. *Pediatrics.* 2009;123(2):483–493

70. Krause KM, Lovelady CA, Peterson BL, Chowdhury N, Østbye T. Effect of breastfeeding on weight retention at 3 and 6 months postpartum: data from the North Carolina WIC Programme. *Public Health Nutr.* 2010;13(12):2019–2026

71. Stuebe AM, Rich-Edwards JW, Willett WC, Manson JE, Michels KB. Duration of lactation and incidence of type 2 diabetes. *JAMA.* 2005;294(20):2601–2610

72. Schwarz EB, Brown JS, Creasman JM, et al. Lactation and maternal risk of type 2 diabetes: a population-based study. *Am J Med.* 2010;123(9):863.e1–.e6

73. Karlson EW, Mandl LA, Hankinson SE, Grodstein F. Do breast-feeding and other reproductive factors influence future risk of rheumatoid arthritis? Results from the Nurses' Health Study. *Arthritis Rheum.* 2004;50(11):3458–3467

74. Schwarz EB, Ray RM, Stuebe AM, et al. Duration of lactation and risk factors for maternal cardiovascular disease. *Obstet Gynecol.* 2009;113(5):974–982

75. Stuebe AM, Willett WC, Xue F, Michels KB. Lactation and incidence of premenopausal breast cancer: a longitudinal study. *Arch Intern Med.* 2009;169(15): 1364–1371

76. Collaborative Group on Hormonal Factors in Breast Cancer. Breast cancer and breastfeeding: collaborative reanalysis of individual data from 47 epidemiological studies in 30 countries, including 50302 women with breast cancer and 96973 women without the disease. *Lancet.* 2002; 360(9328):187–195

77. Lipworth L, Bailey LR, Trichopoulos D. History of breast-feeding in relation to breast cancer risk: a review of the epidemiologic literature. *J Natl Cancer Inst.* 2000;92(4):302–312

78. World Health Organization. The optimal duration of exclusive breastfeeding: report of an expert consultation. Available at: hwww.who.int/nutrition/publications/ optimal_duration_of_exc_bfeeding_report_ eng.pdf. Accessed December 12, 2011

79. Institute of Medicine. Early childhood obesity prevention policies. June 23, 2011. Available at: www.iom.edu/obesityyoungchildren. Accessed December 12, 2011

80. Kramer MS, Kakuma R. Optimal duration of exclusive breastfeeding [review]. *The*

Cochrane Library. January 21, 2009. Available at: http://onlinelibrary.wiley. com/doi/10.1002/14651858.CD003517/full. Accessed December 12, 2011

81. Peterson AE, Perez-Escamilla R, Labbok MH, Hight V, von Hertzen H, Van Look P. Multicenter study of the lactational amenorrhea method (LAM) III: effectiveness, duration, and satisfaction with reduced client-provider contact. *Contraception.* 2000;62 (5):221–230

82. Agostoni C, Decsi T, Fewtrell M, et al; ESPGHAN Committee on Nutrition. Complementary feeding: a commentary by the ESPGHAN Committee on Nutrition. *J Pediatr Gastroenterol Nutr.* 2008;46(1):99–110

83. Cattaneo A, Williams C, Pallás-Alonso CR, et al. ESPGHAN's 2008 recommendation for early introduction of complementary foods: how good is the evidence? *Matern Child Nutr.* 2011;7(4):335–343

84. Gonçalves DU, Proietti FA, Ribas JG, et al. Epidemiology, treatment, and prevention of human T-cell leukemia virus type 1-associated diseases. *Clin Microbiol Rev.* 2010;23(3):577–589

85. Arroyo Carrera I, López Rodríguez MJ, Sapiña AM, López Lafuente A, Sacristán AR. Probable transmission of brucellosis by breast milk. *J Trop Pediatr.* 2006;52(5): 380–381

86. American Academy of Pediatrics. Tuberculosis. In: Pickering LK, Baker CJ, Kimberlin DW, Long SS, eds. Red Book: 2009 Report of the Committee on Infectious Diseases. 28th ed. Elk Grove Village, IL: American Academy of Pediatrics; 2009: 680–701

87. American Academy of Pediatrics. Varicella-zoster infections. In: Pickering LK, Baker CJ, Kimberlin DW, Long SS, eds. Red Book: 2009 Report of the Committee on Infectious Diseases. 28th ed. Elk Grove Village, IL: American Academy of Pediatrics; 2009:714-727

88. Centers for Disease Control and Prevention. 2009 H1N1 Flu (Swine Flu) and Feeding your Baby: What Parents Should Know. Available at: http://www.cdc.gov/h1n1flu/ infantfeeding.htm?s_cid=h1n1Flu_outbreak_ 155. Accessed January 22, 2010

89. Horvath T, Madi BC, Iuppa IM, Kennedy GE, Rutherford G, Read JS. Interventions for preventing late postnatal mother-to-child transmission of HIV. *Cochrane Database Syst Rev.* 2009;21(1):CD006734

90. Chasela CS, Hudgens MG, Jamieson DJ, et al; BAN Study Group. Maternal or infant antiretroviral drugs to reduce HIV-1 transmission. *N Engl J Med.* 2010;362(24): 2271–2281

91. Shapiro RL, Hughes MD, Ogwu A, et al. Antiretroviral regimens in pregnancy and breast-feeding in Botswana. *N Engl J Med.* 2010;362(24):2282–2294

92. Hamele M, Flanagan R, Loomis CA, Stevens T, Fairchok MP. Severe morbidity and mortality with breast milk associated cytomegalovirus infection. *Pediatr Infect Dis J.* 2010; 29(1):84–86

93. Kurath S, Halwachs-Baumann G, Müller W, Resch B. Transmission of cytomegalovirus via breast milk to the prematurely born infant: a systematic review. *Clin Microbiol Infect.* 2010;16(8):1172–1178

94. Maschmann J, Hamprecht K, Weissbrich B, Dietz K, Jahn G, Speer CP. Freeze-thawing of breast milk does not prevent cytomegalovirus transmission to a preterm infant. *Arch Dis Child Fetal Neonatal Ed.* 2006;91 (4):F288–F290

95. Hamprecht K, Maschmann J, Müller D, et al. Cytomegalovirus (CMV) inactivation in breast milk: reassessment of pasteurization and freeze-thawing. *Pediatr Res.* 2004;56(4):529–535

96. Jansson LM; Academy of Breastfeeding Medicine Protocol Committee. ABM clinical protocol #21: Guidelines for breastfeeding and the drug-dependent woman. *Breastfeed Med.* 2009;4(4):225–228

97. Garry A, Rigourd V, Amirouche A, Fauroux V, Aubry S, Serreau R. Cannabis and breastfeeding. *J Toxicol.* 2009;2009:596149

98. Little RE, Anderson KW, Ervin CH, Worthington-Roberts B, Clarren SK. Maternal alcohol use during breast-feeding and infant mental and motor development at one year. *N Engl J Med.* 1989;321(7):425–430

99. Mennella JA, Pepino MY. Breastfeeding and prolactin levels in lactating women with a family history of alcoholism. *Pediatrics.* 2010;125(5). Available at: www.pediatrics. org/cgi/content/full/125/5/e1162

100. Subcommittee on Nutrition During Lactation, Institute of Medicine, National Academy of Sciences. *Nutrition During Lactation.* Washington, DC: National Academies Press; 1991:113–152

101. Koren G. Drinking alcohol while breastfeeding. Will it harm my baby? *Can Fam Physician.* 2002;48:39–41

102. Guedes HT, Souza LS. Exposure to maternal smoking in the first year of life interferes in breast-feeding protective effect against the onset of respiratory allergy from birth to 5 yr. *Pediatr Allergy Immunol.* 2009;20(1):30–34

103. Liebrechts-Akkerman G, Lao O, Liu F, et al. Postnatal parental smoking: an important risk factor for SIDS. *Eur J Pediatr.* 2011; 170(10):1281–1291

104. Yilmaz G, Hizli S, Karacan C, Yurdakök K, Coskun T, Dilmen U. Effect of passive smoking on growth and infection rates of breast-fed and non-breast-fed infants. *Pediatr Int.* 2009;51(3):352–358

105. Vio F, Salazar G, Infante C. Smoking during pregnancy and lactation and its effects on breast-milk volume. *Am J Clin Nutr.* 1991; 54(6):1011–1016

106. Hopkinson JM, Schanler RJ, Fraley JK, Garza C. Milk production by mothers of premature infants: influence of cigarette smoking. *Pediatrics.* 1992;90(6):934–938

107. Butte NF. Maternal nutrition during lactation. *Pediatric Up-to-Date.* 2010. Available at: http://www.uptodate.com/contents/maternal-nutrition-during-lactation?source=search_result&search=maternal+nutrition&selectedTitle=2%7E150. Accessed October 29, 2010

108. Zeisel SH. Is maternal diet supplementation beneficial? Optimal development of infant depends on mother's diet. *Am J Clin Nutr.* 2009;89(2):685S–687S

109. Picciano MF, McGuire MK. Use of dietary supplements by pregnant and lactating women in North America. *Am J Clin Nutr.* 2009;89(2):663S–667S

110. Whitelaw A. Historical perspectives: perinatal profiles: Robert McCance and Elsie Widdowson: pioneers in neonatal science. *NeoReviews.* 2007;8(11):e455–e458

111. Simopoulos AP, Leaf A, Salem N Jr. Workshop on the essentiality of and recommended dietary intakes for omega-6 and omega-3 fatty acids. *J Am Coll Nutr.* 1999; 18(5):487–489

112. Carlson SE. Docosahexaenoic acid supplementation in pregnancy and lactation. *Am J Clin Nutr.* 2009;89(2):678S–684S

113. Koletzko B, Cetin I, Brenna JT; Perinatal Lipid Intake Working Group; ; Child Health Foundation; ; Diabetic Pregnancy Study Group; ; European Association of Perinatal Medicine; ; European Society for Clinical Nutrition and Metabolism; ; European Society for Paediatric Gastroenterology, Hepatology and Nutrition, Committee on Nutrition; ; International Federation of Placenta Associations; ; International Society for the Study of Fatty Acids and Lipids. Dietary fat intakes for pregnant and lactating women. *Br J Nutr.* 2007;98(5):873–877

114. Drugs and Lactation Database. 2010. Available at: http://toxnet.nlm.nih.gov/cgi-bin/sis/htmlgen?LACT. Accessed September 17, 2009

115. Committee on Drugs, American Academy of Pediatrics. The transfer of drugs and other chemicals into human milk. *Pediatrics.* 2011. In press

116. Fortinguerra F, Clavenna A, Bonati M. Psychotropic drug use during breastfeeding: a review of the evidence. *Pediatrics.* 2009;124(4). Available at: www.pediatrics.org/cgi/content/full/124/4/e547

117. US Nuclear Regulatory Commission. Control of access to high and very high radiation areas in nuclear power plants. USNRC Regulatory Guide 8.38. June 1993. Available at: www.nrc.gov/reading-rm/doc-collections/reg-guides/occupational-health/rg/8-38/08-038.pdf.

118. International Commission on Radiological Protection. Doses to infants from ingestion of radionuclides in mother's milk. ICRP Publication 95. *Ann ICRP.* 2004;34(3–4):1-27

119. Stabin MG, Breitz HB. Breast milk excretion of radiopharmaceuticals: mechanisms, findings, and radiation dosimetry. *J Nucl Med.* 2000;41(5):863–873

120. Kaplan M, Hammerman C. Severe neonatal hyperbilirubinemia. A potential complication of glucose-6-phosphate dehydrogenase deficiency. *Clin Perinatol.* 1998;25(3):575–590, viii

121. World Health Organization. *Evidence for the Ten Steps to Successful Breastfeeding.* Geneva, Switzerland: World Health Organization; 1998

122. World Health Organization; United Nations Children's Fund. *Protecting, Promoting, and Supporting Breastfeeding: The Special Role of Maternity Services.* Geneva, Switzerland: World Health Organization; 1989

123. Philipp BL, Merewood A, Miller LW, et al. Baby-friendly hospital initiative improves breastfeeding initiation rates in a US hospital setting. *Pediatrics.* 2001;108(3):677–681

124. Murray EK, Ricketts S, Dellaport J. Hospital practices that increase breastfeeding duration: results from a population-based study. *Birth.* 2007;34(3):202–211

125. Centers for Disease Control and Prevention. Breastfeeding-related maternity practices at hospitals and birth centers—United States, 2007. *MMWR Morb Mortal Wkly Rep.* 2008;57(23):621–625

126. Dewey KG, Nommsen-Rivers LA, Heinig MJ, Cohen RJ. Risk factors for suboptimal infant breastfeeding behavior, delayed onset of lactation, and excess neonatal weight loss. *Pediatrics.* 2003;112(3 pt 1):607–619

127. The Joint Commission. Specifications Manual for Joint Commission National Quality Core Measures. Available at: http://manual.jointcommission.org/releases/TJC2011A/. Accessed January 12, 2011

128. O'Connor NR, Tanabe KO, Siadaty MS, Hauck FR. Pacifiers and breastfeeding:

Appendix B: American Academy of Pediatrics Policy Statement: Breastfeeding and the Use of Human Milk

a systematic review. *Arch Pediatr Adolesc Med.* 2009;163(4):378–382

129. Hauck FR, Omojokun OO, Siadaty MS. Do pacifiers reduce the risk of sudden infant death syndrome? A meta-analysis. *Pediatrics.* 2005;116(5). Available at: www.pediatrics. org/cgi/content/full/116/5/e716

130. American Academy of Pediatrics Task Force on Sudden Infant Death Syndrome. The changing concept of sudden infant death syndrome: diagnostic coding shifts, controversies regarding the sleeping environment, and new variables to consider in reducing risk. *Pediatrics.* 2005;116(5): 1245–1255

131. Li DK, Willinger M, Petitti DB, Odouli R, Liu L, Hoffman HJ. Use of a dummy (pacifier) during sleep and risk of sudden infant death syndrome (SIDS): population based case-control study. *BMJ.* 2006;332(7532):18–22

132. American Academy of Pediatrics Committee on Fetus and Newborn. Controversies concerning vitamin K and the newborn. *Pediatrics.* 2003;112(1 pt 1):191–192

133. Wagner CL, Greer FR; American Academy of Pediatrics Section on Breastfeeding; ; American Academy of Pediatrics Committee on Nutrition. Prevention of rickets and vitamin D deficiency in infants, children, and adolescents. *Pediatrics.* 2008;122(5): 1142–1152

134. American Academy of Pediatric Dentistry. Guidelines for Fluoride Therapy, Revised 2000. Available at: http://www.aapd.org/pdf/ fluoridetherapy.pdf. Accessed September 17, 2009

135. Garza C, de Onis M. Rationale for developing a new international growth reference. *Food Nutr Bull.* 2004;25(suppl 1):S5–S14

136. de Onis M, Garza C, Onyango AW, Borghi E. Comparison of the WHO child growth standards and the CDC 2000 growth charts. *J Nutr.* 2007;137(1):144–148

137. Grummer-Strawn LM, Reinold C, Krebs NF; Centers for Disease Control and Prevention. Use of World Health Organization and CDC growth charts for children aged 0–59 months in the United States. *MMWR Recomm Rep.* 2010;59(RR-9):1–15

138. Grummer-Strawn LM, Reinold C, Krebs NFCenters for Disease Control and Prevention. Use of World Health Organization and CDC growth charts for children aged 0-59 months in the United States. *MMWR Recomm Rep.* 2010;59(RR-9):1–15

139. Schanler RJ. The pediatrician supports breastfeeding. *Breastfeed Med.* 2010;5(5): 235–236

140. Feldman-Winter LB, Schanler RJ, O'Connor KG, Lawrence RA. Pediatricians and the promotion and support of breastfeeding. *Arch Pediatr Adolesc Med.* 2008;162(12):1142–1149

141. American Academy of Pediatrics. American Academy of Pediatrics Breastfeeding Initiatives. 2010. Available at: http://www. aap.org/breastfeeding. Accessed September 17, 2009

142. Academy of Breastfeeding Medicine Protocol Committee. Clinical Protocols. Available at http://www.bfmed.org/Resources/ Protocols.aspx. Accessed January 22, 2010

143. American Academy of Pediatrics Subcommittee on Hyperbilirubinemia. Management of hyperbilirubinemia in the newborn

infant 35 or more weeks of gestation. *Pediatrics.* 2004;114(1):297–316

144. American Academy of Pediatrics, Committee on Practice and Ambulatory Medicine and Bright Futures Steering Committee. Recommendations for preventive pediatric health care. *Pediatrics.* 2007;120(6):1376

145. Cohen R, Mrtek MB, Mrtek RG. Comparison of maternal absenteeism and infant illness rates among breast-feeding and formula-feeding women in two corporations. *Am J Health Promot.* 1995;10(2):148–153

146. Ortiz J, McGilligan K, Kelly P. Duration of breast milk expression among working mothers enrolled in an employer-sponsored lactation program. *Pediatr Nurs.* 2004;30(2): 111–119

147. Tuttle CR, Slavit WI. Establishing the business case for breastfeeding. *Breastfeed Med.* 2009;4(suppl 1):S59–S62

148. US Department of Health and Human Services Office on Women's Health. Business case for breast feeding. 2010. Available at: www.womenshealth.gov/breastfeeding/ government-in-action/business-case-for-breastfeeding. Accessed September 24, 2010

149. Patient Protection and Affordable Care Act 2010, Public Law 111-148. Title IV, §4207, USC HR 3590, (2010)

150. Hurst NM, Myatt A, Schanler RJ. Growth and development of a hospital-based lactation program and mother's own milk bank. *J Obstet Gynecol Neonatal Nurs.* 1998;27(5):503–510

151. Schanler RJ, Fraley JK, Lau C, Hurst NM, Horvath L, Rossmann SN. Breastmilk cultures and infection in extremely premature infants. *J Perinatol.* 2011;31(5):335–338

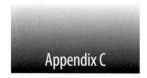

Appendix C

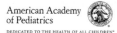

American Academy
of Pediatrics

DEDICATED TO THE HEALTH OF ALL CHILDREN®

CLINICAL REPORT

The Transfer of Drugs and Therapeutics Into Human Breast Milk: An Update on Selected Topics

Hari Cheryl Sachs, MD, FAAP* and COMMITTEE ON DRUGS

KEY WORD
human milk

ABBREVIATIONS
AAP—American Academy of Pediatrics
FDA—Food and Drug Administration
HBV—hepatitis B vaccine
HPV—human papillomavirus vaccine
NSAID—nonsteroidal antiinflammatory drug

This document is copyrighted and is property of the American Academy of Pediatrics and its Board of Directors. All authors have filed conflict of interest statements with the American Academy of Pediatrics. Any conflicts have been resolved through a process approved by the Board of Directors. The American Academy of Pediatrics has neither solicited nor accepted any commercial involvement in the development of the content of this publication.

The guidance in this report does not indicate an exclusive course of treatment or serve as a standard of medical care. Variations, taking into account individual circumstances, may be appropriate.

*The recommendations in this review are those of the authors and do not represent the views of the US Food and Drug Administration.

abstract

Many mothers are inappropriately advised to discontinue breastfeeding or avoid taking essential medications because of fears of adverse effects on their infants. This cautious approach may be unnecessary in many cases, because only a small proportion of medications are contraindicated in breastfeeding mothers or associated with adverse effects on their infants. Information to inform physicians about the extent of excretion of a particular drug into human milk is needed but may not be available. Previous statements on this topic from the American Academy of Pediatrics provided physicians with data concerning the known excretion of specific medications into human milk. More current and comprehensive information is now available on the Internet, as well as an application for mobile devices, at LactMed (http://toxnet.nlm.nih.gov). Therefore, with the exception of radioactive compounds requiring temporary cessation of breastfeeding, the reader will be referred to LactMed to obtain the most current data on an individual medication. This report discusses several topics of interest surrounding lactation, such as the use of psychotropic therapies, drugs to treat substance abuse, narcotics, galactogogues, and herbal products, as well as immunization of breastfeeding women. A discussion regarding the global implications of maternal medications and lactation in the developing world is beyond the scope of this report. The World Health Organization offers several programs and resources that address the importance of breastfeeding (see http://www.who.int/topics/breastfeeding/en/). *Pediatrics* 2013;132:1–14

INTRODUCTION

Lactating women can be exposed to medications or other therapeutics, either on a limited or long-term basis, depending on the need to treat acute or chronic conditions. Many women are advised to discontinue nursing or avoid taking necessary medications because of concerns about possible adverse effects in their infants.[1] Such advice is often not based on evidence, because information about the extent of drug excretion into human milk may be unavailable, and for many drugs, information is limited to data from animal studies, which may not correlate with human experience. In addition, not all drugs are excreted in clinically significant amounts into human milk, and the presence of a drug in human milk may not pose a risk for the infant. To weigh the risks and benefits of breastfeeding, physicians need to consider multiple factors. These factors include the need for the drug by the mother, the potential effects of

www.pediatrics.org/cgi/doi/10.1542/peds.2013-1985

doi:10.1542/peds.2013-1985

All clinical reports from the American Academy of Pediatrics automatically expire 5 years after publication unless reaffirmed, revised, or retired at or before that time.

PEDIATRICS (ISSN Numbers: Print, 0031-4005; Online, 1098-4275).

Copyright © 2013 by the American Academy of Pediatrics

the drug on milk production, the amount of the drug excreted into human milk, the extent of oral absorption by the breastfeeding infant, and potential adverse effects on the breastfeeding infant. The age of the infant is also an important factor in the decision-making process, because adverse events associated with drug exposure via lactation occur most often in neonates younger than 2 months and rarely in infants older than 6 months.[2] In the near future, pharmacogenetics may also provide important guidance for individualized decisions.

In large part because of efforts by Cheston Berlin, Jr, MD, a statement by the American Academy of Pediatrics (AAP) on the transfer of drugs and chemicals into human milk was first published in 1983[3] and underwent several subsequent revisions,[4,5] the most recent of which was published in 2001.[6] Previous editions were intended to list drugs potentially used during lactation and to describe possible effects on the infant and/or on lactation. Revisions for the statement can no longer keep pace with the rapidly changing information available via the Internet, published studies, and new drug approvals. A more comprehensive and current database is available at LactMed (http://toxnet. nlm.nih.gov). LactMed includes up-to-date information on drug levels in human milk and infant serum, possible adverse effects on breastfeeding infants, potential effects on lactation, and recommendations for possible alternative drugs to consider. Common herbal products are also included. For this reason, with the exception of radioactive compounds that require temporary or permanent cessation of breastfeeding, the reader will be referred to LactMed to obtain the most current data on an individual medication.

This statement reviews proposed changes in US Food and Drug Administration (FDA) labeling that are designed to provide useful information to the physician and to outline general

---

LactMed is part of the National Library of Medicine's Toxicology Data Network (TOXNET)

Each record includes the following information:

- Generic name: refers to US-adopted name of active portion of the drug
- Scientific name: genus and species of botanical products (when applicable)
- Summary of use during lactation (includes discussion of conflicting recommendations and citations)
- Drug levels
  - Maternal levels: based on studies that measure concentration in breast milk; includes relative infant dose (weight-adjusted percentage of maternal dose) when possible
  - Infant levels: serum or urine concentrations from the literature
- Effects in breastfed infants: adverse events with Naranjo* assessment of causality (definite, probably, possibly, unlikely)
- Possible effects on lactation: if known, including effects on infants that may interfere with nursing (eg, sedation)
- Alternative drugs to consider: may not be comprehensive
- References
- Chemical Abstracts Service Registry Number
- Drug class
- LactMed record number
- Last revision date

Primary Author: Philip O. Anderson, PharmD

Contributor: Jason Sauberan, PharmD

Peer Review Panel:

Cheston M. Berlin, Jr, MD
Shinya Ito, MD
Kathleen Uhl, MD
Sonia Neubauer, MD

* The Naranjo probability scale is a method used to estimate the probability that an adverse event is caused by a drug.[7]

Appendix C: American Academy of Pediatrics:
The Transfer of Drugs and Therapeutics Into Human Breast Milk

considerations for individual risk/benefit counseling. An update regarding the use of antidepressants, anxiolytics, and antipsychotics in the lactating woman is also provided, because the use of psychotropic agents during lactation is still debated. Since publication of the last statement, numerous questions have been raised regarding the use of methadone in the lactating woman. For this reason, therapies for substance abuse and smoking cessation are discussed. Given the finding that codeine use may be associated with toxicity in patients, including neonates with ultrarapid metabolism, a brief review of alternative agents to treat pain in the lactating woman is provided. The use of galactagogues is also reviewed because more women now endeavor to breastfeed adopted infants or preterm neonates. The increasing use of herbal products has invited a discussion of the merits of these alternative therapies in the nursing woman. Finally, immunization of breastfeeding women and their infants will be reviewed to assist pediatricians in encouraging immunization when needed in lactating women and addressing parental reluctance to immunize breastfed infants.

GENERAL CONSIDERATIONS

Several factors should be considered when advising a woman regarding a decision to breastfeed her infant while she is on drug therapy. The benefits of breastfeeding for both the infant and mother need to be weighed against the risks of drug exposure to the infant (or to the mother, in the case of agents intended to induce lactation). Many factors affect the individual risk/benefit decision, including specific information about chemical and pharmacologic properties of the drug, which may be available from resources such as LactMed and in product labeling. In

general, chemical properties of a drug, such as lack of ionization, small molecular weight, low volume of distribution, low maternal serum protein binding, and high lipid solubility, facilitate drug excretion into human milk. Drugs with long half-lives are more likely to accumulate in human milk, and drugs with high oral bioavailability are more easily absorbed by the infant.[8] The adverse event profile of the drug is another property that affects the individual risk/benefit ratio. Use of a drug with a significant adverse effect in a lactating woman (such as an arrhythmia) may be acceptable to treat a serious illness in the mother; however, use of the same drug to increase milk production would not be acceptable. For drugs with an adverse event profile that correlates with increasing dosage, higher maternal doses may be associated with greater neonatal toxicity. In addition, the timing of exposure and the duration of therapy are other important considerations. A decision to breastfeed when continuing treatment with an agent for which in utero exposure also has occurred differs from a decision to initiate a novel therapy in the early postpartum period. Similarly, the risks of a single-dose therapy or short-term treatment may differ from those of a chronic therapy.

In addition to pharmacokinetic or chemical properties of the drug, the infant's expected drug exposure is influenced by infant and maternal factors beyond basic known pharmacokinetic and chemical properties of the drug itself. For example, the risk of adverse reactions in a preterm infant or an infant with underlying chronic medical conditions may be higher than that for a more mature or healthier infant. Certain drugs may accumulate in the breastfed infant because of reduced clearance or immaturity of metabolic pathways. However, for other

drugs (eg, acetaminophen), the immaturity of these same pathways may protect an infant from toxic drug metabolites. Similarly, patients with specific genotypes may experience drug toxicity, as evidenced by fatalities observed in individuals who demonstrate ultrarapid metabolism of codeine.[9] Finally, certain infant conditions, such as metabolic diseases, and maternal health conditions may preclude nursing (eg, HIV) or require multiple therapies that are particularly toxic (eg, cancer treatment).

CHANGES IN DRUG LABELING

In the past, the lactation section in FDA-approved labeling was often limited to statements that advise caution or contain an admonition to discontinue breastfeeding or discontinue therapy, depending on the importance to the mother. In 2008, the FDA published a proposed revision to the regulations, which affects the pregnancy and lactation sections of labeling. The agency is currently working on the final rule, which is intended to provide a clinically oriented framework for placement of pregnancy and lactation information into drug labeling and to permit the patient and physician to explore the risk/benefit on the basis of the best available data. Under the proposed rule, the current Nursing Mothers section is replaced by a section called Lactation. The Lactation section of labeling will contain 3 subsections: Risk Summary, Clinical Considerations, and Data. The Risk Summary section will include a summary of what is known about the excretion of the drug into human milk and potential effects on the breastfed infant, as well as maternal milk production. The Clinical Considerations section will include methods to minimize exposure of the breastfed infant to the drug when applicable, as well as information about monitoring for expected adverse drug effects on the infant. The Data component will provide a detailed overview of the existing data that forms the evidence base for the other 2 sections.

In addition to the proposed rule, the FDA published "Guidance for Industry: Clinical Lactation Studies: Study Design, Data Analysis, and Recommendations for Labeling."[10] Along with outlining recommendations regarding lactation study design as well as the timing and indications for these studies, this draft guidance includes advice on parameters (several of which are used in LactMed) that can be used to inform physicians about the extent of drug exposure. Using these parameters, drug exposure to the infant may be measured directly in infant serum or estimated on the basis of pharmacokinetic parameters. These estimates of infant exposure (for example, relative infant dose) can be expressed as a percent of weight-adjusted maternal or, when known, weight-adjusted pediatric dose.

ESTIMATES OF DRUG EXPOSURE

Daily Infant Dosage (mg/day) =

$\sum$(drug concentration in each milk collection × expreesed volume in each milk collection)

OR

C_{milk}[average drug concentration in milk(mg/mL)] × V_{milk}(volume in mL of milk ingested in 24 hours)

Note: V_{milk} is typically estimated to be 150 mL/kg/day

Relative Infant Dose

% Maternal Dose= [Daily Infant Dosage (mg/kg/day) ÷ Maternal Dose (mg/kg/day)] × 100

% Infant or Pediatric Dose= [Daily Infant Dosage (mg/kg/day) ÷ Infant or Pediatric dose(mg/kg/day)] × 100

ANTIDEPRESSANTS, ANXIOLYTICS, AND ANTIPSYCHOTICS

Previous statements from the AAP categorized the effect of psychoactive drugs on the nursing infant as "unknown but may be of concern." Although new data have been published since 2001, information on the long-term effects of these compounds is still limited. Most publications regarding psychoactive drugs describe the pharmacokinetics in small numbers of lactating women with short-term observational studies of their infants. In addition, interpretation of the effects on the infant from the small number of longer-term studies is confounded by prenatal treatment or exposure to multiple therapies. For these reasons, the long-term effect on the developing infant is still largely unknown.[11,12]

Many antianxiety drugs, antidepressants, and mood stabilizers appear in low concentrations in human milk, with estimated relative infant doses less than 2% of weight-adjusted maternal dose and/or milk-plasma ratios less than 1.[13] However, the percentage of maternal doses that approach clinically significant levels (10% or more) have been reported for bupropion,[14] diazepam,[13] fluoxetine,[15] citalopram,[16] lithium,[17] lamotrigine,[18] and venlafaxine.[19] Data on drug excretion in human milk are not available for up to one-third of psychoactive therapies.[13]

Because of the long half-life of some of these compounds and/or their metabolites, coupled with an infant's immature hepatic and renal function, nursing infants may have measurable amounts of the drug or its metabolites in plasma and potentially in neural tissue. Infant plasma concentrations that exceed 10% of therapeutic maternal plasma concentrations have been reported for a number of selective serotonin reuptake inhibitors,

TABLE 1 Psychoactive Drugs With Infant Serum Concentrations Exceeding 10% of Maternal Plasma Concentrations[a]

Agent	Reference
Citalopram	Weissman 2004[20]
Clomipramine	Schimmell 1991[21]
Diazepam	Wesson 1985[22]
Doxepin	Moretti 2009[16]
Fluoxetine	Weissman 2004,[20] product labeling
Fluvoxamine	Weissman 2004[20]
Lamotrigine	Newport 2008,[18] Fotopoulou 2009[23]
Lithium	Viguerra 2007,[24] Grandjean 2009,[25] Bogen 2012[26]
Mirtazapine	Tonn 2009[27]
Nortriptyline	Weissman 2004[20]
Olanzapine	Whitworth 2008[28]
Sertraline	Hendrick 2001,[29] Stowe 2003[30]
Venlafaxine	Newport 2009[19]

[a] Based on individual maternal-infant pair(s); may include active metabolites.

antipsychotics, anxiolytics, and mood stabilizers (see Table 1).

Mothers who desire to breastfeed their infant(s) while taking these agents should be counseled about the benefits of breastfeeding as well as the potential risk that the infant may be exposed to clinically significant levels and that the long-term effects of this exposure are unknown. Consideration should be given to monitoring growth and neurodevelopment of the infant.

DRUGS FOR SMOKING CESSATION OR TO TREAT SUBSTANCE ABUSE/ ALCOHOL DEPENDENCE

Although many women are appropriately advised to refrain from smoking, drinking, and using recreational drugs during and after pregnancy, in part because of adverse effects on their infants (see Table 2), some are unable to do so and may seek assistance after delivery. Maternal smoking is not an absolute contraindication to breastfeeding.[31] Nonetheless, for multiple reasons, including the association of sudden infant death syndrome with

FROM THE AMERICAN ACADEMY OF PEDIATRICS

TABLE 2 Drugs of Abuse for Which Adverse Effects on the Breastfeeding Infant Have Been Reported[a]

Drug	Reported Effect or Reason for Concern	Reference
Alcohol	Impaired motor development or postnatal growth, decreased milk consumption, sleep disturbances.	Koren 2002,[34] Backstrand 2004,[35] Mennella 2007[36]
	Note: Although binge drinking should be avoided, occasional, limited ingestion (0.5 g of alcohol/kg/d; equivalent to 8 oz wine or 2 cans of beer per day) may be acceptable.	National Academy of Sciences 1991[37]
Amphetamines	Hypertension, tachycardia, and seizures.	Product labeling
	In animal studies of postnatal exposure, long-term behavioral effects, including learning and memory deficits and altered locomotor activity, were observed.	
Benzodiazepines	Accumulation of metabolite, prolonged half-life in neonate or preterm infant is noted; chronic use not recommended.	Jain 2005,[38] Malone 2004[39]
	Apnea, cyanosis, withdrawal, sedation, cyanosis, and seizures.	
Cocaine	Intoxication, seizures, irritability, vomiting, diarrhea, tremulousness.	Chasnoff 1987,[40] Winecker 2001[41]
Heroin	Withdrawal symptoms, tremors, restlessness, vomiting, poor feeding.	vandeVelde 2007[42]
LSD	Potent hallucinogen.	
Methamphetamine	Fatality, persists in breast milk for 48 h.	Ariagno 1995,[43] Bartu 2009[44]
Methylene dioxy-methamphetamine (ecstasy)	Closely related products (amphetamines) are concentrated in human milk.	
Marijuana (cannabis)	Neurodevelopmental effects, delayed motor development at 1 y, lethargy, less frequent and shorter feedings, high milk-plasma ratios in heavy users.	Djulus 2005,[45] Campolongo 2009,[46] Garry 2010[47]
Phencyclidine	Potent hallucinogen, infant intoxication.	AAP 2001,[6] Academy of Breastfeeding Medicine[48]

[a] Effect on maternal judgment or mood may affect ability to care for infant.

tobacco exposure,[32,33] lactating women should be strongly encouraged to stop smoking and to minimize secondhand exposure. Exposure to alcohol or recreational drugs may impair a mother's judgment and interfere with her care of the infant and can cause toxicity to the breastfeeding infant (see Table 2).

Limited information is available regarding the use of medications in lactating women to treat substance abuse or alcohol dependence or smoking cessation. However, the presence of behaviors, such as continued ingestion of illicit drugs or alcohol, and underlying conditions, such as HIV infection, are not compatible with breastfeeding.[49,50] Patients also require ongoing psychosocial support to maintain abstinence.[48]

Methadone, buprenorphine, and naltrexone are 3 agents approved by the FDA for use in the treatment of opioid dependence. Continued breastfeeding by women undergoing such treatment presumes that the patient remains abstinent, is HIV negative, and is en-

rolled in and closely monitored by an appropriate drug treatment program with significant social support.[48,51]

Potential adverse effects on breast-feeding infants from methadone (according to product labeling) and buprenorphine include lethargy, respiratory difficulty, and poor weight gain.[52] The long-term effects of methadone in humans are unknown. Nonetheless, methadone levels in human milk are low, with calculated infant exposures less than 3% of the maternal weight-adjusted dose.[53,54] Plasma concentrations in infants are also low (less than 3% of maternal trough concentrations) during the neonatal period and up to 6 months postpartum.[55,56] For these reasons, guidelines from the Academy of Breastfeeding Medicine encourage breastfeeding for women treated with methadone who are enrolled in methadone-maintenance programs.[48]

Buprenorphine is excreted into human milk and achieves a level similar to that in maternal plasma.[57] Infant exposure

appears to be up to 2.4% of the maternal weight-adjusted dose.[55,56,58] However, buprenorphine can be abused, and although the significance in humans is unknown, labeling for buprenorphine and buprenorphine/naloxone combinations states that use is not advised by lactating women, because animal lactation studies have shown decreased milk production and viability of the offspring. FDA labeling also advises caution for use of naltrexone in nursing infants of opioid-dependent women. Of note, published information on naltrexone is limited to 1 case report that estimates infant exposure to be low (7 μg/kg/d, or 0.86% of the maternal weight-adjusted dose).[59]

Transferred amounts of methadone or buprenorphine are insufficient to prevent symptoms of neonatal abstinence syndrome.[49,60] Neonatal abstinence syndrome can occur after abrupt discontinuation of methadone.[51,61] Thus, breastfeeding should not be stopped abruptly, and gradual weaning is advised if a decision is made to discontinue breastfeeding.

Limited information is available for disulfiram and naltrexone, agents that are used to treat alcohol dependence. As noted previously, a low relative infant dose (<1%) was observed in a single case report of naltrexone exposure in a 6-week-old breastfed infant.[59] FDA labeling discourages use of disulfiram and both the injectable and oral form of naltrexone in lactating women.

Only one-third of women successfully discontinue smoking without pharmacologic aids.[62] Nicotine replacement therapy, bupropion, and varenicline are agents indicated for use as aids to smoking cessation treatment. Nicotine replacement therapy is compatible with breastfeeding as long as the dose (assuming a cigarette delivers ~1 mg of nicotine) is less than the number of cigarettes typically smoked, because nicotine passes freely into human milk and is orally absorbed as nicotine. Cotinine concentrations are lower than those related to tobacco use. Short-acting products (eg, gum or lozenges) are recommended.[62] Infant exposure decreases proportionally with maternal patch doses.[63]

In contrast, bupropion is excreted into human milk with exposures that may exceed 10% (range, 1.4%–10.6%) of the maternal dose.[14] Although infant levels were not measured, there is a case report of a seizure in a 6-month-old breastfed infant potentially related to bupropion.[64] Limited published information is available for varenicline, but the varenicline label includes a boxed warning for serious neuropsychiatric adverse events, including suicidal ideation or behavior. FDA labeling discourages use of both these agents in lactating women.

PAIN MEDICATIONS

Rarely, normal doses of codeine given to lactating women may result in dangerously high levels of its active metabolite morphine in breastfeeding infants. A fatality has been noted in an infant of a mother with ultrarapid metabolism.[65] In this infant, the postmortem level of morphine (87 ng/mL) greatly exceeded a typical level in a breastfeeding infant (2.2 ng/mL), as well as the therapeutic range for neonates (10–12 ng/mL). In addition, unexplained apnea, bradycardia, cyanosis, and sedation have been reported in nursing infants of mothers receiving codeine.[2,66] Hydrocodone is also metabolized via the CYP2D6 pathway. On the basis of pharmacokinetic data, infants exposed to hydrocodone through human milk may receive up to 9% of the relative maternal dose.[67] Given the reduced clearance of hydrocodone in neonates and the adverse events observed in ultrarapid metabolizers of codeine, caution is advised for use of codeine and hydrocodone in both the mother and nursing infant. Close monitoring for signs and symptoms of neonatal as well as maternal toxicity is recommended. A commercial test to identify ultrarapid metabolizers is not yet widely available. The incidence of this specific CYP2D6 genotype varies with racial and ethnic group as follows: Chinese, Japanese, or Hispanic, 0.5% to 1.0%; Caucasian, 1.0% to 10.0%; African American, 3.0%; and North African, Ethiopian, and Saudi Arabian, 16.0% to 28.0%.[68]

For these reasons, when narcotic agents are needed to treat pain in the breastfeeding woman, agents other than codeine (eg, butorphanol, morphine, or hydromorphone) are preferred. Clinically insignificant levels of butorphanol are excreted into human milk. Morphine appears to be tolerated by the breastfeeding infant, although there is 1 case report of an infant with plasma concentrations within the therapeutic range.[69] Clearance of morphine is decreased in infants younger than 1 month and approaches 80% of adult values by 6 months of age.[70] Limited data suggest that use of hydromorphone for brief periods may be compatible with breastfeeding[71,72]; however, FDA labeling discourages use. Regardless of the choice of therapy, to minimize adverse events for both the mother and her nursing infant, the lowest dose and shortest duration of therapy should be prescribed. Drug delivery via patient-controlled anesthesia or administration by the epidural route may also minimize infant exposure.

Other narcotic agents, such as oxycodone, pentazocine, propoxyphene, and meperidine, are not recommended in the lactating mother. Relatively high amounts of oxycodone are excreted into human milk, and therapeutic concentrations have been detected in the plasma of a nursing infant.[73] Central nervous system depression was noted in 20% of infants exposed to oxycodone during breastfeeding.[74] Thus, use of oxycodone should be discouraged. Limited published data are available about pentazocine. However, respiratory depression and apnea occur frequently in infants, particularly in neonates or in preterm infants, who are treated with pentazocine. Propoxyphene has been associated with unexplained apnea, bradycardia, and cyanosis, as well as hypotonia in nursing infants.[75,76] Moreover, propoxyphene was withdrawn from the market because significant QT prolongation occurred at therapeutic doses.[77] Meperidine use is associated with decreased alertness of the infant and is likely to interfere with breastfeeding.[71] Although estimates of meperidine exposure are low (approximately 2% to 3% of the maternal weight-adjusted dose), the half-life of the active metabolite for meperidine is prolonged, and it may accumulate in infant blood or tissue.[71,72]

When narcotics are not required to relieve mild to moderate pain, other analgesic agents can be used. Presuming that pain relief is adequate, short-acting agents, such as ibuprofen and acetaminophen, are acceptable.[78] Although the half-life of ibuprofen may be prolonged in neonates, particularly in preterm infants (according to product labeling), minimal amounts of ibuprofen are excreted into human milk.[72] Despite reduced clearance of acetaminophen,[79] hepatotoxicity is less common in neonates than in older infants, in part because of low levels of certain cytochrome P-450 enzymes, which convert acetaminophen into toxic metabolites.[80] Acetaminophen is available for both oral and intravenous administration.

Although all nonsteroidal antiinflammatory drugs (NSAIDs) carry a boxed warning regarding gastrointestinal bleeding and potential long-term cardiac toxicity, according to their product labeling and Gardiner et al,[81] celecoxib, flurbiprofen, and naproxen are considered to be compatible with breastfeeding, because less than 1% is excreted into human milk. In addition, a breastfeeding infant would receive less than 1% of the relative pediatric dose of celecoxib prescribed for a 2-year-old (according to product labeling). However, long-term use of naproxen is not recommended because of the drug's long half-life and case reports of gastrointestinal tract bleeding and emesis. Avoiding NSAIDs in breastfeeding infants with ductal-dependent cardiac lesions may be prudent.

Limited published data on other NSAIDs (etodolac, fenoprofen, meloxicam, oxaprozin, piroxicam, sulindac, and tolmetin) are available, and FDA labeling discourages their use for a variety of reasons. Although the implications for humans are unknown, meloxicam concentrations in milk of lactating animals exceed plasma concentrations. Diflunisal has a long half-life and is not recommended because of potential adverse events, including cataracts and fatality, in neonatal animals. Similarly, mefenamic acid has a prolonged half-life in preterm infants. Injectable and oral forms of ketorolac are contraindicated in nursing women, according to product labeling, because of potential adverse effects related to closure of the ductus arteriosus in neonates. Less than 1% of ketorolac nasal spray is excreted into human milk, and unlike the oral and intravenous forms of ketorolac, use is not contraindicated (product labeling).

Carisoprodol and its active metabolite, meprobamate, are concentrated in human milk (2–4 times maternal plasma concentrations). Impaired milk production has been observed, and animal studies suggest maternal use may lead to less effective infant feeding (because of sedation) and/or decreased milk production (according to product labeling).

Low doses (75–162 mg/d) of aspirin may be acceptable[82]; however, use of high-dose aspirin therapy during breastfeeding is not advised, because the serum concentration of salicylate in breastfeeding infants has been reported to reach approximately 40% of therapeutic concentrations. Adverse events, such as rash, platelet abnormalities, bleeding, and metabolic acidosis have also been reported.[71]

GALACTAGOGUES

Galactagogues, or agents to stimulate lactation, are often used to facilitate lactation, particularly for mothers of preterm infants. They also may be used to induce lactation in an adoptive mother. However, evidence to support these agents, including use of dopamine antagonists, such as domperidone and metoclopramide; herbal treatments; and hormonal manipulation, is lacking.[83]

Although a placebo-controlled study (n = 42) suggested that domperidone may increase milk volume in mothers of preterm infants,[84] maternal safety has not been established. The FDA issued a warning in June 2004 regarding use of domperidone in breastfeeding women because of safety concerns based on published reports of arrhythmia, cardiac arrest, and sudden death associated with intravenous therapy. Furthermore, treatment with oral domperidone is associated with QT prolongation in children and infants.[85,86] Domperidone is not an approved product in the United States, and labeling for oral formulations marketed outside the United States do not recommend use during lactation.

Several small trials (each with fewer than 25 subjects) published before 1990 suggested that metoclopramide increases prolactin concentrations and/or milk production in mothers of both term and preterm infants.[87] However, more recent controlled studies do not replicate this finding.[88,89] Human milk concentrations of metoclopramide are similar to therapeutic concentrations in adult plasma,[88] and measurable amounts can be detected in breastfeeding infants.[90] Clearance of metoclopramide in neonates is prolonged, which may result in excessive serum concentrations and the risk of conditions associated with overdose, such as methemoglobinemia. Of concern, prolactin concentrations were increased in 4 of 7 infants exposed to metoclopramide via human milk.[90] The safety profile for metoclopramide includes adverse reactions, such as dystonia, depression, suicidal ideation, and gastrointestinal tract disturbances, as well as a boxed warning about the risk of tardive dyskinesia. These risks to the mother limit the usefulness of this therapy.

Although a pilot study in 8 lactating women performed decades ago suggested that oxytocin nasal spray increased human milk production, a larger placebo-controlled trial in 51 women has not confirmed that observation.[91] Oxytocin nasal spray is no longer marketed in the United States. Similarly, anecdotal reports supporting the use of the herb fenugreek to facilitate lactation have not been confirmed by controlled studies.[92,93] Fenugreek contains coumarin, which may interact with NSAIDs.[94] Use of fenugreek in lactating women also is associated with maple-syrup odor in infants.[95] Available data do not support the routine use of other herbal products, such as fennel, to facilitate lactation.[96]

In summary, galactagogues have a limited role in facilitating lactation and have not been subject to full assessments of safety for the nursing infant. Nursing mothers should seek consultation with a lactation specialist and use non-pharmacologic measures to increase milk supply, such as ensuring proper technique, using massage therapy, increasing the frequency of milk expression, prolonging the duration of pumping, and maximizing emotional support.

COMMONLY USED HERBAL PRODUCTS

Despite the frequent use of herbal products in breastfeeding women (up to 43% of lactating mothers in a 2004 survey),[97] reliable information on the safety of many herbal products is lacking. Herbal products are not subject to the same standards for manufacturing and proven effectiveness and safety as are drug products before they are marketed.[98] In fact, the use of several herbal products may be harmful, including kava and yohimbe. For example, the FDA has issued a warning that links kava supplementation to severe liver damage.[99] Breastfeeding mothers should not use yohimbe because of reports of associated fatalities in children.[100] In addition, from 2008 through 2010, the

FDA recalled 10 or more dietary supplements each year because of the presence of potentially toxic undeclared ingredients in the supplement.[101] Similarly, the US Government Accountability Office found that 16 of 40 common herbal dietary supplements obtained from retail stores contained pesticide residues.[102]

Safety data are lacking for many herbs commonly used during breastfeeding, such as chamomile,[103] black cohosh,[104] blue cohosh,[105] chastetree,[106] echinacea,[107] ginseng,[108] gingko,[109] Hypericum (St John's wort),[110,111] and valerian.[112] Adverse events have been reported in both breastfeeding infants and mothers. For example, St John's wort may cause colic, drowsiness, or lethargy in the breastfed infant even though milk production and infant weight do not appear to be adversely affected[110] and relative maternal dose and infant plasma concentrations are low.[113] Prolonged use of fenugreek may require monitoring of coagulation status and serum glucose concentrations.[114] For these reasons, these aforementioned herbal products are not recommended for use by nursing women.

Although supplementation of nursing mothers with iron and vitamins is safe as long as recommended daily allowances are not exceeded, the use of other nutritional supplements may not be. For instance, L-tryptophan has been associated with eosinophilic myositis.[115] Therefore, physicians should inquire about the use of herbal products and dietary supplements in lactating women and discuss the need for caution because of the paucity of data available.

DIAGNOSTIC IMAGING

When feasible, elective imaging procedures should be delayed until a woman is no longer breastfeeding. For most radiopharmaceuticals, breastfeeding should be interrupted for a time period based on the rate of de-

cline of the agent and dosimetry to avoid infant exposures greater than 1 mSv (100 mrem). For agents that may be concentrated in breast tissue, close contact of the mother with the infant and, consequently, nursing may need to be avoided for a period of time, although expressed milk that has been refrigerated until the radioactivity has decayed may be safe. General guidelines based on Nuclear Regulatory Commission regulations and International Commission on Radiologic Protection guidelines[116] are cited in Tables 3 and 4. However, because there is considerable variability in milk radioactivity, and close contact with an infant may result in additional exposure, consultation with a radiologist should be sought. If deemed necessary, individualized testing of expressed milk may be performed to ensure that radioactivity has reached background levels before breastfeeding is resumed.[117]

Notably, because radiolabeled iodinated products are concentrated in developing thyroid and radioactivity persists after imaging with most ^{131}I and ^{125}I radiopharmaceuticals (with the exception of [125]I- hippurate), breastfeeding should be interrupted for a minimum of 3 weeks. Similarly, [22]Na and [67]Ga (gallium) administration also require a prolonged (3-week) interruption in breastfeeding. Because the lactating breast has a greater ^{131}I affinity than does the nonlactating breast, women should cease breastfeeding at least 4 weeks before whole-body procedures with ^{131}I and should discontinue breastfeeding thereafter. Doing so will reduce the radiation dose and potential cancer risk to maternal breast tissue.

Traditionally, lactating women receiving intravascular gadolinium or iodinated contrast (as opposed to radiolabeled iodine) are advised to discontinue nursing for 24 hours. However, a minimal amount (0.04%) of the intravenous dose reaches human milk, and, of that, less than 1% to

FROM THE AMERICAN ACADEMY OF PEDIATRICS

TABLE 3 Radioactive Compounds That May Require Temporary Cessation of Breastfeeding: Recommendations of the International Commission on Radiologic Protection

Compound	Examples	Example of Procedures	Recommended Time for Cessation of Breastfeeding	Comments
^{14}C-labeled	Triolein, glycocholic acid, urea	*Helicobacter pylori* breath test	None	No approved US products
^{99m}Tc-labeled	DMSA, DTPA, phosphonates (MDP), PYP, tetrofosmin Microspheres, pertechnetate, WBC Sulfur-colloids, RBC in vivo	Multiple: imaging of kidney, bone, lung, heart, tumors	0 to 4 h, as long as no free pertechnetate 12–24 h 6 h	Consider discarding at least 1 meal after procedure Range depends on dose
I-labeled	^{123}I, ^{125}I or ^{131}I-iodo hippurate	Thyroid imaging	12 h	Note: whole-body irradiation with ^{131}I requires prolonged cessation
Others	^{11}C, ^{11}N or ^{11}O-labeled ^{57}Co-labeled vitamin B$_{12}$ ^{18}F-FDG	PET scans Schilling test PET scans	None 24 h None, first feeding should be expressed breast milk to avoid direct contact[120]	Short physical half-life Pomeroy 2005[119] Use alternatives for 10 half-lives (10×109 min= 18 h)[a]
	^{51}Cr-EDTA ^{81m}Kr-gas ^{82}Rb chloride	Renal imaging Pulmonary imaging PET scan of myocardium	None None May resume 1 h after last infusion	No approved US products Half-life 75 s[a]
	^{111}In-octreotide ^{111}In -WBC ^{133}Xe	SPECT, neuroendocrine tumors Cardiac, pulmonary, and cerebral imaging	None 1 wk None	Depends on dose Half-life 5 d[a]

DMSA, dimercaptosuccinic acid; DTPA, diethylenetriaminepentaacetate; EDTA, ethylenediaminetetraacetic acid; FDG, fludeoxyglucose; PET, positron emission tomography; PYP, pyrophosphate; RBC, red blood cell; SPECT, single-photon emission computed tomography; WBC, white blood cell.
[a] FDA-approved drug labeling.

TABLE 4 Radioactive Compounds Requiring Prolonged Cessation of Breastfeeding

Compound	Examples	Example of Procedures	Recommended Time for Cessation of Breastfeeding	Comments
I-labled	^{123}I- BMIPP, -HSA, -IPPA, -MIBG, -NaI, or -HSA ^{131}I-MIBG or -NaI	Imaging of tumors	Greater than 3 wk	Essentially need to stop breastfeeding
Others	^{201}TI-chloride ^{67}Ga-citrate ^{22}Na, ^{75}Se	Cardiac imaging Imaging of tumors	48 h to 2 wk 1 wk to 1 mo Greater than 3 wk	Half-life 73 h[a] Depends on dose Essentially need to stop breastfeeding

Use of expressed human milk recommended because of exposure via direct contact.[120] BMIPP, β-methyl-p-iodophenyl-pentadecanoic acid; HSA, human serum albumin; IPPA, iodophenylpentadecanoic; MIBG, metaiodobenzylguanidine; NaI, sodium iodide.
[a] FDA-approved drug labeling.

2% is absorbed by the infant. Therefore, breastfeeding can be continued without interruption after the use of iodinated contrast or gadolinium.[118]

BREASTFEEDING AND VACCINES

With rare exceptions, maternal immunization does not create any problems for breastfeeding infants, although questions concerning 2 topics often arise regarding lactation and immunization: the effect of lactation on the infant's immune response to a vaccine and a potential adverse effect on the infant from maternal immunization. Breastfeeding does not interfere with

the infant's immune response to most routine immunizations (eg, diphtheria and tetanus toxoids and acellular pertussis vaccine, inactivated poliovirus vaccine, and hepatitis B vaccine [HBV]),[121] despite the presence of maternal antibodies in human milk. Seroconversion rates are also similar between breastfed and formula-fed infants receiving rotavirus vaccine; however, vaccine efficacy for severe rotavirus gastroenteritis appears to be higher in formula-fed infants compared with exclusively breastfed infants, particularly during the second season (98% vs 88%) when breastfeeding has been discontinued.[122] Nonetheless, protection

during the first year is similar. Moreover, breastfeeding enhances the antibody response to pneumococcal and *Haemophilus influenzae* type b vaccines.[123] Breastfeeding may also decrease the incidence of fever after infant immunization.[124] Therefore, the timing of infant feeding (including human milk) relative to immunization is not restricted, even for live vaccines, such as rotavirus.

Lactating women may need to be immunized. Inactivated vaccines (such as tetanus toxoid, reduced diphtheria toxoid, and acellular pertussis vaccine; inactivated poliovirus vaccine; influenza; hepatitis A vaccine; HBV; or human papillomavirus vaccine [HPV]) given to a nursing mother do not pose a risk to the breastfeeding infant. Several vaccines, such as tetanus toxoid, reduced diphtheria toxoid, and acellular pertussis vaccine and influenza vaccine, are recommended for the mother during the postpartum period to protect the infant as well as the mother. Other routine or catch-up vaccines, such as HPV, hepatitis A vaccine, and HBV, can be given to the lactating mother. HPV immunization is recommended for women younger than 27 years. The incidence of adverse reactions in nursing infants within 30 days of maternal immunization with HPV was similar to nursing infants of women receiving the control except for acute respiratory illness (according to Gardasil labeling). Hence, caution is warranted when immunizing mothers of infants who are vulnerable to respiratory illnesses (eg, preterm infants, infants with congenital heart disease or chronic respiratory problems).

Most live vaccines are not associated with virus secretion in human milk. For example, despite maternal seroconversion, neither the varicella virus nor antibody to varicella DNA has been detected in breastfeeding infants.[125] Although attenuated rubella can be secreted into human milk and transmitted to breastfed infants, infections are usually asymptomatic or mild. Consequently, postpartum immunization with measles-mumps-rubella vaccine is recommended for women who lack immunity, especially to rubella.[126] In contrast, infants are considered to be at high risk of developing vaccinia

after exposure to smallpox vaccine or encephalitis after yellow fever vaccine. Two cases of meningoencephalitis in nursing infants whose mothers had been immunized against yellow fever are documented in the literature.[127,128] Therefore, most vaccines, with the exception of smallpox or yellow-fever vaccine, which are contraindicated in nonemergency situations, may be administered during lactation.

SUMMARY

The benefits of breastfeeding outweigh the risk of exposure to most therapeutic agents via human milk. Although most drugs and therapeutic agents do not pose a risk to the mother or nursing infant, careful consideration of the individual risk/benefit ratio is necessary for certain agents, particularly those that are concentrated in human milk or result in exposures in the infant that may be clinically significant on the basis of relative infant dose or detectable serum concentrations. Caution is also advised for drugs and agents with unproven benefits, with long half-lives that may lead to drug accumulation, or with known toxicity to the mother or infant. In addition, specific infants may be more vulnerable to adverse events because of immature organ function (eg, preterm infants or neonates) or underlying medical conditions. Several excellent resources are available for the pediatrician, including product labeling and the peer-reviewed database, LactMed. Consultation with a specialist may be indicated, particularly when the

use of radiopharmaceuticals, oncologic drugs, or other therapies not addressed by LactMed is contemplated. Additional information about topics outside the scope of this report, such as environmental agents, can be obtained from the third edition of the AAP textbook *Pediatric Environmental Health*.[129]

LEAD AUTHOR
Hari Cheryl Sachs, MD, FAAP

COMMITTEE ON DRUGS, 2012–2013
Daniel A. C. Frattarelli, MD, FAAP, Chairperson
Jeffrey L. Galinkin, MD, FAAP
Thomas P. Green, MD, FAAP
Timothy Johnson, DO, FAAP
Kathleen Neville, MD, FAAP
Ian M. Paul, MD, MSc, FAAP
John Van den Anker, MD, PhD, FAAP

FORMER COMMITTEE MEMBERS
Mark L. Hudak, MD, FAAP
Matthew E. Knight, MD, FAAP

LIAISONS
John J. Alexander, MD, FAAP – *Food and Drug Administration*
Sarah J. Kilpatrick, MD, PhD – *American College of Obstetricians and Gynecologists*
Janet D. Cragan, MD, MPH, FAAP – *Centers for Disease Control and Prevention*
Michael J. Rieder, MD, FAAP – *Canadian Pediatric Society*
Adelaide Robb, MD – *American Academy of Child and Adolescent Psychiatry*
Hari Cheryl Sachs, MD, FAAP – *Food and Drug Administration*
Anne Zajicek, MD, PharmD, FAAP – *National Institutes of Health*

CONTRIBUTOR
Ashley Moss, MD, FAAP

STAFF
Tamar Haro, JD
Raymond J. Koteras, MHA

REFERENCES

1. Berlin CM, Briggs GG. Drugs and chemicals in human milk. *Semin Fetal Neonatal Med*. 2005;10(2):149–159

2. Anderson PO, Pochop SL, Manoguerra AS. Adverse drug reactions in breastfed infants: less than imagined. *Clin Pediatr (Phila)*. 2003;42(4):325–340

3. American Academy of Pediatrics, Committee on Drugs. The transfer of drugs and other chemicals into human breast milk. *Pediatrics*. 1983;72(3):375–383

4. American Academy of Pediatrics, Committee on Drugs. The transfer of drugs and other chemicals into human breast milk. *Pediatrics*. 1989;84(5):924–936

5. American Academy of Pediatrics, Committee on Drugs. The transfer of drugs and other chemicals into human breast milk. *Pediatrics*. 1994;93(1):137–150

FROM THE AMERICAN ACADEMY OF PEDIATRICS

6. American Academy of Pediatrics Committee on Drugs. Transfer of drugs and other chemicals into human milk. *Pediatrics.* 2001;108(3):776–789

7. Naranjo CA, Busto U, Sellers EM, et al. A method for estimating the probability of adverse drug reactions. *Clin Pharmacol Ther.* 1981;30(2):239–245

8. Hale TW. Maternal medications during breastfeeding. *Clin Obstet Gynecol.* 2004; 47(3):696–711

9. Berlin CM, Jr, Paul IM, Vesell ES. Safety issues of maternal drug therapy during breastfeeding. *Clin Pharmacol Ther.* 2009; 85(1):20–22

10. Food and Drug Administration. Draft guidance for industry: clinical lactation studies —study design, data analysis, and recommendations for labeling. February 2005. Available at: www.fda.gov/downloads/RegulatoryInformation/Guidances/ucm127505. pdf. Accessed November 26, 2012

11. Gentile S. SSRIs in pregnancy and lactation: emphasis on neurodevelopmental outcome. *CNS Drugs.* 2005;19(7):623–633

12. Gentile S. The safety of newer antidepressants in pregnancy and breastfeeding. *Drug Saf.* 2005;28(2):137–152

13. Fortinguerra F, Clavenna A, Bonati M. Psychotropic drug use during breastfeeding: a review of the evidence. *Pediatrics.* 2009;124(4). Available at: www.pediatrics.org/cgi/content/full/124/4/e547

14. Davis MF, Miller HS, Nolan PE Jr. Bupropion levels in breast milk for 4 mother-infant pairs: more answers to lingering questions. *J Clin Psychiatry.* 2009;70(2):297–298

15. Kristensen JH, Ilett KF, Hackett LP, Yapp P, Paech M, Begg EJ. Distribution and excretion of fluoxetine and norfluoxetine in human milk. *Br J Clin Pharmacol.* 1999;48 (4):521–527

16. Moretti ME. Psychotropic drugs in lactation—Motherisk Update 2008. *Can J Clin Pharmacol.* 2009;16(1):e49–e57

17. Ostrea EM, Jr, Mantaring JB, III, Silvestre MA. Drugs that affect the fetus and newborn infant via the placenta or breast milk. *Pediatr Clin North Am.* 2004;51(3): 539–579, vii

18. Newport DJ, Pennell PB, Calamaras MR, et al. Lamotrigine in breast milk and nursing infants: determination of exposure. *Pediatrics.* 2008;122(1). Available at: www.pediatrics.org/cgi/content/full/122/ 1/e223

19. Newport DJ, Ritchie JC, Knight BT, Glover BA, Zach EB, Stowe ZN. Venlafaxine in human breast milk and nursing infant

plasma: determination of exposure. *J Clin Psychiatry.* 2009;70(9):1304–1310

20. Weissman AM, Levy BT, Hartz AJ, et al. Pooled analysis of antidepressant levels in lactating mothers, breast milk, and nursing infants. *Am J Psychiatry.* 2004;161 (6):1066–1078

21. Schimmell MS, Katz EZ, Shaag Y, Pastuszak A, Koren G. Toxic neonatal effects following maternal clomipramine therapy. *J Toxicol Clin Toxicol.* 1991;29(4):479–484

22. Wesson DR, Camber S, Harkey M, Smith DE. Diazepam and desmethyldiazepam in breast milk. *J Psychoactive Drugs.* 1985; 17(1):55–56

23. Fotopoulou C, Kretz R, Bauer S, et al. Prospectively assessed changes in lamotrigine-concentration in women with epilepsy during pregnancy, lactation and the neonatal period. *Epilepsy Res.* 2009;85 (1):60–64

24. Viguera AC, Newport DJ, Ritchie J, et al. Lithium in breast milk and nursing infants: clinical implications. *Am J Psychiatry.* 2007;164(2):342–345

25. Grandjean EM, Aubry JM. Lithium: updated human knowledge using an evidence-based approach: part III: clinical safety. *CNS Drugs.* 2009;23(5):397–418

26. Bogen DL, Sit D, Genovese A, Wisner KL. Three cases of lithium exposure and exclusive breastfeeding. *Arch Women Ment Health.* 2012;15(1):69–72

27. Tonn P, Reuter SC, Hiemke C, Dahmen N. High mirtazapine plasma levels in infant after breast feeding: case report and review of the literature. *J Clin Psychopharmacol.* 2009;29(2):191–192

28. Whitworth A, Stuppaeck C, Yazdi K, et al. Olanzapine and breast-feeding: changes of plasma concentrations of olanzapine in a breast-fed infant over a period of 5 months. *J Psychopharmacol.* 2010;24(1): 121–123

29. Hendrick V, Fukuchi A, Altshuler L, Widawski M, Wertheimer A, Brunhuber MV. Use of sertraline, paroxetine and fluvoxamine by nursing women. *Br J Psychiatry.* 2001;179:163–166

30. Stowe ZN, Hostetter AL, Owens MJ, et al. The pharmacokinetics of sertraline excretion into human breast milk: determinants of infant serum concentrations. *J Clin Psychiatry.* 2003;64(1):73–80

31. Section on Breastfeeding. Breastfeeding and the use of human milk. *Pediatrics.* 2012;129(3). Available at: www.pediatrics. org/cgi/content/full/129/3/e827

32. Liebrechts-Akkerman G, Lao O, Liu F, et al. Postnatal parental smoking: an important

risk factor for SIDS. *Eur J Pediatr.* 2011; 170(10):1281–1291

33. Moon RY; Task Force on Sudden Infant Death Syndrome. SIDS and other sleep-related infant deaths: expansion of recommendations for a safe infant sleeping environment. *Pediatrics.* 2011;128(5): 1030–1039

34. Koren G. MotherRisk update: drinking alcohol while breastfeeding. *Can Fam Physician.* 2002;48:29–41

35. Backstrand JR, Goodman AH, Allen LH, Pelto GH. Pulque intake during pregnancy and lactation in rural Mexico: alcohol and child growth from 1 to 57 months. *Eur J Clin Nutr.* 2004;58(12):1626–1634

36. Mennella JA, Yourshaw LM, Morgan LK. Breastfeeding and smoking: short-term effects on infant feeding and sleep. *Pediatrics.* 2007;120(3):497–502

37. Institute of Medicine, Subcommittee on Nutrition During Lactation. *Nutrition During Lactation.* Washington, DC: National Academies Press; 1991

38. Jain AE, Lacy T. Psychotropic drugs in pregnancy and lactation. *J Psychiatr Pract.* 2005;11(3):177–191

39. Malone K, Papagni K, Ramini S, Keltner NL. Antidepressants, antipsychotics, benzodiazepines, and the breastfeeding dyad. *Perspect Psychiatr Care.* 2004;40 (2):73–85

40. Chasnoff IJ, Lewis DE, Squires L. Cocaine intoxication in a breast-fed infant. *Pediatrics.* 1987;80(6):836–838

41. Winecker RE, Goldberger BA, Tebbett IR, et al. Detection of cocaine and its metabolites in breast milk. *J Forensic Sci.* 2001;46(5):1221–1223

42. vande Velde S, Verloo P, Van Biervliet S, et al. Heroin withdrawal leads to metabolic alkalosis in an infant with cystic fibrosis. *Eur J Pediatr.* 2007;166(1):75–76

43. Ariagno R, Karch SB, Middleberg R, Stephens BG, Valdès-Dapena M. Methamphetamine ingestion by a breast-feeding mother and her infant's death: People v Henderson. *JAMA.* 1995;274(3):215

44. Bartu A, Dusci LJ, Ilett KF. Transfer of methadone and amphetamine into breast milk following recreational use of methamphetamine. *Br J Clin Pharmacol.* 2009;67(4):455–459

45. Djulus J, Moretti M, Koren G. Marijuana use and breastfeeding. *Can Fam Physician.* 2005;51:349–350

46. Campolongo P, Trezza V, Palmery M, Trabace L, Cuomo V. Developmental exposure to cannabinoids causes subtle and enduring neurofunctional alterations. *Int Rev Neurobiol.* 2009;85:117–133

47. Garry A, Rigourd V, Amirouche A, et al. Cannabis and breastfeeding. *J Toxicol.* 2009;2009:596149

48. Jansson LM; Academy of Breastfeeding Medicine Protocol Committee. ABM clinical protocol #21: guidelines for breastfeeding and the drug-dependent woman. *Breastfeed Med.* 2009;4(4):225–228

49. Jones HE, Martin PR, Heil SH, et al. Treatment of opioid-dependent pregnant women: clinical and research issues. *J Subst Abuse Treat.* 2008;35(3):245–259

50. Centers for Disease Control and Prevention. Human immunodeficiency virus (HIV), and acquired immunodeficiency syndrome (AIDS). Available at: www.cdc.gov/breastfeeding/disease/hiv.htm. Accessed November 3, 2012

51. Jansson LM, Velez M, Harrow C. Methadone maintenance and lactation: a review of the literature and current management guidelines. *J Hum Lact.* 2004;20(1):62–71

52. Hirose M, Hosokawa T, Tanaka Y. Extradural buprenorphine suppresses breast feeding after caesarean section. *Br J Anaesth.* 1997;79(1):120–121

53. Glatstein MM, Garcia-Bournissen F, Finkelstein Y, Koren G. Methadone exposure during lactation. *Can Fam Physician.* 2008;54(12):1689–1690

54. Farid WO, Dunlop SA, Tait RJ, Hulse GK. The effects of maternally administered methadone, buprenorphine and naltrexone on offspring: review of human and animal data. *Curr Neuropharmacol.* 2008;6(2):125–150

55. Jansson LM, Choo R, Velez ML, Lowe R, Huestis MA. Methadone maintenance and long-term lactation. *Breastfeed Med.* 2008;3(1):34–37

56. Jansson LM, Choo R, Velez ML, et al. Methadone maintenance and breastfeeding in the neonatal period. *Pediatrics.* 2008;121(1):106–114

57. Johnson RE, Jones HE, Jasinski DR, et al. Buprenorphine treatment of pregnant opioid-dependent women: maternal and neonatal outcomes. *Drug Alcohol Depend.* 2001;63(1):97–103

58. Lindemalm S, Nydert P, Svensson JO, Stahle L, Sarman I. Transfer of buprenorphine into breast milk and calculation of infant drug dose. *J Hum Lact.* 2009;25(2):199–205

59. Chan CF, Page-Sharp M, Kristensen JH, O'Neil S, Ilett KF. Transfer of naltrexone and its metabolite 6,beta-naltrexol into human milk. *J Hum Lact.* 2004;20(3):322–326

60. Abdel-Latif ME, Pinner J, Clews S, Cooke F, Lui K, Oei J. Effects of breast milk on the severity and outcome of neonatal abstinence syndrome among infants of drug-dependent mothers. *Pediatrics.* 2006;117(6). Available at: www.pediatrics.org/cgi/content/full/117/6/e1163

61. Malpas TJ, Darlow BA. Neonatal abstinence syndrome following abrupt cessation of breastfeeding. *N Z Med J.* 1999;112(1080):12–13

62. Molyneux A. Nicotine replacement therapy. *BMJ.* 2004;328(7437):454–456

63. Ilett KF, Hale TW, Page-Sharp M, Kristensen JH, Kohan R, Hackett LP. Use of nicotine patches in breast-feeding mothers: transfer of nicotine and cotinine into human milk. *Clin Pharmacol Ther.* 2003;74(6):516–524

64. Chaudron LH, Schoenecker CJ. Bupropion and breastfeeding: a case of a possible infant seizure. *J Clin Psychiatry.* 2004;65(6):881–882

65. Madadi P, Shirazi F, Walter FG, Koren G. Establishing causality of CNS depression in breastfed infants following maternal codeine use. *Paediatr Drugs.* 2008;10(6):399–404

66. Madadi P, Koren G, Cairns JU, et al. Safety of codeine during breastfeeding: fatal morphine poisoning in the breastfed neonate of a mother prescribed codeine. *Can Fam Physician.* 2007;53(1):33–35

67. Sauberan JB, Anderson PO, Lane JR, et al. Breast milk hydrocodone and hydromorphone levels in mothers using hydrocodone for postpartum pain. *Obstet Gynecol.* 2011;117(3):611–617

68. Food and Drug Administration. FDA Alert. Information for healthcare professionals: use of codeine products in nursing mothers. August 17, 2007. Available at: www.fda.gov/drugs/drugsafety/postmarketdrugsafetyinformationforpatientsandproviders/ucm124889.htm. Accessed November 26, 2012

69. Robieux I, Koren G, Vandenbergh H, Schneiderman J. Morphine excretion in breast milk and resultant exposure of a nursing infant. *J Toxicol Clin Toxicol.* 1990;28(3):365–370

70. Bouwmeester NJ, Anderson BJ, Tibboel D, Holford NH. Developmental pharmacokinetics of morphine and its metabolites in neonates, infants and young children. *Br J Anaesth.* 2004;92(2):208–217

71. Bar-Oz B, Bulkowstein M, Benyamini L, et al. Use of antibiotic and analgesic drugs during lactation. *Drug Saf.* 2003;26(13):925–935

72. Spigset O, Hägg S. Analgesics and breastfeeding: safety considerations. *Paediatr Drugs.* 2000;2(3):223–238

73. Seaton S, Reeves M, McLean S. Oxycodone as a component of multimodal analgesia for lactating mothers after Caesarean section: relationships between maternal plasma, breast milk and neonatal plasma levels. *Aust N Z J Obstet Gynaecol.* 2007;47(3):181–185

74. Lam J, Kelly L, Ciszkowski C, et al. Central nervous system depression of neonates breastfed by mothers receiving oxycodone for postpartum analgesia. *J Pediatr.* 2011;160(1):33.e2–37.e2

75. Rigourd V, Amirouche A, Tasseau A, Kintz P, Serreau R. Retrospective diagnosis of an adverse drug reaction in a breastfed neonate: liquid chromatography-tandem mass spectrometry quantification of dextropropoxyphene and norpropoxyphene in newborn and maternal hair. *J Anal Toxicol.* 2008;32(9):787–789

76. Naumburg EG, Meny RG. Breast milk opioids and neonatal apnea. *Am J Dis Child.* 1988;142(1):11–12

77. Food and Drug Administration. Medwatch Safety Information. Propoxyphene: withdrawal – risk of cardiac toxicity. November 19, 2010. Available at: www.fda.gov/Safety/MedWatch/SafetyInformation/SafetyAlertsforHumanMedicalProducts/ucm234389.htm. Accessed November 26, 2012

78. Spencer J, Gonzalez L, Barnhart D. Medications in the breastfeeding mother. *Am Fam Physician.* 2001;64(1):119–126

79. Jacqz-Aigrain E, Serreau R, Boissinot C, et al. Excretion of ketoprofen and nalbuphine in human milk during treatment of maternal pain after delivery. *Ther Drug Monit.* 2007;29(6):815–818

80. van der Marel CD, Anderson BJ, van Lingen RA, et al. Paracetamol and metabolite pharmacokinetics in infants. *Eur J Clin Pharmacol.* 2003;59(3):243–251

81. Gardiner SJ, Doogue MP, Zhang M, Begg EJ. Quantification of infant exposure to celecoxib through breast milk. *Br J Clin Pharmacol.* 2006;61(1):101–104

82. Bell AD, Roussin A, Cartier R, et al; Canadian Cardiovascular Society. The use of antiplatelet therapy in the outpatient setting: Canadian Cardiovascular Society guidelines. *Can J Cardiol.* 2011;27(suppl A):S1–S59

83. Academy of Breastfeeding Medicine Protocol Committee. ABM Clinical Protocol #9: use of galactogogues in initiating or augmenting the rate of maternal secretion. *Breastfeed Med.* 2011;6(1):41–49

84. Campbell-Yeo ML, Allen AC, Joseph KS, et al. Effect of domperidone on the composition of preterm human breast milk. *Pediatrics.* 2010;125(1). Available at: www.pediatrics.org/cgi/content/full/125/1/e107

FROM THE AMERICAN ACADEMY OF PEDIATRICS

85. Collins KK, Sondheimer JM. Domperidone-induced QT prolongation: add another drug to the list. *J Pediatr.* 2008;153(5):596–598

86. Djeddi D, Kongolo G, Lefaix C, Mounard J, Léké A. Effect of domperidone on QT interval in neonates. *J Pediatr.* 2008;153(5):663–666

87. Zuppa AA, Sindico P, Orchi C, Carducci C, Cardiello V, Romagnoli C. Safety and efficacy of galactogogues: substances that induce, maintain and increase breast milk production. *J Pharm Pharm Sci.* 2010;13(2):162–174

88. Hansen WF, McAndrew S, Harris K, Zimmerman MB. Metoclopramide effect on breastfeeding the preterm infant: a randomized trial. *Obstet Gynecol.* 2005;105(2):383–389

89. Fife S, Gill P, Hopkins M, Angello C, Boswell S, Nelson KM. Metoclopramide to augment lactation, does it work? A randomized trial. *J Matern Fetal Neonatal Med.* 2011;24(11):1317–1320

90. Kauppila A, Arvela P, Koivisto M, Kivinen S, Ylikorkala O, Pelkonen O. Metoclopramide and breast feeding: transfer into milk and the newborn. *Eur J Clin Pharmacol.* 1983;25(6):819–823

91. Fewtrell MS, Loh KL, Blake A, Ridout DA, Hawdon J. Randomised, double blind trial of oxytocin nasal spray in mothers expressing breast milk for preterm infants. *Arch Dis Child Fetal Neonatal Ed.* 2006;91(3):F169–F174

92. Betzold CM. Galactagogues. *J Midwifery Womens Health.* 2004;49(2):151–154

93. Ulbricht C, Basch E, Burke D, et al. Fenugreek (*Trigonella foenum-graecum* L. Leguminosae): an evidence-based systematic review by the natural standard research collaboration. *J Herb Pharmacother.* 2007;7(3-4):143–177

94. Abebe W. Herbal medication: potential for adverse interactions with analgesic drugs. *J Clin Pharm Ther.* 2002;27(6):391–401

95. Korman SH, Cohen E, Preminger A. Pseudo-maple syrup urine disease due to maternal prenatal ingestion of fenugreek. *J Paediatr Child Health.* 2001;37(4):403–404

96. Jackson PC. Complementary and alternative methods of increasing breast milk supply for lactating mothers of infants in the NICU. *Neonatal Netw.* 2010;29(4):225–230

97. Nordeng H, Havnen GC. Use of herbal drugs in pregnancy: a survey among 400 Norwegian women. *Pharmacoepidemiol Drug Saf.* 2004;13(6):371–380

98. Denham BE. Dietary supplements—regulatory issues and implications for public health. *JAMA.* 2011;306(4):428–429

99. Food and Drug Administration. Consumer advisory: kava-containing dietary supplements may be associated with severe liver injury. March 25, 2002. Available at: www.fda.gov/Food/ResourcesForYou/Consumers/ucm085482.htm. Accessed November 26, 2012

100. Medline Plus. Yohimbe. Available at: www.nlm.nih.gov/medlineplus/druginfo/natural/759.html. Accessed November 26, 2012

101. Food and Drug Administration. Safety alerts for human medical products 2008-2010. Available at: www.fda.gov/Safety/MedWatch/SafetyInformation/default.htm. Accessed November 26, 2012

102. US Government Accountability Office. Herbal dietary supplements: examples of deceptive or questionable marketing practices and potentially dangerous advice. May 26, 2010. Available at: www.gao.gov/products/GAO-10-662T. Accessed November 26, 2012

103. Gardiner P. Complementary, holistic, and integrative medicine: chamomile. *Pediatr Rev.* 2007;28(4):e16–e18

104. Dugoua JJ, Seely D, Perri D, Koren G, Mills E. Safety and efficacy of black cohosh (*Cimicifuga racemosa*) during pregnancy and lactation. *Can J Clin Pharmacol.* 2006;13(3):e257–e261

105. Dugoua JJ, Perri D, Seely D, Mills E, Koren G. Safety and efficacy of blue cohosh (*Caulophyllum thalictroides*) during pregnancy and lactation. *Can J Clin Pharmacol.* 2008;15(1):e66–e73

106. Dugoua JJ, Seely D, Perri D, Koren G, Mills E. Safety and efficacy of chastetree (*Vitex agnus-castus*) during pregnancy and lactation. *Can J Clin Pharmacol.* 2008;15(1):e74–e79

107. Perri D, Dugoua JJ, Mills E, Koren G. Safety and efficacy of echinacea (*Echinacea angustafolia, E. purpurea* and *E. pallida*) during pregnancy and lactation. *Can J Clin Pharmacol.* 2006;13(3):e262–e267

108. Seely D, Dugoua JJ, Perri D, Mills E, Koren G. Safety and efficacy of panax ginseng during pregnancy and lactation. *Can J Clin Pharmacol.* 2008;15(1):e87–e94

109. Dugoua JJ, Mills E, Perri D, Koren G. Safety and efficacy of ginkgo (*Ginkgo biloba*) during pregnancy and lactation. *Can J Clin Pharmacol.* 2006;13(3):e277–e284

110. Dugoua JJ, Mills E, Perri D, Koren G. Safety and efficacy of St. John's wort (hypericum) during pregnancy and lactation. *Can J Clin Pharmacol.* 2006;13(3):e268–e276

111. Budzynska K, Gardner ZE, Dugoua JJ, Low Dog T, Gardiner P. Systematic review of breastfeeding and herbs. *Breastfeed Med.* 2012;7(6):489–503

112. Drugs and Lactation Database (LactMed). Available at: http://toxnet.nlm.nih.gov/cgi-bin/sis/htmlgen?LACT. Accessed May 8, 2013

113. Klier CM, Schmid-Siegel B, Schäfer MR, et al. St. John's wort (*Hypericum perforatum*) and breastfeeding: plasma and breast milk concentrations of hyperforin for 5 mothers and 2 infants. *J Clin Psychiatry.* 2006;67(2):305–309

114. Tiran D. The use of fenugreek for breast feeding women. *Complement Ther Nurs Midwifery.* 2003;9(3):155–156

115. Dourmishev LA, Dourmishev AL. Activity of certain drugs in inducing of inflammatory myopathies with cutaneous manifestations. *Expert Opin Drug Saf.* 2008;7(4):421–433

116. ICRP. Radiation dose to patients from radiopharmaceuticals. Addendum 3 to ICRP Publication 53. ICRP Publication 106. Approved by the Commission in October 2007. *Ann ICRP.* 2008;38(1-2):1–197

117. Stabin MG, Breitz HB. Breast milk excretion of radiopharmaceuticals: mechanisms, findings, and radiation dosimetry. *J Nucl Med.* 2000;41(5):863–873

118. Chen MM, Coakley FV, Kaimal A, Laros RK Jr. Guidelines for computed tomography and magnetic resonance imaging use during pregnancy and lactation. *Obstet Gynecol.* 2008;112(2 pt 1):333–340

119. Pomeroy KM, Sawyer LJ, Evans MJ. Estimated radiation dose to breast feeding infant following maternal administration of 57Co labelled to vitamin B12. *Nucl Med Commun.* 2005;26(9):839–841

120. Devine CE, Mawlawi O. Radiation safety with positron emission tomography and computed tomography. *Semin Ultrasound CT MR.* 2010;31(1):39–45

121. Atkinson WL, Pickering LK, Schwartz B, Weniger BG, Iskander JK, Watson JC; Centers for Disease Control and Prevention. General recommendations on immunization. Recommendations of the Advisory Committee on Immunization Practices (ACIP) and the American Academy of Family Physicians (AAFP). *MMWR Recomm Rep.* 2002;51(RR-2):1–35

122. Vesikari T, Prymula R, Schuster V, et al. Efficacy and immunogenicity of live-attenuated human rotavirus vaccine in breast-fed and formula-fed European infants. *Pediatr Infect Dis J.* 2012;31(5):509–513

123. Silfverdal SA, Ekholm L, Bodin L. Breastfeeding enhances the antibody response

to Hib and Pneumococcal serotype 6B and 14 after vaccination with conjugate vaccines. *Vaccine.* 2007;25(8):1497–1502

124. Pisacane A, Continisio P, Palma O, Cataldo S, De Michele F, Vairo U. Breastfeeding and risk for fever after immunization. *Pediatrics.* 2010;125(6). Available at: www.pediatrics.org/cgi/content/full/125/6/e1448

125. Bohlke K, Galil K, Jackson LA, et al. Postpartum varicella vaccination: is the vaccine virus excreted in breast milk? *Obstet Gynecol.* 2003;102(5 pt 1):970–977

126. Kroger AT, Atkinson WL, Marcuse EK, Pickering LK; Advisory Committee on Immunization Practices (ACIP) Centers for Disease Control and Prevention (CDC). General recommendations on immunization: recommendations of the Advisory Committee on Immunization Practices (ACIP). *MMWR Recomm Rep.* 2006;55(RR-15):1–48

127. Centers for Disease Control and Prevention (CDC). Transmission of yellow fever vaccine virus through breast-feeding -

Brazil, 2009. *MMWR Morb Mortal Wkly Rep.* 2010;59(5):130–132

128. Traiber C, Coelho-Amaral P, Ritter VR, Winge A. Infant meningoencephalitis caused by yellow fever vaccine virus transmitted via breastmilk. *J Pediatr (Rio J).* 2011;87(3): 269–272

129. American Academy of Pediatrics, Council on Environmental Health. In: Etzel RA, Balk SJ, eds. *Pediatric Environmental Health.* 3rd ed. Elk Grove Village, IL: American Academy of Pediatrics; 2012

ACOG COMMITTEE OPINION

Number 361 • February 2007

Breastfeeding: Maternal and Infant Aspects

Committee on Health Care for Underserved Women

Committee on Obstetric Practice

The Committees would like to thank Sharon Mass, MD, for her contributions to the development of this document.

The American College of Obstetricians and Gynecologists
Women's Health Care Physicians

ABSTRACT: Evidence continues to mount regarding the value of breastfeeding for both women and their infants. The American College of Obstetricians and Gynecologists strongly supports breastfeeding and calls on its Fellows, other health care professionals caring for women and their infants, hospitals, and employers to support women in choosing to breastfeed their infants. Obstetrician–gynecologists and other health care professionals caring for pregnant women should provide accurate information about breastfeeding to expectant mothers and be prepared to support them should any problems arise while breastfeeding.

Research in the United States and throughout the world indicates that breastfeeding and human milk provide benefits to infants, women, families, and society. In 1971, only 24.7% of mothers left the hospital breastfeeding. Since then, breastfeeding initiation rates have been increasing because of a growing awareness of the advantages of breast milk over formula, but they have not yet reached the goal set by the U.S. Public Health Service for Healthy People 2010 (1). In 2005, 72.9% of new U.S. mothers initiated breastfeeding (2). Although this is close to the target rate of 75% in the early postpartum period, there is still a long way to go to achieve target breastfeeding rates of 50% at 6 months and 25% at 12 months (1). Improvement in breastfeeding initiation rates has been uneven as women attempt to overcome practical obstacles. Women and infants who could benefit most from breastfeeding are often within population groups (geographic, racial, economic, and educational) with low rates of breastfeeding. Education and support services can improve rates among these as well as other women. Breastfeeding education and support are an economical investment for health plans and employers because there are lower rates of illness among infants who are breastfed.

Breastfeeding is the preferred method of feeding for newborns and infants. Nearly every woman can breastfeed her child. Exceptions are few and include those women who take street drugs or do not control alcohol use, have an infant with galactosemia, are infected with human immunodeficiency virus (HIV) or human T-cell lymphotropic virus type I or type II, and have active untreated tuberculosis or varicella or active herpes simplex virus with breast lesions (3, 4).

The American College of Obstetricians and Gynecologists strongly supports breastfeeding and calls upon its Fellows, other health care professionals caring for women and their infants, hospitals, and employers to support women in choosing to breastfeed their infants. All should work to facilitate the continuation of breastfeeding in the workplace and public facilities. Health care professionals have a wide range of opportunities to serve as a primary resource to the public and their patients regarding the benefits of breastfeeding and the knowledge, skills, and support needed for successful breastfeeding (5). In addition to providing supportive clinical care for their own patients, obstetrician–gynecologists should be in the forefront of fostering changes in the public environment that will support breastfeeding, whether through change in hospital practices, through community efforts, or through supportive legislation.

The advice and encouragement of the obstetrician–gynecologist during preconception, prenatal, postpartum, and interconception care are critical in making the decision to breastfeed. Good hospital practices surrounding childbirth are significant factors in enabling women to breastfeed. Health care providers should be aware that the giving of gift packs with formula to breastfeeding women is commonly a deterrent to continuation of breastfeeding (4). A professional recommendation of the care and feeding products in the gift pack is implied. For this reason, physicians may conclude that noncommercial educational alternatives or gift packs without health-related items are preferable. After discharge, the obstetrician–gynecologist's office should be a resource for 24-hour assistance, or provide links to other resources in the community. Breastfeeding problems, including breast and nipple pain, should be evaluated and treated promptly. Clinical breast examinations are recommended for breastfeeding women. If any mass or abnormality is detected, it should be fully evaluated.

Contraception is an important topic for early discussion and follow-up for breastfeeding women. Women should be encouraged to consider their future plans for contraception and childbearing during prenatal care and be given information and services that will help them meet their goals. Options that should be explained in detail include nonhormonal methods, hormonal methods, and the lactational amenorrhea method.

Women should be supported in integrating breastfeeding into their daily lives in the community and in the workplace to enable them to continue breastfeeding as long as possible. Maintaining milk supply depends largely on frequency and adequacy of maternal stimulation through breastfeeding and through pumping when mother and baby are separated. The American College of Obstetricians and Gynecologists recommends that exclusive breastfeeding be continued until the infant is approximately 6 months old. A longer breastfeeding experience is, of course, beneficial. The professional objectives are to encourage and enable as many women as possible to breastfeed and to help them continue as long as possible (3, 4). Physicians' offices can set the example in encourag-

ing and welcoming breastfeeding through staff training, office environment, awareness and educational materials, and supportive policies (3, 4).

More detailed information on breastfeeding and practical strategies for support can be found in the *ACOG Clinical Review* "Special Report From ACOG, Breastfeeding: Maternal and Infant Aspects" and in the American Academy of Pediatrics and ACOG resource, *Breastfeeding Handbook for Physicians* (3, 4).

References

1. U.S. Department of Health and Human Services. Increase in the proportion of mothers who breastfeed their babies. In: Healthy people 2010: objectives for improving health. 2nd ed. Washington, DC: U.S. Government Printing Office; 2000. p. 16–46.

2. Centers for Disease Control and Prevention. Breastfeeding: data and statistics: breastfeeding practices—results from the 2005 National Immunization Survey. Atlanta (GA): CDC. Available at: http://www.cdc.gov/breastfeeding/data/NIS_data/data_2005.htm. Retrieved November 14, 2006.

3. American Academy of Pediatrics, American College of Obstetricians and Gynecologists. Breastfeeding handbook for physicians. Elk Grove Village (IL): AAP; Washington, DC: ACOG; 2006.

4. American College of Obstetricians and Gynecologists. Breastfeeding: maternal and infant aspects. Special report from ACOG. ACOG Clin Rev 2007;12(suppl):1S–16S.

5. American College of Obstetricians and Gynecologists. Breastfeeding. ACOG Executive Board Statement. Washington, DC; ACOG: 2003. Available at: http://www.acog.org/departments/underserved/breastfeedingStatement.pdf. Retrieved November 1, 2006.

Breastfeeding: maternal and infant aspects. ACOG Committee Opinion No. 361. American College of Obstetricians and Gynecologists. Obstet Gynecol 2007;109:479–80.

12345/10987

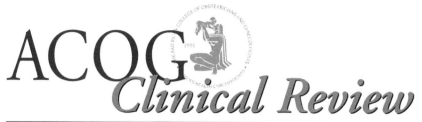

Appendix E

Volume 12 • Issue 1 (Supplement)   January–February 2007

SPECIAL REPORT FROM ACOG

Breastfeeding: Maternal and Infant Aspects

Committee on Health Care for Underserved Women
Committee on Obstetric Practice

The promotion of breastfeeding has been an ongoing priority of the College. Working with national and international groups dedicated to promoting the health of infants worldwide, ACOG has participated in an interdisciplinary group effort to formulate guidelines for breastfeeding. These guidelines were developed by the ACOG Committee on Health Care for Underserved Women and the ACOG Committee on Obstetric Practice and are presented in this special report in an effort to give them the widest possible exposure and eventually reach those who would benefit most—mothers and their babies. These guidelines, as well as additional information, can be found at www.acog.org.

Ralph W. Hale, MD
ACOG Executive Vice President

ABSTRACT: *Evidence continues to mount regarding the value of breastfeeding for both women and their infants. Human milk provides developmental, nutritional, and immunologic benefits to the infant that cannot be duplicated by formula feeding. Breastfeeding also provides significant benefits to women. It is critical that women make an informed choice in deciding what is best for them, their families, and their babies. The American College of*

Obstetricians and Gynecologists strongly supports breastfeeding and calls on its Fellows, other health care professionals caring for women and their infants, hospitals, and employers to support women in choosing to breastfeed their infants. Specifically, obstetrician–gynecologists and other health care professionals caring for pregnant women should regularly impart accurate information about breastfeeding to expectant mothers and be prepared to support them should any problems arise while breastfeeding.

BACKGROUND

With the development of iron-fortified formula, breastfeeding rates began to decrease in the late 1950s as formula feeding gained popularity. In 1971, only 24.7% of mothers left the hospital breastfeeding. Since that time, breastfeeding initiation rates have been increasing fairly consistently, but they have not yet reached the goal set by the U.S. Public Health Service for Healthy People 2010 (1). In 2005, 72.9% of all U.S. mothers initiated breastfeeding (2). Although this is close to the target rate of 75% in the early postpartum period, there is still a long way to go to achieve breastfeeding rates of 50% at 6 months, and 25% at 12 months (1).

The increase in the proportion of women initiating breastfeeding reflects a growing awareness of the advantages of breast milk over formula. Improvement in breastfeeding initiation rates, however, has been uneven, as women attempt to overcome practical obstacles. Breastfeeding initiation rates are lowest among non-Hispanic black women, women younger than 20 years, women enrolled in WIC (Special Supplemental Nutrition Program for Women, Infants, and Children), and those who completed high school or less. Breastfeeding initiation rates vary considerably by state with the lowest rates (less than 55%) occurring in Arkansas, Kentucky, Louisiana, Mississippi, and West Virginia (2).

In 2005, the rate of any breastfeeding at 6 months reached 39.1%, the highest rate in the nearly 35 years such data have been collected. The lowest 6-month rates are among mothers with the same demographic and socioeconomic characteristics as those who have the lowest breastfeeding initiation rates (2).

The sharpest decrease in breastfeeding (approximately 20%) occurs within the first month after discharge. Accounting for this precipitous decrease, the most common reasons given for

ACOG
Clinical Review

Morton A. Stenchever, MD
Editor

Ralph W. Hale, MD
Associate Editor

Nancy Rowe
Managing Editor

🍃

The ACOG Committee on Health Care for Underserved Women and the ACOG Committee on Obstetric Practice would like to thank Sharon Mass, MD, for her contributions to the development of this document.

🍃

premature discontinuation are insufficient milk production, difficulty with attachment (latch-on and infant suckling), and lack of maternal confidence (3–6). Some concentrated educational efforts have had a statistical impact in specific populations (7). Compared with other demographic groups, the breastfeeding initiation rates increased most rapidly among black women between 1993 and 2003. However, despite this welcome trend, the breastfeeding rates at hospital discharge in 2003 remained lowest among black women at 48.3% compared with national rates of 66.0%. Additionally, women enrolled in WIC are among those with the most rapid increases in rates of breastfeeding, although their rates remain well below national averages (8).

This document addresses primarily breastfeeding by healthy mothers with healthy infants born at term. Human milk and breastfeeding are recommended for premature newborns and mother–infant pairs with other special needs; however, specific information in this regard is beyond the scope of this document.

BENEFITS OF BREASTFEEDING

Research in the United States and throughout the world indicates that breastfeeding and human milk provide benefits to infants, women, families, and society. This research has been conducted in a variety of settings, resulting in information derived from culturally and economically diverse populations.

In 2005, the American Academy of Pediatrics (AAP) published a revised policy statement, "Breastfeeding and the Use of Human Milk" (9). The statement was developed by the AAP Section on Breastfeeding, which evaluated the considerable amount of research literature on relationships between breastfeeding and infant health and development. The statement summarizes established infant protective effects, as well as positive associations that require further study (see box). Many of the benefits of breastfeeding for both the mother and infant are

recognized to be enhanced by exclusivity and duration (9). Early studies, which failed to account for these factors, led to inconsistent conclusions. Obstetrician–gynecologists who review these sources of evidence for infant benefit will be better prepared to care for the women in their practices.

Infants

The benefits of breastfeeding for the infant have been established in the following areas. Human milk provides species-specific and age-specific nutrients for the infant (10). Colostrum, the fluid secreted from the breast immediately after the infant's birth, conveys a high level of immune protection, particularly secretory immunoglobulin A (IgA). During the first 4–7 days after birth, protein and mineral concentrations decrease, and water, fat, and lactose increase. Milk composition continues to change to match infant nutritional needs. In addition to the right balance of nutrients and immunologic factors, human milk contains factors that act as biologic signals for promoting cellular growth and differentiation. Human milk also contains multiple substances with antimicrobial properties, which protect against infection (10, 11). However, human milk alone may not provide adequate iron for infants older than 6 months, infants whose mothers have low iron stores, and premature infants at all ages (11).

Women

The benefits of breastfeeding for women are well documented. Benefits start in the immediate postpartum period with the release of oxytocin during milk letdown. This results in increased uterine contractions aiding with uterine involution and a decrease in maternal blood loss (12). Additionally, evidence exists that oxytocin and prolactin contribute to the mother's feelings of relaxation and of her attachment to her baby. Breastfeeding also is associated with a decreased risk of developing ovarian and breast cancer (13–15). Moreover, breastfeeding delays postpartum ovulation, supporting birth spacing (16–18).

Research on Established and Potential Protective Effects of Human Milk and Breastfeeding on Infants

According to the American Academy of Pediatrics' policy statement, "Breast-feeding and the Use of Human Milk," the findings of extensive research suggest various benefits of breastfeeding as indicated in the following excerpt.

Infectious Diseases
Research in developed and developing countries of the world, including middle-class populations in developed countries, provides strong evidence that human milk feeding decreases the incidence and/or severity of a wide range of infectious diseases including bacterial meningitis, bacteremia, diarrhea, respiratory tract infection, necrotizing enterocolitis, otitis media, urinary tract infection, and late-onset sepsis in preterm infants. In addition, postneonatal infant mortality rates in the United States are reduced by 21% in breastfed infants.

Other Health Outcomes
Some studies suggest decreased rates of sudden infant death syndrome in the first year of life and reduction in incidence of insulin-dependent (type 1) and non-insulin-dependent (type 2) diabetes mellitus, lymphoma, leukemia, and Hodgkin disease, overweight and obesity, hypercholesterolemia, and asthma in older children and adults who were breastfed, compared with individuals who were not breastfed. Additional research in this area is warranted.

Neurodevelopment
Breastfeeding has been associated with slightly enhanced performance on tests of cognitive development. Breastfeeding during a painful procedure such as a heel-stick for newborn screening provides analgesia to infants.

Breastfeeding and the use of human milk. AAP Policy Statement. American Academy of Pediatrics. Section on Breastfeeding. Pediatrics 2005;115:496–506.

(To review the full-text AAP document online with complete references, go to http://pediatrics. aappublications.org/cgi/reprint/115/2/496.)

Although breastfeeding causes some bone demineralization, studies indicate that "catch-up" remineralization occurs after weaning. Importantly, clinical studies have demonstrated a protective effect of breastfeeding, such as a lower incidence of osteoporosis and hip fracture after menopause (19, 20).

Families and Society

Studies indicate that the breastfed child has fewer illnesses and, therefore, fewer visits to the doctor and hospital (21). This translates into lower medical expenses and, for women who work outside the home, less absenteeism from work. Because women now constitute a large portion of the workforce, improvement in work productivity may be significant for society as well. More than 60% of all women return to outside employment during the first year after birth of a child.

Breastfeeding, while demanding maternal time and attention, can save families and public programs consider-able money compared with formula feeding (22). Society may benefit as well when the ecologic issues of disposal of formula cans, bottles, and bottle liners are considered.

OBSTACLES TO BREASTFEEDING

Women need to know that breastfeeding, like other aspects of having a new baby, has its demands as well as its rewards. Women who initiate breastfeeding should be assured that they will have support and that there are options for problem solving and professionals available to help address the difficulties they may encounter. Any doubts a woman has regarding her ability or willingness to continue or potential barriers to breastfeeding should be discussed and she should be encouraged to try breastfeeding. Physicians and other health professionals should recognize the potential effectiveness of applying their knowledge and skills to encourage and support women in initiating and continuing breastfeeding. Studies support the influence of the physician's recommendation to breastfeed exclusively, even when mothers have not made a clear choice to do so. For example, physicians who express support for exclusive breast-feeding have a higher percentage of mothers who breastfeed for an extended period (4, 23).

Modern society has created obstacles to breastfeeding that may contribute to the low percentage of mothers (13.9% in 2005) breastfeeding exclusively at 6 months postpartum (2). Short hospital stays make the teaching of breastfeeding a challenge. Lack of spousal or partner support and family customs may discourage breastfeeding. Although some employers recognize that encouraging breastfeeding as a policy improves employee morale and decreases absenteeism (24, 25), having to return to work may still be an obstacle. An unfriendly social environment may also make it difficult to breastfeed in public. Although the effect of these obstacles can be mitigated by educating the families, employers, and society, some women will decide that the challenges outweigh the benefits for themselves and their babies.

WHO CAN BREASTFEED

Nearly every woman can breastfeed her child. Mother and newborn can more easily learn the basics and how to deal with the challenges if they have skilled and experienced support. The patient population for maternity services has changed dramatically over the past decade with an increase in the percentage of mother–infant dyads with risk factors for breastfeeding problems. These include mothers who have cesarean deliveries, have multiple births, have near term infants, had breast surgery, or have been separated from their infants (6, 26, 27). Women who have cesarean deliveries should be reassured that they can breastfeed their newborns as well as women who have vaginal deliveries. With early identification and proactive management, additional support can be focused on promoting the three key factors: the establishment of adequate milk production, attachment (latch-on and infant suckling), and maternal confidence. With an increase in the percentage of mothers with risk factors for breastfeeding problems, physicians should recognize opportunities in the early postpartum period for preventive management.

Some women are incorrectly informed, or assume, they cannot breastfeed because of their anatomy or other special circumstances, such as women who have inverted nipples or have had breast surgery. In reality, these circumstances do not necessarily prevent breastfeeding. True inverted nipples are rare. If milk production can be established by means of hand or electrical expression, inverted nipples should not preclude breast-milk feeding or direct breastfeeding with the use of a silicone nipple shield. Most women with nipples that appear flat or inverted can breastfeed given appropriate assistance in the early days of lactation. Pumping for a minute or two before offering the breast to the newborn has been shown to facilitate latch-on (10). Lactation is possible for women who have had breast surgery unless it involved the complete severing of the lactiferous ducts. Women may breastfeed after reduction mammoplasty, depending on the degree of interruption to the ductile system (28). Those who have had augmentation mammoplasty may facilitate breastfeeding through frequent emptying during the time of lactogenesis. Breast biopsies involving an areolar incision have the potential to be problematic, but women can compensate by augmenting production on the uninvolved side. Women with periareolar incisions and women who have had breast reductions should be counseled about monitoring infant growth because they are at increased risk of producing an insufficient supply of milk. Pierced nipples have not been associated with breastfeeding difficulties unless there is infection or scarring. Nipple devices should be removed before feeding to avoid the risk of infant choking (29). Women with hypoplastic or tubular breasts may have difficulty producing suf-

ficient milk and should seek specialized advice; this condition is rare.

Some babies with cleft lips or palates may be able to breastfeed. The soft breast tissue may fill the defect and enable the infant to develop a seal. Sometimes a palatal obturator allows the infant to breastfeed and not aspirate milk. Mothers with premature infants can breastfeed. However, a premature infant has special nutritional needs. In all of these situations, evaluation by experts may be beneficial.

WHO SHOULD NOT BREASTFEED

Although it is true that most women can breastfeed, there are exceptional circumstances. All clinicians should understand these exceptions so that a patient's frustration and disappointment can be minimized. The contraindications to breastfeeding are few (9, 30). Women who should not breastfeed are those who:

- Take street drugs or do not control alcohol use (9)
- Have an infant with galactosemia (9)
- Have certain infections, such as human immunodeficiency virus (HIV); human T-cell lymphotropic virus type I or type II; active, untreated tuberculosis or varicella; or active herpes simplex with breast lesions (10)
- Are taking antineoplastic, thyrotoxic, and immunosuppressive agents (9, 10, 31)
- Take certain medications or are undergoing treatment for breast cancer (10, 31)

Drugs ingested by a woman can be transmitted to her newborn through breastfeeding. If the effect of the drug on the newborn is detrimental, or questionable, it should be avoided. This is especially true of alcohol and illicit drugs. Alcohol is a toxin. A woman who drinks significant amounts of alcohol should not breastfeed (11). Information on infant exposure to street drugs in breast milk, such as cocaine, 3,4-methylenedioxymethamphetamine (MDMA), lysergic acid diethylamide (LSD), phencyclidine (PCP), and heroin, can be found in

ACOG's resource *Special Issues in Women's Health* (32). There is evidence that women who participate in a successful methadone maintenance program may breastfeed (31).

Infants with galactosemia should neither breastfeed nor consume any formula containing lactose (eg, cows' milk) because doing so will exacerbate the condition. These infants should be fed special lactose-free formula.

Some infections contraindicate breastfeeding; others require precautions. Approaches to breastfeeding vary according to the infection and the environment. Information about breastfeeding in relation to common maternal infections is available for further reference (10). Highlights of this information follow.

Women in the United States who have human immunodeficiency virus (HIV) or human T-cell lymphotropic virus infections should not breastfeed because breast milk can transmit these infections to the infant. In some countries with high infant mortality rates, however, the benefits of breastfeeding in providing nutrition and preventing infections may still outweigh the risks of transmitting HIV or human T-cell lymphotropic virus.

If a woman has active pulmonary tuberculosis, the repeated and prolonged close contact involved in feeding exposes the infant to risk of airborne infection. Therefore, the woman should not be in contact with her baby until she has been adequately treated and is considered to be noncontagious. The infant can be given the mother's expressed breast milk because it does not contain *Mycobacterium tuberculosis* (10).

A woman with active varicella (chickenpox) lesions should neither breastfeed nor bottle-feed her infant. She should be isolated from the infant while she is clinically infectious. Once the infant has received varicella-zoster immune globulin (10), the woman can provide expressed breast milk for the infant if there are no skin lesions on the breasts. She can resume breastfeeding when she is no longer clinically infectious. An immunocompetent woman who develops herpes zoster infection (shingles) can continue breastfeeding if lesions are covered and are not on the breast. Maternal antibodies delivered through the placenta and breast milk will prevent the disease or diminish its severity. An infant may be given varicella-zoster immune globulin to reduce risk of transmission (10). Breastfeeding also is contraindicated in women who have active herpes simplex infections on the breast until the lesions are cleared.

Hepatitis infections do not preclude breastfeeding. With appropriate immunoprophylaxis, including hepatitis B immune globulin and hepatitis vaccine, breastfeeding of babies born to women positive for hepatitis B surface antigen poses no additional risk for the transmission of hepatitis B virus (33). If a woman has acute hepatitis A infection, her infant can breastfeed after receiving immune serum globulin and vaccine (10). The average rate of hepatitis C virus (HCV) infection reported in infants born to HCV-positive women is 4% for both breastfed and bottle-fed infants. Therefore, maternal HCV is not considered a contraindication to breastfeeding (34).

In women with cytomegalovirus infection, both the virus and maternal antibodies are present in breast milk. Because of this, otherwise healthy infants born at term with congenital or acquired cytomegalovirus infections usually are not affected by the virus if they are breastfed. A study of infants who developed infections during breastfeeding found that the infants also developed an immune response, did not develop the disease, and rarely manifested symptoms (30).

Many medications are compatible with breastfeeding (31). Information about the current data on the transfer of drugs and other chemicals in human milk can be found in the AAP/ACOG resource *Breastfeeding Handbook for Physicians* (see "Resources"). There is also a new online National Library of Medicine database on drugs and lactation available at http://toxnet.nlm.nih.gov/. Generally, breastfeeding is contraindicated for women taking antineoplastic, thyrotoxic, and immunosuppressive agents. Similarly, women who are receiving therapeutic radioactive isotopes or undergoing chemotherapy or radiation therapy should not breastfeed (31, 33, 35). Medications with relative contraindications may sometimes be used cautiously by timing doses to immediately follow a feeding (35). Diagnostic radioactive isotopes require temporary interruption of breastfeeding. For additional information, refer to guidelines developed by the Nuclear Regulatory Commission (36).

PRECONCEPTION AND PRENATAL EDUCATION ON BREASTFEEDING

The health benefits of breastfeeding and the health risks of not breastfeeding warrant professional cooperation and coordination among all health care workers to educate and encourage women and their families to choose breastfeeding. Patient education materials can reinforce the message (see "Resources"). The obstetrician–gynecologist has many opportunities during periodic gynecologic examinations and prenatal visits to promote breastfeeding, allay a woman's anxieties, and suggest solutions or resources to make breastfeeding a practical choice for the patient and her family.

Periodic Gynecologic Examinations

Obstetrician–gynecologists can advocate breastfeeding to all reproductive-aged women by mentioning breastfeeding during the breast examination portion of routine gynecologic visits, if appropriate. Women whose breast anatomy appears to be normal can be told that if they decide to have a baby, there are no structural impediments to breastfeeding.

Prenatal Visits

Teaching the pregnant woman and her partner about childbirth and breastfeeding is an integral part of good prenatal care. Other family members who could support breastfeeding may be included. Education can occur in the physician's office or clinic. The advice and encouragement of the obstetrician–gynecologist are critical in making the decision to breastfeed. Other health professionals, such as pediatricians, nurses, and certified lactation specialists, also play an important role. Alternatively, hospitals and other organizations, including mother-to-mother groups and other lay organizations, can provide education for pregnant women and their partners.

Some women who choose to breastfeed were breastfed themselves or had a sibling who was breastfed, which established it as normal behavior in their household. These women would probably benefit from some education and reinforcement concerning breastfeeding. Women whose family and friends have not shared breastfeeding experiences also approach pregnancy with a desire to do what is healthiest for their babies. Guidance and consideration of life situations are important in helping these women and their families make a decision about feeding their infants. Information about the benefits and challenges of breastfeeding compared with the use of formula will help them make good decisions.

The initial prenatal visit is an optimal time to encourage or reinforce the decision to breastfeed. Most patients seek information and guidance from their physicians, and the importance of the physician's recommendation should never be underestimated. A large percentage of women make decisions about infant feeding before pregnancy or in the first trimester. The first visit is, therefore, an ideal time to emphasize the advantages of breastfeeding compared with formula feeding, as well as the advantages of exclusive breastfeeding. Mothers who intend to combine breastfeeding and bottle-feeding rather than exclusively breastfeeding are less likely to reach their own breastfeeding goals (37). Some experts suggest replacing the question, "Are you planning to bottle-feed or breastfeed?" with statements that do not equate the two feeding methods. Suggested statements that would promote discussion include, "Have you noticed your breasts are changing in preparation for feeding your baby?" or "What have you heard about breastfeeding?" Barriers should be explored to determine if they can be addressed in such a way as to encourage breastfeeding. During the breast examination, the physician can perform a breastfeeding-specific examination and answer any questions about the usual pattern of changes in the breasts during pregnancy and breastfeeding. If there are no structural problems, the woman can be reassured about her ability to breastfeed. If her nipples appear to be inverted, she should know that appearance is not necessarily prognostic and she may be able to breastfeed. The techniques to assist in nipple eversion, however, are not recommended during pregnancy because there is no evidence to support their effectiveness (10). Any abnormal breast masses noted on this examination should be adequately explored with the use of technology such as ultrasonography and, possibly, biopsy as indicated.

Prenatal Breastfeeding Instruction

Today, with shorter postpartum hospital stays, it is important for pregnant women to come to the hospital for delivery with a good foundation of knowledge gained during the antepartum period. Prenatal education groups have been shown to be particularly effective in increasing duration of breastfeeding (38). Education in the hospital can then focus on operational aspects of breastfeeding such as latch-on and feeding techniques.

A woman who is appropriately counseled on breastfeeding options and chooses not to breastfeed should be reassured that her milk production will abate during the first few days after delivery. Hormone treatment to stop milk production is no longer recommended. Current recommendations include a well-fitted support bra, analgesics, and ice packs to relieve the pain. She also can be assured that if she changes her mind, she may still be able to initiate breastfeeding within the first few days postpartum. Several hospital protocols and practices have been shown to increase rates of successful breastfeeding (see the box) (39).

LABOR

Certain pain management interventions in labor may decrease breastfeeding initi-

ation rates. To support a mother's desire to breastfeed, pain management should be balanced to ensure pain relief for the mother while avoiding excessive amounts of medication, particularly narcotics that can adversely affect the infant's ability to breastfeed effectively. Although cesarean delivery may make breastfeeding more challenging (29), patients who have a cesarean delivery should still be encouraged to breastfeed. Women undergoing cesarean deliveries using a regional anesthetic or under nonemergent situations are more likely to initiate and continue breastfeeding than those who have undergone an emergency cesarean delivery or received general anesthesia (40).

DELIVERY

The immediate postpartum period should allow the woman and her newborn to experience optimal bonding with immediate physical contact, preferably skin to skin. Separation may lead to complications such as hypothermia and hypoglycemia, increasing the likelihood

of supplementation. The initial feeding should occur as soon after birth as possible, preferably in the first hour when the baby is awake, alert, and ready to suckle. The longer the interval between birth and the first feeding, the more likely the use of supplementation (41). Newborn eye prophylaxis, weighing, measuring, and other such examinations should be deferred until after the first feeding or until they can take place without separating the infant from the mother (9). Such procedures usually can be performed later in the woman's room.

POSTPARTUM SUPPORT FOR BREASTFEEDING

All hospitals should have trained personnel available to provide breastfeeding support and should offer 24-hour rooming-in to maximize the interaction between the woman and the newborn. Rooming-in allows the mother to begin recognizing her infant's hunger cues. Rooming-in and promoting skin-to-skin contact have numerous advantages for

---

Ten Hospital Practices to Encourage and Support Breastfeeding*

1. Maintain a [supportive] written breastfeeding policy that is communicated to all health care staff.
2. Train all pertinent health care staff in skills necessary to implement this policy.
3. Inform all pregnant women about the benefits of breastfeeding.
4. Offer all mothers the opportunity to initiate breastfeeding within 1 hour of birth.
5. Show breastfeeding mothers how to breastfeed and how to maintain lactation even if they are separated from their infants.
6. Give breastfeeding infants only breast milk unless medically indicated.
7. Facilitate rooming-in; encourage all mothers and infants to remain together during their hospital stay.
8. Encourage unrestricted breastfeeding when baby exhibits hunger cues or signals or on request of mother.
9. Encourage exclusive suckling at the breast by providing no pacifiers or artificial nipples.
10. Refer mothers to established breastfeeding and/or mothers' support groups and services, and foster the establishment of those services when they are not available.

*The 1994 report of the Healthy Mothers, Healthy Babies National Coalition Expert Work Group recommended that the UNICEF-WHO Baby Friendly Hospital Initiative be adapted for use in the United States as the United States Breastfeeding Health Initiative, using the adapted 10 steps above.

Healthy Mothers, Healthy Babies National Coalition. Baby friendly hospital initiative feasibility study: final report. Alexandria (VA): HMHB; 1994.

both the infant and mother. Infants cry less, sleep more, and become adept at breastfeeding sooner (41, 42). Mothers also sleep better and have increased milk production (43, 44). Separation of a breastfeeding woman and newborn should be avoided whenever possible. Most newborn care and procedures, including bathing, blood drawing, physical examinations, and administration of medication and phototherapy, can be performed in the mother's room (9). In this way, mother and baby can benefit together from the nursing care available.

POSTPARTUM EDUCATION ON BREASTFEEDING

Instruction During Hospital Stay

Hospital personnel should have adequate time allotted to each patient, no matter when the delivery occurs, and provide a specific program on practical aspects of breastfeeding that women master before discharge. Trained staff should assess breastfeeding behavior of the woman and newborn during the first 24–48 hours after birth for correct nursing positions, latch-on, and adequacy of newborn milk transfer (9). They also should ensure that the woman is skilled in the technique of manual expression of milk. Milk expressed by hand into a plastic spoon can be fed to the infant. This simple skill can help augment milk production and feed the sleepy baby or one who latches poorly. If the mother becomes engorged at home, she will know from this instruction how to soften the breast, feed the baby, and preserve production. During a rooming-in experience, a woman can learn to observe and respond to her newborn's signs of hunger, such as increased alertness or activity, mouthing, or rooting. She should understand that crying is a late sign of hunger. Personnel should teach mothers that newborns need to be breastfed on demand approximately 8–12 times every 24 hours until satiety (9); time at the breast varies and often is 10–15 minutes on each breast, and breastfeeding should not be limited unless a mother experiences soreness.

Instructions should indicate that breastfeeding should not be painful, but minor discomfort is common during the first 2 weeks. Discomfort may occur temporarily as the woman's milk is beginning to be produced. A physician should assess any significant pain or tenderness promptly. Generally, painful breastfeeding almost always results from poor positioning or latch-on, which should be immediately corrected, rather than from breastfeeding "too long." ACOG's "Breastfeeding Your Baby" pamphlet is a resource that can be used to help women with positioning and latch-on (see "Resources"). Latch-on is one of the most important steps to successful breastfeeding (see the box). Several helpful approaches are reviewed in greater depth in the *Breastfeeding Handbook for Physicians* (see "Resources").

Instructions for the First Week of Breastfeeding

Before discharge the woman should be educated about indicators of adequate intake and informed that for most breastfeeding infants, no water is required. She also should be educated about age-appropriate elimination patterns of her newborn during the first week after birth. At least six urinations per day and three to four bowel movements per day are to be expected by 5–7 days of age. She can be shown how to keep simple records for the first few weeks, noting the frequency and length of feedings and the number of bowel movements and wet diapers, for discussion with her health care providers. Although new, more absorbent diapers make it difficult to assess frequency of urination, a simple gage of adequate breast-milk intake is loose, bright-yellow bowel movements by day 5. She should understand expected patterns of newborn weight loss and gain. Before gaining weight, the breastfeeding newborn may lose 5–7% of birth weight in the first week. When the loss is greater than 5–7% or reaches that level in the first 3 days, a clinician should evaluate the breastfeeding process to address any problems before they become serious. A weight loss of up to 10% is the maximum that is acceptable only if all else is going well and the physical examination findings are negative for problems. Follow-up should confirm that the newborn is beginning to regain weight after the first week (10). Continued meconium elimination by

---

Positioning and Latch-On for Breastfeeding

When observing an infant being breastfed, take note of the following:

- Position of mother, body language, and tension. Pillows may provide support for the arms or the infant.
- Position of infant: Ventral surface should be to mother's ventral surface, with lower arm, if not swaddled, around mother's thorax. Infant cannot swallow if head has to turn to breast, and grasp of areola will be poor. Infant's head should be in crook of arm and moved toward breast by the mother's arm movement if cradle hold is used.
- Position of mother's hand on breast not in way of proper grasp by infant
- Position of infant's lips on areola about 1–1½ inches (2.5–3.7 cm) from base of nipple
- Lips flanged and lower lip not folded in so that infant does not suck it
- Actual events around the presenting breast to assist infant in latching on
- The infant's response to lower lip stimulus by opening mouth wide
- The motions of the masseter muscle during suckling and sounds of swallowing indicative of appropriate suckling
- Ratio of sucks to swallows becomes 1:1 as feeding progresses
- Mother comfortable with no breast pain

Modified from Lawrence RA, Lawrence RM. Breastfeeding: a guide for the medical profession. 6th ed. Philadelphia (PA): Elsevier Mosby; 2005, with permission from Elsevier.

day 5 also should prompt further evaluation of the breastfeeding process.

Phone-In Resource

The departure of a woman and her newborn from the hospital can be a joyous but daunting experience. The family is now responsible for the care and feeding of the newborn. Whether or not they have a support system at home, a phone-in resource is needed for ongoing instruction and advice. The obstetrician–gynecologist's office, the place where the woman has received most of her care, should be that resource or at least provide links to other resources in the community, such as lactation specialists and support groups. Many times these specialists and groups are available through local hospitals.

POSTPARTUM CARE

All breastfeeding women and their babies should be seen by a pediatrician or other knowledgeable health care practitioner when the baby is 3–5 days old (9). Timing depends in part on time of discharge from the hospital and other risk factors such as those for hyperbilirubinemia (45). This early visit is important in order to evaluate health status of the newborn (eg, weight, hydration, and hyperbilirubinemia) at this critical age, as well as to observe the woman and newborn during breastfeeding. Breastfeeding infants should have a second ambulatory care visit at 2–3 weeks of age to further monitor weight gain and provide ongoing support to the mother (9).

Women can be reassured that eating a well-balanced diet generally will provide the nutrients their infants need. One exception is that many individuals do not synthesize adequate amounts of vitamin D from the sunlight. Furthermore, unprotected exposure to sunlight is not recommended. For this reason vitamin D is added to milk for general consumption and to infant formula. Breastfed babies should also receive vitamin D supplementation (200 international units of oral drops daily) beginning in the first 2 months of life and continuing until daily consumption of vitamin D forti-

fied milk or formula is 500 mL (9, 46, 47) or vitamin D supplemented foods are added. Vitamin D supplementation for a woman will not significantly increase the content of vitamin D in her breast milk. In general, mothers can be reassured that the quantitative and caloric value of their breast milk will not be affected with dieting and exercise (48).

On average, it is estimated that women will need approximately 500 kcal per day more than recommended levels for nonpregnant and nonlactating women. Additional maternal food intake generally will provide additional needed vitamins and minerals (with the possible exceptions of calcium and zinc). Women of childbearing age need to maintain a calcium intake of 1,000 mg per day at all times, including during pregnancy and lactation (1,300 mg for adolescents through 18 years of age). Dietary intake is the preferred source of all needed nutrients. However, many women breastfeed on a lower calorie intake level than suggested, consuming bodily stores instead. The resultant weight loss of the mother usually does not affect breastfeeding but may result in the woman having deficiencies of magnesium, vitamin B_6, folate, calcium, and zinc (11, 47). Corrective measures can be suggested by a nutritionist for improving nutrient intakes of women with extreme or restrictive eating patterns (11). Women should be encouraged to drink plenty of fluids to satisfy their thirst and maintain adequate hydration. However, fluid intake does not affect milk volume. Breastfeeding women need not avoid spicy or strong flavored foods unless the infant seems to react negatively to specific foods.

The spouse or partner can play a vital support role for the breastfeeding woman by doing such things as bringing the newborn to her for feeding, changing the newborn, holding the newborn, and offering encouragement. Couples should be encouraged to discuss emotional adjustments to their new family status. Couples may find that caring for a baby can complicate their own rela-

tionship, including a desired resumption of sexual intercourse. Health care providers should address contraceptive needs, and the emotional adjustments, as well as physical problems of soreness, fatigue, and vaginal dryness secondary to lactation.

CONTRACEPTION

Women should be encouraged to consider their future plans for contraception and childbearing during prenatal care and be given information and services that will help them meet their goals. Many women resume intercourse before they return for their postpartum checkup and may be at risk of becoming pregnant. Avoiding unintended pregnancy is important for a woman who is breastfeeding because there will be fewer variables that can affect her milk production and nutrition status if the next pregnancy is delayed until she has completed breastfeeding (10). Most women desire a birth interval of greater than 1 year, so a discussion of contraception with both breastfeeding and nonbreastfeeding women is important. For more information on contraception and breastfeeding refer to the *Breastfeeding Handbook for Physicians* (see "Resources").

The average time to first ovulation is 45 days postpartum (range, 25–72 days) for a woman who does not breastfeed (49). In contrast, ovulation in women who breastfeed exclusively can be delayed 6 months. When carefully defined criteria are met, this can be used as a reliable natural form of family planning or birth spacing temporarily (see section on "Lactational Amenorrhea").

Nonhormonal Methods

Nonhormonal contraceptive options neither affect breastfeeding nor pose a risk to the infant. Such methods include intrauterine devices, condoms, diaphragms, or cervical caps. Intrauterine devices may be particularly well suited to breastfeeding women because they often desire highly effective long-term contraception, they are parous, and they desire a method that has no impact on breastfeeding. Diaphragms and cervical caps may need to be refitted postpartum. Prelubricated latex condoms have noncontraceptive advantages in helping to prevent sexually transmitted diseases and to relieve vaginal dryness. Female sterilization or vasectomy may be considered by couples desiring permanent birth control (49).

Hormonal Methods

Limited data exist about the impact of hormonal contraception on breastfeeding. Although some studies suggest that estrogen-containing hormonal contraceptives may decrease the amount of breastmilk produced, no well-designed randomized controlled trials have proved this association. Evidence related to the effect of progestin-only methods is similarly lacking. Package inserts recommend delaying or avoiding hormonal contraception. This reflects early concerns that have not been supported by subsequent research and experience. A recent Cochrane review concluded that evidence is insufficient to reach conclusions about the impact of hormonal contraception on breastfeeding (50). Based on clinical experience in the absence of conclusive data, ACOG makes the following practical recommendations for hormonal contraception in breastfeeding women:

* Progestin-only oral contraceptives can be prescribed or dispensed at discharge from the hospital to be started 2–3 weeks postpartum (eg, the first Sunday after the newborn is 2 weeks old).

* Depot medroxyprogesterone acetate can be initiated at 6 weeks postpartum.

* Hormonal implants can be inserted at 6 weeks postpartum.

* The levonorgestrel intrauterine system can be inserted at 6 weeks postpartum.

* Combined estrogen–progestin contraceptives, if prescribed, typically should not be started before 6 weeks postpartum, and only when lactation is well established and the infant's nutritional status is appropriate.

There are certain clinical situations in which earlier initiation might be con-

sidered, such as uncertainty about the opportunities for follow-up. Given the overall lack of data, health care providers may consider earlier initiation of progestin-only methods (eg, before hospital discharge) and initiation of estrogen-containing hormonal contraception after the period of hypercoagulability associated with pregnancy has resolved (eg, 2–4 weeks).

Lactational Amenorrhea

Women who breastfeed can make use of the natural contraceptive effect of lactation. The lactational amenorrhea method is most appropriate for women who plan to breastfeed exclusively for 6 months. If the baby is fed only breast milk or is given supplemental non-breast-milk feedings only to a minor

extent and the woman has not experienced her first postpartum menses, breastfeeding provides greater than 98% protection from pregnancy in the first 6 months after delivery (49, 51, 52). Four prospective clinical trials of the contraceptive effect of the lactational amenorrhea method demonstrated cumulative 6-month life-table, perfect-use pregnancy rates of 0.5%, 0.6%, 1.0%, and 1.5% among women who relied solely on it. To suspend fertility, women should be advised that intervals between feedings should not exceed 4 hours during the day or 6 hours at night (Fig. 1). Supplemental feedings should not exceed 5–10% of the total (53–57). For example, more than one supplemental feeding out of every 10 might increase the likelihood of returning fertility.

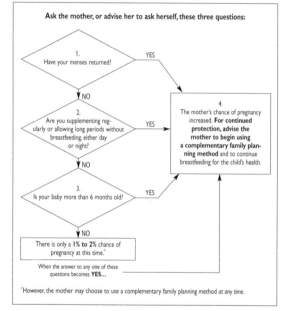

Ask the mother, or advise her to ask herself, these three questions:

1. Have your menses returned? — YES
NO ↓

2. Are you supplementing regularly or allowing long periods without breastfeeding, either day or night? — YES
NO ↓

3. Is your baby more than 6 months old? — YES
NO ↓

There is only a 1% to 2% chance of pregnancy at this time.*

When the answer to any one of these questions becomes YES...

4. The mother's chance of pregnancy increased. **For continued protection, advise the mother to begin using a complementary family planning method** and to continue breastfeeding for the child's health.

*However, the mother may choose to use a complementary family planning method at any time.

Figure 1. Algorithm for lactational amenorrhea method (LAM). (Labbok M, Cooney K, Coly S. Guidelines: breastfeeding, family panning, and the lactational amenorrhea method—LAM. Washington, DC: Institute for Reproductive Health, Georgetown University; 1994.)

Feeding practices other than direct breastfeeding, insofar as they may reduce the vigor and frequency of suckling and the maternal neuroendocrine response, increase the probability of returning ovulation (58). If there is uncertainty regarding the extent to which a woman is breastfeeding, it would be prudent to recommend additional methods of family planning.

VACCINATION

Neither inactivated nor live vaccines administered to a lactating woman affect the safety of breastfeeding for mothers or infants. Breastfeeding does not adversely affect immunization and is not a contraindication for any vaccine. Although live vaccines multiply within the mother's body, most have not been demonstrated to be excreted in human milk. Inactivated, recombinant, subunit, polysaccharide, conjugate vaccines, and toxoids pose no risk for mothers who are breastfeeding or for their infants (59). For information on vaccines, refer to *Medications and Mother's Milk* (see "Resources").

MAINTAINING MILK SUPPLY

Regular breastfeeding generally ensures adequate milk supply. As the baby grows and requires more milk, the woman's supply increases to accommodate the baby's needs. This matching of supply with demand may extend even to situations such as multiple births and continuing to breastfeed a child along with a subsequently delivered infant (tandem feeding). Avoiding unintended pregnancy is important for a woman who breastfeeds because variations in her milk production and nutrition status are minimized if she is not simultaneously breastfeeding and pregnant (10). Galactagogues, which are intended to enhance milk supply, should be used only with caution. Although some have been studied (35, 60–62), they also are used primarily outside of FDA regulation regarding content, safety, strength, and effectiveness.

BOTTLE SUPPLEMENTS AND PACIFIERS

The use of pacifiers and supplemental bottle-feeding are considered by many to be deterrents to sustained breastfeeding. However, evidence is not clear that a direct effect on breastfeeding exists (6, 63–66). Poor breastfeeding outcomes and the use of bottles and pacifiers may be common results of behaviors such as extending intervals between feedings and beginning weaning. Because introduction of a pacifier or bottle has the potential to disrupt the development of effective breastfeeding behavior, their use should be minimized until breastfeeding is well established. It is important to help mothers understand that substituting for or delaying breastfeedings may ultimately reduce milk supply because of the reduction in stimulation derived from infant suckling. Encouraging good breastfeeding practices should be the primary focus of counseling along with increasing the mother's understanding that the use of pacifiers and bottles often has been associated with reduced breastfeeding (6, 65, 66).

INTERRUPTION OF BREASTFEEDING

Separation of mother and infant should be avoided whenever possible, especially during the early establishment of lactation (first 3 weeks). If it is known in advance that hospitalization or a trip, for example, will require the mother to be separated from the infant for more than a day, careful planning can ensure that the ability to breastfeed will be preserved and breast milk will be available for the infant. During the separation, regular pumping of the breasts should be sufficient to maintain the milk supply. The milk may be saved for feeding the infant. When the separation is because of hospitalization, the milk should be discarded if it is judged to contain drugs that are contraindicated. Anesthetics are not contraindicated (67). When the mother and infant are reunited, the reestablishment of normal breastfeeding generally progresses well.

BREAST PAIN

Breast and nipple pain is a common problem for the breastfeeding woman, and is the second most common factor leading to cessation of breastfeeding (68). The cause should be diagnosed and treated promptly. Breast pain may result from engorgement, nipple pain, or mastitis.

Engorgement

Engorgement results from ineffective or infrequent removal of milk from the breast and leads to full, hard, and tender breasts. This may result from mother and infant separation, a sleepy baby, sore nipples, or improper breastfeeding technique. Prevention involves ensuring proper latch-on and milk removal and encouraging on-demand feeding (10, 68).

Nipple Pain

Sore nipples are the most common complaint raised by mothers in the immediate postpartum period. Soreness usually results from poor positioning or latch-on. Trauma, plugged ducts, candidiasis, harsh breast cleansing, or use of potentially irritating products, and skin disorders also may contribute to nipple pain. The first-line treatment should be counseling about basic latch-on techniques (69). Purified lanolin cream and breast shells (to protect the nipples from friction between feedings) may be suggested to facilitate healing (68, 70).

Mastitis

Mastitis occurs in 2–9.5% of breastfeeding women (71, 72). It most commonly occurs between the second and third weeks postpartum but may be seen any time throughout the first year (73). Mastitis is manifested by a sore, reddened area on one breast and often is accompanied by chills, fever, and malaise. The fever can be as high as 40°C. A segment of the breast becomes hard and erythematous.

The differential diagnosis includes clogged milk duct, marked breast engorgement, and a rare but lethal condition, inflammatory breast carcinoma. Clogged milk ducts present as localized

ISSN 1085-6862

tender masses. They respond to warm wet compresses and manual massage of the loculated milk toward the nipple. Breast engorgement is always bilateral with generalized involvement. It occurs most commonly in the first 2 weeks postpartum. The major feature that differentiates mastitis from inflammatory breast cancer is the knowledge of previous negative breast examination results during the pregnancy. If examination results have been normal, breast engorgement is the more likely diagnosis (71). Inflammatory breast cancer presents as unilateral erythema, heat, and induration that is more diffuse and recurrent (74).

The most common causative agent in mastitis is *Staphylococcus aureus*, occurring in 40% of cases (75). It also is the most common cause of abscess. Other common organisms in mastitis include *Haemophilus influenzae* and *H parainfluenzae*, *Escherichia coli*, *Enterococcus faecalis*, *Klebsiella pneumoniae*, *Enterobacter cloacae*, *Serratia marcescens*, group B streptococci, and *Pseudomonas pickettii* (74, 76–78).

The condition usually can be treated successfully with narrow-spectrum antibiotics (the first choice for women who are not allergic is dicloxacillin, 500 mg, four times daily for 10–14 days), hydration, bed rest, and analgesics such as acetaminophen or ibuprofen. The mother should continue to breastfeed or express the milk from both breasts because it is important to empty the affected breast. Discarding the milk from the affected breast is not recommended when a mother with mastitis is being treated, except in unusual circumstances. It does not pose a risk for the healthy, term infant. Breast milk from the unaffected breast may be used under any circumstance. The antibiotics commonly used to treat mastitis and anti-inflammatory agents, such as ibuprofen, are safe to use when breastfeeding (33, 79).

If mastitis is not treated aggressively, it may become chronic or an abscess may develop. Treatment is successful in curing mastitis if started early; the most common cause of recurrent mastitis is inadequate treatment. Delayed administration of antibiotics is associated with an increased incidence of breast abscesses. Many staphylococcal infections are caused by organisms sensitive to penicillin or a cephalosporin. Empirical treatment with dicloxacillin may be started (75, 80). Women who are allergic to penicillin may be given erythromycin. If the infection is caused by resistant, penicillinase-producing staphylococci, an antibiotic such as vancomycin or cefotetan can be used. All antibiotics should be continued until 2 days after the infection subsides, a minimum of 10–14 days.

Abscess

An abscess is diagnosed by the presence of a palpable mass or fever that fails to abate within 48–72 hours of antibiotic therapy. Generally, abscesses have been treated with incision and drainage. Multiple abscesses may require multiple incisions, with a finger inserted to break down the locules. Breast milk should be discarded for the first 24 hours after surgery, with breastfeeding resuming thereafter if there is no drainage into the breast milk (10). Recently, ultrasonographically guided needle aspiration was shown to be successful in treating abscesses (81, 82).

WORKING MOTHERS AND TIME AWAY

Many mothers are employed outside the home. In some situations they can feed their infants at work, but this is not common. Health care professionals can help the mother consider the method by which she plans to feed her infant when she returns to work. Employers are increasingly supportive of accommodating the needs of their breastfeeding employees (24). If a woman wants to continue to breastfeed or breast-milk feed, she should plan to pump her breasts to maintain her milk supply and to provide stored milk for the caregiver to feed the infant in her absence. A mother can be reassured that breastfeeding has already benefited her infant and that continuing breastfeeding and the use of breast milk to whatever degree she finds possible will be of further benefit. She also should be assured that professional support is available to help her continue breastfeeding. The physician should continue to support the woman, ultimately helping her choose the best alternative possible for feeding her infant if she chooses to stop breastfeeding.

Expressing Milk

Several methods are available to collect milk. Health care professionals should ensure that breastfeeding women can successfully express milk by hand. Because use of a breast pump is more efficient, rental or purchase of a pump can be considered. In general, electric pumps are more efficient than hand pumps. Pumping both breasts simultaneously is more effective and saves time.

On occasion, women have to educate employers about the necessity of time and location to pump breasts during the workday. The influence of the physician in creating a better environment should not be underestimated. A physician's letter or telephone call to the employer explaining how simple but vital the breastfeeding employee's needs are can be effective. Women who pump milk should have clean pumping and washing facilities available and, ideally, a refrigerator to store milk.

Storage of Milk

Human milk should be stored in a cool, safe place to maximize its preservation and minimize contamination. Breast milk can be stored in the refrigerator or on ice in glass or plastic containers. The use of refrigerated milk within 2 days is recommended, which is well before appreciable bacterial growth usually occurs. Breast milk intended for longer storage should be frozen as soon as possible and kept at the lowest and most constant temperatures available; for example, a deep freezer is preferable to a refrigerator freezer with a self-defrost cycle. Frozen milk can be stored for 3–6 months. Milk should be dated and used in date order to avoid loss of beneficial properties over time. Frozen milk can be thawed quickly under running water or gradually in the refrigerator. It should not be left out at room temperature for

ISSN 1085-6862

more than 4–8 hours, exposed to very hot water, or put in the microwave. Once the milk has thawed, it should be used within 24 hours or discarded (10, 83).

BREASTFEEDING EXPECTATIONS IN DAILY LIFE

There is an increased level of acceptance of breastfeeding nationally, but sporadic instances of authorities forbidding breastfeeding in public remain. Supportive laws and policies are becoming the norm. Recently, breastfeeding mothers have had increasing success in leading active lives. Couples commonly take their babies with them to meetings, outings, restaurants, and while traveling. Women who wish to be unobtrusive while breastfeeding their babies in public can do so.

Physicians' offices and other health care facilities should welcome and encourage breastfeeding by providing educational material and an atmosphere receptive to breastfeeding women. All staff members should be aware of the

value and importance of breastfeeding and understand that their contacts with patients can help them decide to breastfeed and encourage them to continue (see the box).

Health care providers should be aware that the giving of gift packs with formula to breastfeeding women is commonly a deterrent to continuation of breastfeeding (84, 85). A professional recommendation of the care and feeding products in the gift pack is implied. It should be recognized and explained to new mothers that formula companies try to attract the interest of pregnant women with these gift packs. Physicians may conclude that noncommercial educational alternatives or gift packs without health-related items are preferable.

HOW LONG TO BREASTFEED

During the first 6 months of life, exclusive breastfeeding is the preferred feeding approach for the healthy infant born at term. It provides optimal nutrients for

growth and development of the infant. The American College of Obstetricians and Gynecologists recommends that exclusive breastfeeding be continued until the infant is approximately 6 months old. A longer breastfeeding experience is, of course, beneficial. The professional objectives are to encourage and enable as many women as possible to breastfeed and to help them continue as long as possible. Gradual introduction of iron-enriched solid foods in the second half of the first year should complement the breast-milk diet. The AAP recommends that breastfeeding continue for at least 12 months, and thereafter for as long as is mutually desired (9). Although some women continue breastfeeding during and after a subsequent pregnancy, the mother may wish to wean when a subsequent pregnancy occurs or the infant may wean naturally. Weaning creates a hormonal milieu conducive to remineralization of bone and maternal replenishment. This may be a consideration favoring delay of the next pregnancy until the mother has completed breastfeeding.

There are no rules about when to wean. Various situations and preferences may influence the timing. Whenever possible, the weaning process should be gradual. Eliminating a feeding every 2–3 days will achieve a comfortable transition for the infant and prevent engorgement in the mother. An infant weaned before 12 months should receive iron-fortified infant formula rather than cows' milk (9). If an infant is younger than 6 months, weaning can be accomplished by substituting a bottle or cup for a breastfeeding. If an infant is 6 months or older, he or she may use a cup and substitute other foods for breastfeeding. It should be recognized that the baby may wean by itself abruptly or gradually.

Abrupt weaning can be difficult for the mother and the baby, but certain measures can be helpful. The mother should wear a support bra. She does not need to restrict fluids. She may manually express just enough milk to relieve the engorgement. Cool compresses will reduce engorgement. Hormonal therapy is not recommended.

Office Tips

- Make ACOG Patient Education Pamphlets and other patient education materials available in waiting and examination rooms.
- Offer a call-in telephone number for advice—yours or another health care resource available in the community or hospital of birth.
- Provide information about and telephone numbers of lactation consultants and resources such as La Leche League in your community.
- Show videos on breastfeeding; if women's health videos normally play in the waiting room, include those on breastfeeding so all patients see them, not just pregnant or breastfeeding patients.
- Provide seating, such as pillows and a rocking chair for women with infants, that keeps breastfeeding in mind.
- Have pumps and an appropriate room for employees and patients. If in a medical office complex with other practices, make its availability known to other employees (they may be your patients) or collaborate in setting up a room elsewhere in the building.
- Identify a staff member interested in being a special resource on breastfeeding in the office and facilitate further training for the individual in order to assist you, other staff, and patients.
- Develop breastfeeding statistics for your practice and encourage staff by showing changes over time on displays in staff areas.
- Ask about hospital policies and practices and offer to help with staff training and patient orientation materials.
- Find out about breastfeeding skills, interests, and services of family physician and pediatric colleagues in the community. Encourage women and parents to choose a supportive caregiver for the infant and meet with him or her during pregnancy.

BREAST CANCER DETECTION

Clinical breast examination and breast self-examination are recommended for breastfeeding women, just as for all women aged 19 years and older. Because of normal changes in the breasts during pregnancy and lactation, cancer detection by palpation becomes more difficult. Studies indicate there are delays in the diagnosis of breast cancer during pregnancy and lactation, including greater intervals between palpation of a lesion and diagnosis. These delays result in an increased risk of metastatic disease at diagnosis and a reduced chance of diagnosis at stage I (86). If a mass or other abnormality is detected during lactation, it should be fully evaluated, including biopsy, if indicated. Breastfeeding can continue during the evaluation. Although the milk is not affected by a mammogram, a woman may want to breastfeed her infant just before the procedure to reduce discomfort. During lactation, mammograms are less reliable because of the associated increase in breast tissue density, which may make the test more difficult to interpret (74). Ultrasound examination can provide further assistance in evaluating palpable breast masses (solid or fluid-filled) during lactation (29).

Clinical breast examinations of women who may become pregnant are especially important. Increasing age is one of many risk factors for breast cancer; this concern is especially important for women who are having babies in their late 30s and early 40s. Although regular breast examinations should continue during the 1- or 2-year period of pregnancy and lactation, detection of abnormalities may be more difficult during that time. Therefore, some women and their health care providers may consider a screening mammogram before age 40 years for women planning pregnancies in their late 30s.

EMERGING ISSUES

Environmental Toxins

Numerous national organizations have evaluated the issue of environmental contaminants in human milk. These environmental sources include food, water, air, cleaning products, and other daily exposures. Although additional research is needed, to date, there is little or no evidence of morbidity in a nursing infant from common chemical agents even though most of these substances are detectable in breast milk, including some persistent organic pollutants (87, 88).

Milk Banks

Some women who cannot breastfeed look to donor breast milk rather than formula to nourish their infants. Donor human milk is particularly beneficial for infants in neonatal intensive care units, primarily very low birth weight infants and those with gastrointestinal pathology (89). The Human Milk Bank Association of North America (HMBANA) is the only professional membership association for milk banks in Canada, Mexico, and the United States, and sets the standards and guidelines for donor screening, storage, sterilization of milk, and modern distribution methods. For more information, refer to the Human Milk Banking Association of North America at http://www.hmbana.org. In the United States, these banks have been able to meet the needs of neonatal intensive care units throughout most of the country, although priority is given to the most vulnerable infants. Locations of milk banks include Raleigh, North Carolina; San Jose, California; Denver, Colorado; Newark, Delaware; Iowa City, Iowa; and Austin, Texas. Informal sources, including Internet sites, for matching donors and families in need of human milk generally should not be recommended for safety reasons, such as transmission of infection caused by improper screening, sterilization, and storage.

CONCLUSION

In addition to supportive clinical care for their own patients, obstetrician–gynecologists should be in the forefront of fostering changes in the public environment that will support breastfeeding, whether through change in hospital practices, through community efforts, or through supportive legislation. The American College of Obstetricians and Gynecologists' Executive Board has indicated that "The American College of Obstetricians and Gynecologists strongly supports breastfeeding and calls upon its Fellows, other health professionals caring for women and their infants, hospitals, and employers to support women in choosing to breastfeed their infants. All should work to facilitate the continuation of breastfeeding in the work place and public facilities. Breastfeeding is the preferred method of feeding for newborns and infants. Health professionals have a wide range of opportunities to serve as a primary resource to the public and their patients regarding the benefits of breastfeeding and the knowledge, skills, and support needed for successful breastfeeding" (90).

With the cooperation of many dedicated health care providers, it appears that the Healthy People 2010 goals may be achievable. However, even if 75% of women initiate breastfeeding, two thirds of them will need to continue breastfeeding to reach the proposed target of 50% of all women breastfeeding at 6 months. This will be a challenge given that in 2004, the rate of any breastfeeding at 6 months was 36.2% (2). The greatest benefits for mother and infant and the best continuation rates accrue with exclusive breastfeeding in approximately the first 6 months. Obstetrician–gynecologists should ensure that women have the correct information to make an informed decision and, together with pediatricians, they should ensure that each woman has the help and support necessary to continue to breastfeed successfully (91, 92). The combined efforts of all health care providers will be necessary to meet these goals.

References

1. U.S. Department of Health and Human Services. Increase in the proportion of mothers who breastfed their babies. In: Healthy people 2010: objectives for improving health. 2nd ed. Washington, DC: U.S. Government Printing Office; 2000. p. 16-46–16-48.

2. Centers for Disease Control and Prevention. Breastfeeding: data and statistics: breastfeeding practices—results from the 2005 National Immunization Survey. Atlanta (GA): CDC. Available at: http://www.cdc.gov/breastfeeding/data/NIS_data/data_2005.htm. Retrieved November 14, 2006.

3. Ertem IO, Votto N, Leventhal JM. The timing and predictors of early termination of breastfeeding. Pediatrics 2001;107:543–8.

4. Taveras EM, Capra AM, Braveman PA, Jensvold NG, Escobar GJ, Lieu TA. Clinician support and psychosocial risk factors associated with breastfeeding discontinuation. Pediatrics 2003;112:108–15.

5. Kuan LW, Britto M, Decolongon J, Schoettker PJ, Atherton JD, Kotagal UR. Health system factors contributing to breastfeeding success. Pediatrics 1999; 104(3):e28.

6. Dewey KG, Nommsen-Rivers LA, Heinig MJ, Cohen RJ. Risk factors for suboptimal infant breastfeeding behavior, delayed onset of lactation, and excess neonatal weight loss. Pediatrics 2003;112:607–19.

7. Ryan AS. The resurgence of breastfeeding in the United States. Pediatrics 1997;99:E12.

8. Ross Products Division of Abbott Laboratories. Breastfeeding trends—2003. Columbus (OH): Abbott Laboratories. Available at: http://www.ross.com/images/library/BF_Trends_2003.pdf. Retrieved August 17, 2006.

9. Breastfeeding and the use of human milk. AAP Policy Statement. American Academy of Pediatrics. Section on Breastfeeding. Pediatrics 2005;115:496–506.

10. Lawrence RA, Lawrence RM. Breastfeeding: a guide for the medical profession. 6th ed. Philadelphia (PA): Elsevier Mosby; 2005.

11. Institute of Medicine (US). Nutrition during lactation. Washington, DC: National Academy Press; 1991.

12. Chua S, Arulkumaran S, Lim I, Selamat N, Ratnam SS. Influence of breastfeeding and nipple stimulation on postpartum uterine activity. Br J Obstet Gynaecol 1994;101:804–5.

13. Rosenblatt KA, Thomas DB. Lactation and the risk of epithelial ovarian cancer. The WHO Collaborative Study of Neoplasia and Steroid Contraceptives. Int J Epidemiol 1993;22:192–7.

14. Newcomb PA, Storer BE, Longnecker MP, Mittendorf R, Greenberg ER, Clapp RW, et al. Lactation and a reduced risk of premenopausal breast cancer. N Engl J Med 1994;330:81–7.

15. Breast cancer and breastfeeding: collaborative reanalysis of individual data from 47 epidemiological studies in 30 countries, including 50302 women with breast cancer and 96973 women without the disease. Collaborative Group on Hormonal Factors in Breast Cancer. Lancet 2002;360:187–95.

16. Kennedy KI, Visness CM. Contraceptive efficacy of lactational amenorrhoea. Lancet 1992;339:227–30.

17. Gray RH, Campbell OM, Apelo R, Eslami SS, Zacur H, Ramos RM, et al. Risk of ovulation during lactation. Lancet 1990;335:25–9.

18. Labbok MH, Colie C. Puerperium and breast-feeding. Curr Opin Obstet Gynecol 1992;4:818–25.

19. Melton LJ 3d, Bryant SC, Wahner HW, O'Fallon WM, Malkasian GD, Judd HL, et al. Influence of breastfeeding and other reproductive factors on bone mass later in life. Osteoporos Int 1993;3:76–83.

20. Cumming RG, Klineberg RJ. Breastfeeding and other reproductive factors and the risk of hip fractures in elderly women [published erratum appears in Int J Epidemiol 1993;22:962]. Int J Epidemiol 1993;22:684–91.

21. Ball TM, Wright AL. Health care costs of formula-feeding in the first year of life. Pediatrics 1999;103:870–6.

22. Montgomery DL, Splett PL. Economic benefit of breast-feeding infants enrolled in WIC. J Am Diet Assoc 1997;97:379–85.

23 Taveras EM, Li R, Grummer-Strawn L, Richardson M, Marshall R, Rego VH, et al. Opinions and practices of clinicians associated with continuation of exclusive breastfeeding. Pediatrics 2004;113:e283–90.

24. Washington Business Group on Health. Business, babies and the bottom line: corporate innovations and best practices in maternal and child health. Washington, DC: WBGH; 1996.

25. Cohen R, Mrtek MB, Mrtek RG. Comparison of maternal absenteeism and infant illness rates among breast-feeding and formula-feeding women in two corporations. Am J Health Promot 1995;10:148–53.

26. Sarici SU, Serdar MA, Korkmaz A, Erdem G, Oran O, Tekinalp G, et al. Incidence, course, and prediction of hyperbilirubinemia in near-term and term newborns. Pediatrics 2004;113:775–80.

27. Powers NG, Bloom B, Peabody J, Clark R. Site of care influences breastmilk feedings at NICU discharge. J Perinatol 2003; 23:10–13.

28. Souto GC, Giugliani ER, Giugliani C, Schneider MA. The impact of breast reduction surgery on breastfeeding performance. J Hum Lact 2003;19:43–9; quiz 66–9, 120.

29. American Academy of Pediatrics, American College of Obstetricians and Gynecologists. Breastfeeding handbook for physicians. Elk Grove Village (IL): AAP; Washington, DC: ACOG; 2006.

30. Lawrence RA. A review of the medical benefits and contraindications to breastfeeding in the United States. Maternal and Child Health Technical Information Bulletin. Arlington (VA): National Center

for Education in Maternal and Child Health; 1997.

31. The transfer of drugs and other chemicals into human milk. American Academy of Pediatrics Committee on Drugs. Pediatrics 2001;108:776–89.

32. American College of Obstetricians and Gynecologists. Special issues in women's health. Washington, DC: ACOG; 2005.

33. American Academy of Pediatrics, American College of Obstetricians and Gynecologists. Guidelines for perinatal care. 5th ed. Elk Grove Village (IL): AAP; Washington, DC: ACOG; 2002.

34. Recommendations for prevention and control of hepatitis C virus (HCV) infection and HCV-related chronic disease. Centers for Disease Control and Prevention. MMWR Recomm Rep 1998;47 (RR-19):1–39.

35. Hale TW. Maternal medications during breastfeeding. Clin Obstet Gynecol 2004; 47:696–711.

36. U.S. Nuclear Regulatory Commission. Table U.3. Activities of radiopharmaceuticals that require instructions and records when administered to patients who are breast-feeding an infant or child. In: Consolidated guidance about materials licenses. Program-specific guidance about medical use licenses. Final report. Vol. 9, Rev. 1. Washington, DC: NRC; 2005. p. U-9–U-10. Publication No. NUREG-1556. Available at: http://www.nrc.gov/reading-rm/doc-collections/nuregs/staff/sr1556/v9/r1/sr1556v9r1.pdf. Retrieved September 19, 2006.

37. Chezem J, Friesen C, Boettcher J. Breastfeeding knowledge, breastfeeding confidence, and infant feeding plans: effects on actual feeding practices. J Obstet Gynecol Neonatal Nurs 2003;32:40–7.

38. Pugin E, Valdes V, Labbok MH, Perez A, Aravena R. Does prenatal breastfeeding skills group education increase the effectiveness of a comprehensive breastfeeding promotion program? J Hum Lact 1996;12:15–9.

39. Healthy Mothers, Healthy Babies National Coalition. Baby friendly hospital initiative feasibility study: final report. Alexandria (VA): HMHB; 1994.

40. Mathur GP, Pandey PK, Mathur S, Sharma S, Agnihotri M, Bhalla M, et al. Breastfeeding in babies delivered by cesarean section. Indian Pediatr 1993;30:1285–90.

41. Kurinij N, Shiono PH. Early formula supplementation of breast-feeding. Pediatrics 1991;88:745–50.

42. Ferber SG, Makhoul IR. The effect of skin-to-skin contact (kangaroo care) shortly after birth on the neurobehavioral responses of the term newborn: a randomized, controlled trial. Pediatrics 2004; 113:858–65.

43. Quillan SI, Glenn LL. Interaction between feeding method and co-sleeping

on maternal-newborn sleep. J Obstet Gynecol Neonatal Nurs 2004;33:580–8.

44. Hurst N. Breastfeeding after breast augmentation. J Hum Lact 2003;19:70–1.

45. Management of hyperbilirubinemia in the newborn infant 35 or more weeks of gestation [published erratum appears in Pediatrics 2004;114:1138]. Pediatrics 2004;114:297–316.

46. Institute of Medicine (US). Dietary reference intakes for calcium, phosphorus, magnesium, vitamin D, and fluoride. Washington, DC: National Academy Press; 1997.

47. Gartner LM, Greer FR. Prevention of rickets and vitamin D deficiency: new guidelines for vitamin D intake. Section on Breastfeeding and Committee on Nutrition. American Academy of Pediatrics. Pediatrics 2003;111:908–10.

48. Dewey K. Effects of maternal caloric restriction and exercise during lactation. J Nutr 1998;128 (suppl):386S–389S.

49. Hatcher RA, Trussell J, Stewart FH, Nelson AL, Cates W Jr, Guest F, et al. Contraceptive technology. 18th ed. New York (NY): Ardent Media, Inc; 2004.

50. Truitt ST, Fraser A, Gallo MF, Lopez LM, Grimes DA, Schulz KF. Combined hormonal versus nonhormonal versus progestin-only contraception in lactation. Cochrane Database of Systematic Reviews 2003, Issue 2. Art. No.: CD003988. DOI: 10.1002/14651858.CD003988.

51. Kennedy KI, Rivera R, McNeilly AS. Consensus statement on the use of breastfeeding as a family planning method. Contraception 1989;39:477–96.

52. The World Health Organization multinational study of breast-feeding and lactational amenorrhea. III. Pregnancy during breast-feeding. World Health Organization. Task Force on Methods for the Natural Regulation of Fertility. Fertil Steril 1999;72;431–40.

53. Perez A, Labbok MH, Queenan JT. Clinical study of the lactational amenorrhoea method for family planning. Lancet 1992;339:968–70.

54. Ramos R, Kennedy KI, Visness CM. Effectiveness of lactational amenorrhoea in prevention of pregnancy in Manila, the Philippines: non-comparative prospective trial. BMJ 1996;313:909–12.

55. Labbok MH, Hight-Laukaran V, Peterson AE, Fletcher V, von Hertzen H, Van Look PF. Multicenter study of the Lactational Amenorrhea Method (LAM): I. Efficacy, duration, and implications for clinical application. Contraception 1997;55: 327–36.

56. Kazi A, Kennedy KI, Visness CM, Khan T. Effectiveness of the lactational amenorrhea method in Pakistan. Fertil Steril 1995;64:717–23.

57. Labbok MH, Cooney K, Coly S. Guidelines: breastfeeding, family planning, and the lactational amenorrhea method— LAM. Washington, DC: Institute for Reproductive Health; 1994.

58. Campbell OM, Gray RH. Characteristics and determinants of postpartum ovarian function in women in the United States. Am J Obstet Gynecol 1993;169:55–60.

59. Atkinson WL, Pickering LK, Schwartz B, Weniger BG, Iskander JK, Watson JC. General recommendations on immunization. Recommendations of the Advisory Committee on Immunization Practices (ACIP) and the American Academy of Family Physicians (AAFP). Centers for Disease Control and Prevention. MMWR Recomm Rep 2002;51(RR-2):1–35.

60. Academy of Breastfeeding Medicine. Protocol #9: use of galactogogues in initiating or augmenting maternal milk supply. Available at: http://www.bfmed.org/acefiles/protocol/prot9galactogoguesEnglish.pdf. Retrieved August 18, 2006.

61. Betzold CM. Galactogogues. J Midwifery Womens Health 2004;49:151–4.

62. FDA warns against using unapproved drug, domperidone, to increase milk production. FDA talk paper. Rockville (MD): U.S. Food and Drug Administration; 2004. Available at: http://www.fda.gov/bbs/topics/ANSWERS/2004/ANS01292.html. Retrieved August 29, 2006.

63. Howard CR, Howard FM, Lanphear B, deBlieck EA, Eberly S, Lawrence RA. The effects of early pacifier use on breastfeeding duration. Pediatrics 1999;103:E33.

64. Schubiger G, Schwarz U, Tonz O. UNICEF/WHO baby-friendly hospital initiative: does the use of bottles and pacifiers in the neonatal nursery prevent successful breastfeeding? Neonatal Study Group. Eur J Pediatr 1997;156:874–7.

65. Ekstrom A, Widstrom AM, Nissen E. Duration of breastfeeding in Swedish primiparous and multiparous women. J Hum Lact 2003;19:172–8.

66. Howard CR, Howard FM, Lanphear B, Eberly S, deBlieck AW, Oakes D, et al. Randomized clinical trial of pacifier use and bottle-feeding or cupfeeding and their effect on breastfeeding. Pediatrics 2003; 111:511–8.

67. Hale TW. Medications and mother's milk. 12th ed. Amarillo (TX): Hale Publishing; 2006.

68. Mass S. Breast pain: engorgement, nipple pain and mastitis. Clin Obstet Gynecol 2004;47:676–82.

69. American College of Obstetricians and Gynecologists. Breastfeeding your baby. ACOG Patient Education Pamphlet AP029. Washington, DC: ACOG; 2001.

70. Brent N, Rudy SJ, Redd B, Rudy TE, Roth LA. Sore nipples in breast-feeding women: a clinical trial of wound dressings vs conventional care. Arch Pediatr Adolesc Med 1998;152:1077–82.

71. Stehman FB. Infections and inflammations of the breast. In: Hindle WH, editor. Breast disease for gynecologists. Norwalk (CT): Appleton & Lange; 1990. p.151–4.

72. Foxman B, D'Arcy H, Gillespie B, Bobo JK, Schwartz K. Lactation mastitis: occurrence and medical management among

946 breastfeeding women in the United States. Am J Epidemiol 2002;155:103–14.

73. Niebyl JR, Spence MR, Parmley TH. Sporadic (nonepidemic) puerperal mastitis. J Reprod Med 1978;20:97–100.

74. Snyder R, Zahn C. Breast disease during pregnancy and lactation. In: Gilstrap LC 3rd, Cunningham FG, VanDorsten JP, editors. Operative obstetrics. 2nd ed. New York (NY): McGraw-Hill; 2002.

75. Matheson I, Aursnes I, Horgen M, Aabo O, Melby K. Bacteriological findings and clinical symptoms in relation to clinical outcome in puerperal mastitis. Acta Obstet Gynecol Scand 1988;67:723–6.

76. Osterman KL, Rahm VA. Lactation mastitis: bacterial cultivation of breast milk, symptoms, treatment, and outcome. J Hum Lact 2000;16:297–302.

77. Kotiw M, Zhang GW, Daggard G, Reiss-Levy E, Tapsall JW, Numa A. Late-onset and recurrent neonatal Group B streptococcal disease associated with breast-milk transmission. Pediatr Dev Pathol 2003;6: 251–6.

78. Dinger J, Muller D, Pargac N, Schwarze R. Breast milk transmission of group B streptococcal infection. Pediatr Infect Dis J 2002;21:567–8.

79. American Academy of Pediatrics. Red book. Report of the Committee on Infectious Diseases. 27th ed. Elk Grove Village (IL): AAP; 2006.

80. Hindle WH. Other benign breast problems. Clin Obstet Gynecol 1994;37: 916–24.

81. Karstrup S, Solvig J, Nolsoe CP, Nilsson P, Khattar S, Loren I, et al. Acute puerperal breast abscesses: US-guided drainage. Radiology 1993;188:807–9.

82. Christensen AF, Al-Suliman N, Nielsen KR, Vejborg I, Severinsen N, Christensen H, et al. Ultrasound-guided drainage of breast abscesses: results in 151 patients. Br J Radiol 2005;78;186–8.

83. Human Milk Banking Association of North America. Recommendations for collection, storage, and handling of a mother's milk for her own infant in the hospital setting. 3rd ed. Denver (CO): HMBANA; 1999.

84. Howard C, Howard F, Lawrence R, Andresen E, DeBlieck E, Weitzman M. Office prenatal formula advertising and its effect on breast-feeding patterns. Obstet Gynecol 2000;95:296–303.

85. Perez-Escamilla R, Pollitt E, Lonnerdal B, Dewey KG. Infant feeding policies in maternity wards and their effect on breast-feeding success: an analytical overview. Am J Public Health 1994;84:89–97.

86. Zemlickis D, Lishner M, Degendorfer P, Panzarella T, Burke B, Sutcliffe SB, et al. Maternal and fetal outcome after breast cancer in pregnancy. Am J Obstet Gynecol 1992;166:781–7.

87. PCBs in breast milk. American Academy of Pediatrics Committee on Environmental Health. Pediatrics 1994;94:122–3.

88. American Academy of Pediatrics. Pediatric environmental health. 2nd ed. Elk Grove Village (IL): AAP; 2003.

89. Schanler RJ. The use of human milk for premature infants. Pediatr Clin North Am 2001;48:207–19.

90. American College of Obstetricians and Gynecologists. Breastfeeding. ACOG Executive Board Statement. Washington, DC: ACOG; 2003. Available at: http://www.acog.org/departments/underserved/breastfeedingStatement.pdf.

91. Freed GL, Clark SJ, Cefalo RC, Sorenson JR. Breast-feeding education of obstetrics-gynecology residents and practitioners. Am J Obstet Gynecol 1995;173:1607–13.

92. Power ML, Locke E, Chapin J, Klein L, Schulkin J. The effort to increase breast-feeding: do obstetricians, in the forefront, need help? J Reprod Med 2003;48:72–8.

Resources

Patient Education Materials

American Academy of Pediatrics. Ten steps to support parents' choice to breastfeed their baby. Elk Grove Village (IL): AAP; 1999. Available at: http://www.aap.org/breastfeeding/tenSteps.pdf. Retrieved August 22, 2006.

American College of Obstetricians and Gynecologist. Breastfeeding your baby. ACOG Patient Education Pamphlet AP029. Washington, DC: ACOG; 2001. Available for purchase at http://sales.acog.org.

Breastfeeding: loving support for a bright future. Q & A. In: Physicians' breastfeeding support kit. Tampa (FL): Best Start Social Marketing; 1998. Available for purchase at http://www.beststart-inc.org/professional_education_materials.asp. Retrieved September 8, 2006.

National Healthy Mothers, Healthy Babies Coalition. Working & breastfeeding. Can you do it? Yes, you can! Alexandria (VA): NHMHB; 1997. Available for sale at http://www.hmhb.org/pub_breast.html.

References for Health Care Professionals and Patients

American Academy of Pediatrics, American College of Obstetricians and Gynecologists. Breastfeeding handbook for physicians. Elk Grove Village (IL): AAP; Washington, DC: ACOG; 2006.

American Academy of Pediatrics, American College of Obstetricians and Gynecologists. Guidelines for perinatal care. 5th ed. Elk Grove Village (IL): AAP; Washington, DC: ACOG; 2002.

Academy of Breastfeeding Medicine. Breastfeeding Medicine. New Rochelle (NY): ABM. Subscribing information is available at http://www.bfmed.org. Retrieved August 30, 2006.

Breastfeeding and the use of human milk. American Academy of Pediatrics Section on Breastfeeding. Pediatrics 2005;115:496–506.

Hale TW. Medications and mother's milk. 12th ed. Amarillo (TX): Hale Publishing; 2006.

Lawrence RA, Lawrence RM. Breastfeeding: a guide for the medical profession. 6th ed. Philadelphia (PA): Elsevier Mosby; 2005.

Physicians' breastfeeding support kit. Tampa (FL): Best Start Social Marketing; 1998. Available for purchase at http://www.beststart-inc.org/professional_education_materials.asp. Retrieved September 8, 2006.

Transfer of drugs and other chemicals into human milk. American Academy of Pediatrics Committee on Drugs. Pediatrics 2001;108:776–89.

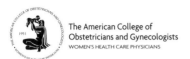

The American College of
Obstetricians and Gynecologists
WOMEN'S HEALTH CARE PHYSICIANS

COMMITTEE OPINION

Number 570 • August 2013

Committee on Health Care for Underserved Women
This information should not be construed as dictating an exclusive course of treatment or procedure to be followed.

Breastfeeding in Underserved Women: Increasing Initiation and Continuation of Breastfeeding

ABSTRACT: Maternal and infant benefits from breastfeeding are well documented and are especially important to underserved women. Underserved women are disproportionately likely to experience adverse health outcomes that may improve with breastfeeding. They face unique barriers and have low rates of initiation and continuation of breastfeeding. Through a multidisciplinary approach that involves practitioners, family members, and child care providers, obstetrician–gynecologists can help underserved women overcome obstacles and obtain the benefits of breastfeeding for themselves and their infants.

The American College of Obstetricians and Gynecologists (the College) strongly supports breastfeeding as the preferred method of feeding for newborns and infants and recommends exclusive breastfeeding until the infant is approximately 6 months of age. A longer breastfeeding experience, with gradual introduction of iron-enriched solid foods in the second half of the first year of life, is beneficial. The College calls on its Fellows, other health care professionals who provide care for women and their infants, hospitals, and employers to support women in choosing to breastfeed their infants. All should work to facilitate continuation of breastfeeding in the workplace and public facilities, and advocate for changes to the public environment that support breastfeeding locally and nationally. Although most women can breastfeed, some women will choose not to breastfeed or cannot breastfeed. Health care providers should be sensitive to the needs of women, regardless of whether or not they choose to breastfeed. Health care providers should aim to support women in the vulnerable postpartum period and encourage and assist women who choose to breastfeed and accept the decision of women who choose not to breastfeed. Additionally, health care providers should help women recognize when their newborns are getting enough nutrition and hydration through breast milk so they can confidently continue exclusive breastfeeding or seek assistance if there is a concern.

According to the 2012 Breastfeeding Report Card, 76.9% of infants in the United States were ever breastfed. However, 47.2% of infants were breastfed at 6 months, which decreased to 25.5% at 12 months (1). Although breastfeeding rates have increased over the past several years, Healthy People 2020 goals include increasing the rate of continued breastfeeding as well as improving the rate of exclusive breastfeeding (see Box 1).

Maternal and infant benefits from breastfeeding include protection from infections (2), biologic signals for promoting cellular growth and differentiation (2), decrease in maternal postpartum blood loss (3), and a reduction in the risk of ovarian and breast cancer (4–6). Despite the benefits of breastfeeding, cultural and societal barriers to breastfeeding exist at all levels; from hospitals to the workplace. Underserved women, those who are unable to obtain quality health care by virtue of poverty, cultural differences, race and ethnicity, geographic region, or other factors that contribute to health care disparities, may face greater barriers in the initiation and continuation of breastfeeding.

Overall, national estimates for breastfeeding initiation meet the Healthy People 2010 target of 75%. However, significant disparities exist with breastfeeding initiation among African American women and women in the Special Supplemental Program for Women, Infants and Children (WIC); 58.9% and 66.1% respectively (7, 8).

Age disparities also exist with initiation rates of 53.0% for women younger than 20 years compared with initiation rates of 69.0% for women aged 20–29 years and 77.5% for women aged 30 years and older (7).

Barriers to Breastfeeding

Barriers to breastfeeding are multifactorial and include socioeconomic status, education, misperceptions, and social norms. Low-income women have lower rates of breastfeeding because they are more likely to return to work sooner after giving birth and are employed in positions that make breastfeeding at work more difficult than women with higher incomes (9). The Affordable Care Act supports breastfeeding through an amendment to the Fair Labor Standards Act or federal wage and hour law. The amendment, which took effect on March 23, 2010, requires employers to provide reasonable break time and a private place, other than a bathroom, for breastfeeding mothers to express breast milk during the workday for 1 year after the infant's birth (10, 11). The absence of such requirements has been noted previously as a substantial obstacle to breastfeeding. It should be noted that employers with fewer than 50 employees may be exempt from this requirement if they are able to show that compliance would cause them undue hardship (11).

Women with a high school diploma or less are also less likely to breastfeed (12) and may be unaware of the specific benefits of breastfeeding, as well as less familiar with techniques for successful breastfeeding. Poor family and social support also can be a barrier (13). Adolescents often have their own misperceptions about breastfeeding. Common myths, such as "it creates dependency," have

been demonstrated as reasons for failure of adolescents to initiate breastfeeding (14).

Social norms also present additional barriers to breastfeeding (13). Breastfeeding in public is not a widely accepted practice. In a focus group study conducted in three major U.S. cities, both women and men expressed their disapproval of breastfeeding in public (15). Nearly all states, the District of Columbia, and the Virgin Islands have laws to support breastfeeding in public (16). Health care providers should be aware of their state or territory laws to inform and empower patients to feel comfortable breastfeeding in public. A listing of U.S. laws by state and territory is available at www.ncsl.org/issues-research/health/breastfeeding-state-laws.aspx. The social belief that formula feeding is the norm is influenced by the marketing efforts of companies that produce infant formula. Many hospitals give new mothers gift packs that include formula, and many hospitals have not developed lactation programs to provide education and support for breastfeeding. Health care providers should be aware that the giving of gift packs with formula to breastfeeding women is commonly a deterrent to continuation of breastfeeding (17). A professional recommendation of the care and feeding products in the gift pack is implied. For this reason, health care providers may conclude that noncommercial educational alternatives or gift packs without health-related items are preferable.

The effects of social norms in the United States are further demonstrated when breastfeeding rates among immigrant women are compared with those of women born in the United States. Even after controlling for socioeconomic and demographic differences, immigrant women have higher rates of initiation and duration of breastfeeding than women born in the United States (18).

Importance of Breastfeeding for Underserved Women, Children, and Society

The benefits of breastfeeding apply to all women, but particularly to underserved women (see Box 2). Underserved women have a disproportionate share of adverse health outcomes, such as obesity, diabetes, and cardiovascular disease, which may improve with breastfeeding. The prevalence of obesity is increasing nationally (19). These increases are seen particularly among underserved women and children. Women who exclusively breastfeed experience greater total body weight loss in the postpartum period than women who breastfeed and formula feed (20, 21). Some studies have suggested that the rate of childhood obesity may be decreased in children who were breastfed as infants (22). According to the Centers for Disease Control and Prevention, 12.6 million women or 10.8% of all women aged 20 years and older have diabetes, with a significant prevalence among minority populations (23). In a large prospective, longitudinal study of two cohorts of women, a reduced incidence of type 2

301

Appendix F: ACOG Committee Opinion #570: Breastfeeding in Underserved Women:
Increasing Initiation and Continuation of Breastfeeding

Box 2. Benefits of Breastfeeding ⇐

- Decreased rate of common childhood infections, such as ear infection and infection that causes diarrhea, which results in decreased parental absenteeism from work
- Decreased rates of childhood obesity in children who were breastfed as infants
- Decreased rates of hypertension, hyperlipidemia, diabetes, and cardiovascular disease among women who breastfed their infants
- Decreased rates of ovarian and breast cancer in women who breastfed their infants
- Increased bonding between mother and infant
- Lower risk of postpartum depression
- Increased postpartum weight loss
- Decreased unintended pregnancy

Data from Lawrence RA, Lawrence RM. Breastfeeding: a guide for the medical profession. 7th ed. Maryland Heights (MO): Elsevier Mosby; 2011; Chua S, Arulkumaran S, Lim I, Selamat N, Ratnam SS. Influence of breastfeeding and nipple stimulation on postpartum uterine activity. Br J Obstet Gynaecol 1994;101: 804–5; Rosenblatt KA, Thomas DB. Lactation and the risk of epithelial ovarian cancer. The WHO Collaborative Study of Neoplasia and Steroid Contraceptives. Int J Epidemiol 1993;22:192–7; Newcomb PA, Storer BE, Longnecker MP, Mittendorf R, Greenberg ER, Clapp RW, et al. Lactation and a reduced risk of premenopausal breast cancer. N Engl J Med 1994;330:81–7; and Breast cancer and breastfeeding: collaborative reanalysis of individual data from 47 epidemiological studies in 30 countries, including 50,302 women with breast cancer and 96,973 women without the disease. Collaborative Group on Hormonal Factors in Breast Cancer. Lancet 2002;360:187–95.

diabetes was associated with a longer duration of breastfeeding (24). Underserved women are also disproportionately affected by cardiovascular disease (25). Some studies indicate that women who have breastfed have lower rates of hypertension, hyperlipidemia, and cardiovascular disease compared with women who have not breastfed (26, 27).

The rate of unintended pregnancy is also higher among underserved women (28). Exclusive breastfeeding delays ovulation and increases the interval between offspring (29). Health care providers should review with patients when breastfeeding can be considered a reliable form of contraception.

Breastfeeding has a societal and socioeconomic benefit. One study estimates that $3.6 billion would be saved annually in the cost of treating some childhood illnesses if breastfeeding rates were increased (30). Children who were breastfed as infants have fewer childhood illnesses and fewer visits to the pediatrician's office, which leads to decreased parental absenteeism from work. In addition, the estimated cost of formula (up to $1,200 per year) is four times that of breastfeeding (approximately $300 per year for increased food for a lactating woman) (31).

Approaches to Improve Breastfeeding Initiation and Continuation

All practitioners, family members, and child care providers involved with the care of mothers and infants can improve rates of breastfeeding initiation and continuation. The benefits of breastfeeding, as well as patient education, counseling, and support strategies, should be emphasized during training of residents in obstetrics and gynecology, family medicine, and pediatrics. Ongoing education also should be promoted for all women's health care providers and hospital staff involved in childbirth.

Several resources are available to educate practitioners to provide breastfeeding assistance for their patients. The American Academy of Pediatrics has developed a curriculum that incorporates didactics, evaluation tools, and resources to help educate obstetrics and gynecology, pediatric, and family medicine residents in breastfeeding (www2.aap.org/breastfeeding/curriculum/). Well Start International, a non-profit organization that has promoted and supported breastfeeding for more than 25 years, offers self-study modules on lactation (www. wellstart.org). The *Breastfeeding Handbook for Physicians* provides guidance for physicians in all specialties (17). The handbook represents the collaborative efforts of the American Academy of Pediatrics and the American College of Obstetricians and Gynecologists.

Obstetrician–gynecologists should counsel patients during prenatal care about the benefits of breastfeeding, starting as early as the first trimester. Counseling to encourage breastfeeding also should involve the patient's partner, a practice shown to improve breastfeeding rates (32). Acknowledging challenges involved in breastfeeding and the difficulties many women experience while breastfeeding, and recognizing that these experiences are risk factors for postpartum depression (33), is critical. Because lack of social support can be a barrier to breastfeeding, especially among the underserved population, health care provider support and knowledge of resources are important to encourage breastfeeding. Health care providers should be aware of community resources, including prenatal lactation classes; lactation consultants; home visiting providers; and support groups, such as La Leche League, WIC peer counselors, and phone support. It is helpful for patients to learn about these resources at the time of discharge or during prenatal care. A campaign to support African American women and breastfeeding has been developed by the Office of Women's Health in the U.S. Department of Health and Human Services (www.womenshealth. gov/itsonlynatural/). The web site contains videos of African American mothers who discuss their real-life experiences with breastfeeding, as well as facts about breastfeeding and a guide to breastfeeding.

Several hospital protocols and practices have been shown to increase rates of successful breastfeeding (see Box 3) (34, 35) and should be the basis for hospital and

---

Box 3. Ten Hospital Practices to Encourage and Support Breastfeeding* ⇦

1. Maintain a (supportive) written breastfeeding policy that is communicated to all health care staff.
2. Train all pertinent health care staff in the skills necessary to implement this policy.
3. Inform all pregnant women about the benefits of breastfeeding.
4. Offer all mothers the opportunity to initiate breast feeding within 1 hour of giving birth.
5. Show breastfeeding mothers how to breastfeed and how to maintain lactation, even if they are separated from their newborns.
6. Give breastfeeding newborns only breast milk, unless medically indicated.
7. Facilitate rooming in and encourage all mothers and newborns to remain together during their hospital stay.
8. Encourage unrestricted breastfeeding when the newborn exhibits hunger cues or signals or on request of the mother.
9. Encourage exclusive suckling at the breast by providing no pacifiers or artificial nipples†.
10. Refer mothers to established breastfeeding support groups and services and foster the establishment of these services when they are not available.

Data from Healthy Mothers, Healthy Babies National Coalition. Baby friendly hospital initiative feasibility study: final report. Washington, DC: HMHBNC; 1994 and Breastfeeding and the use of human milk. Section on Breastfeeding. Pediatrics 2012;129:e827–41.

*The 1994 report of the Healthy Mothers, Healthy Babies National Coalition Expert Work Group recommended that the UNICEF-WHO Baby Friendly Hospital Initiative be adapted for use in the United States as the United States Breastfeeding Health Initiative, using the adapted 10 steps above.

†The American Academy of Pediatrics endorsed the UNICEF-WHO *Ten Steps to Successful Breastfeeding* but does not support a categorical ban on pacifiers because of their role in reducing the risk of sudden infant death syndrome and their analgesic benefit during painful procedures when breastfeeding cannot provide the analgesia.

---

nancy, or in the postpartum period, or both) in the first plan year that begins on or after August 1, 2012 (36). This also applies to the essential benefits baseline for plans sold inside the exchanges, which in turn serves as the baseline for the Medicaid benchmark plans for the new expansion population (37). Patients should be educated about this coverage.

To address lower breastfeeding rates among minorities who participate in the WIC program, WIC has introduced programs and campaigns to increase the rate of breastfeeding among its participants. As a result, from 2010 to 2011, there was a 1.5% increase in the number of WIC infants reported by WIC as being breastfed (38). This was associated with a decrease in the rate of subscription to the WIC food packages that included formula and an increase in the subscription to exclusive breastfeeding packages (39).

Summary

Breast milk is well established as the best source of nutrition for newborns and infants. Breastfeeding has many maternal, infant, and societal benefits. Although national rates of breastfeeding initiation are acceptable, the United States falls short of goals for continuation of breastfeeding, particularly among underserved populations. The College supports efforts to educate patients on the benefits and mechanics of breastfeeding, and encourages health care providers, nursing staff, and government assistance agencies to remain strong advocates for breastfeeding, including lactation programs within hospitals. A multidisciplinary approach that involves community, family, patients, and all involved clinicians will strengthen the support for and feasibility of the desired Healthy People 2020 breastfeeding goals.

References

1. Centers for Disease Control and Prevention. Breastfeeding report card—United States, 2012. Atlanta (GA): CDC; 2012. Available at: http://www.cdc.gov/breastfeeding/pdf/2012 BreastfeedingReportCard.pdf. Retrieved May 17, 2013. ⇦

2. Lawrence RA, Lawrence RM. Breastfeeding: a guide for the medical profession. 7th ed. Maryland Heights (MO): Elsevier Mosby; 2011. ⇦

3. Chua S, Arulkumaran S, Lim I, Selamat N, Ratnam SS. Influence of breastfeeding and nipple stimulation on postpartum uterine activity. Br J Obstet Gynaecol 1994;101: 804–5. [PubMed] ⇦

4. Rosenblatt KA, Thomas DB. Lactation and the risk of epithelial ovarian cancer. The WHO Collaborative Study of Neoplasia and Steroid Contraceptives. Int J Epidemiol 1993;22:192–7. [PubMed] ⇦

5. Newcomb PA, Storer BE, Longnecker MP, Mittendorf R, Greenberg ER, Clapp RW, et al. Lactation and a reduced risk of premenopausal breast cancer. N Engl J Med 1994;330: 81–7. [PubMed] [Full Text] ⇦

6. Breast cancer and breastfeeding: collaborative reanalysis of individual data from 47 epidemiological studies in 30 countries, including 50302 women with breast cancer and

community breastfeeding programs. Lactation consultants should be accessible to women both in the hospital and after discharge. However, the cost of lactation services and the low rate of reimbursement have made such support unobtainable for many women. Additionally, the inclusion of lactation visits in the global prenatal fee has limited the ability of childbirth care providers to provide services after delivery in the absence of a breast infection. The Affordable Care Act addresses this by requiring non-grandfathered plans and issuers to provide coverage without cost sharing (for costs of renting breastfeeding equipment and comprehensive lactation support and counseling by a trained health care provider during preg-

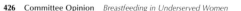

303

Appendix F: ACOG Committee Opinion #570: Breastfeeding in Underserved Women:
Increasing Initiation and Continuation of Breastfeeding

96973 women without the disease. Collaborative Group on Hormonal Factors in Breast Cancer. Lancet 2002;360: 187–95. [PubMed] [Full Text] ⇐

7. Racial and ethnic differences in breastfeeding initiation and duration, by state - National Immunization Survey, United States, 2004–2008. Centers for Disease Control and Prevention (CDC). MMWR Morb Mortal Wkly Rep 2010;59:327–34. [PubMed] [Full Text] ⇐

8. Progress in increasing breastfeeding and reducing racial/ethnic differences - United States, 2000-2008 births. Centers for Disease Control and Prevention (CDC). MMWR Morb Mortal Wkly Rep 2013;62:77–80. [PubMed] [Full Text] ⇐

9. Shealy KR, Li R, Benton-Davis S, Grummer-Strawn LM. Support for breastfeeding in the workplace. In: The CDC guide to breastfeeding interventions. Atlanta (GA): Centers for Disease Control and Prevention; 2005. p. 7–12. Available at: http://www.cdc.gov/breastfeeding/pdf/BF_guide_2.pdf. Retrieved May 17, 2013. ⇐

10. United States Breastfeeding Committee. Workplace accommodations to support and protect breastfeeding. Washington, DC: USBC; 2010. Available at: http://www.usbreastfeeding.org/Portals/0/Publications/Workplace-Background-2010-USBC.pdf. Retrieved May 17, 2013. ⇐

11. Reasonable break time for nursing mothers. 29 U.S.C. 207 (2011). ⇐

12. Centers for Disease Control and Prevention. Provisional breastfeeding rates by socio-demographic factors, among children born in 2007. Available at: http://www.cdc.gov/breastfeeding/data/NIS_data/2007/socio-demographic_any.htm. Retrieved May 17, 2013. ⇐

13. Department of Health and Human Services. The Surgeon General's call to action to support breastfeeding. Washington, DC: Department of Health and Human Services, Office of the Surgeon General; 2011. Available at: http://www.surgeongeneral.gov/library/calls/breastfeeding/calltoactiontosupportbreastfeeding.pdf. Retrieved May 17, 2013. ⇐

14. Nelson AM. Adolescent attitudes, beliefs, and concerns regarding breastfeeding. MCN Am J Matern Child Nurs 2009;34:249–55. [PubMed] ⇐

15. Avery AB, Magnus JH. Expectant fathers' and mothers' perceptions of breastfeeding and formula feeding: a focus group study in three US cities. J Hum Lact 2011;27:147–54. [PubMed] [Full Text] ⇐

16. National Conference of State Legislatures. Breastfeeding laws. Washington, DC: NCSL; 2011. Available at: http://www.ncsl.org/issues-research/health/breastfeeding-state-laws.aspx. Retrieved May 17, 2013. ⇐

17. American Academy of Pediatrics; American College of Obstetricians and Gynecologists. Breastfeeding handbook for physicians. Elk Grove Village (IL): AAP; Washington, DC: ACOG; 2006. ⇐

18. Singh GK, Kogan MD, Dee DL. Nativity/immigrant status, race/ethnicity, and socioeconomic determinants of breastfeeding initiation and duration in the United States, 2003. Pediatrics 2007;119(suppl 1):S38–46. [PubMed] [Full Text] ⇐

19. Centers for Disease Control and Prevention. Obesity: halting the epidemic by making health easier. Atlanta (GA):

CDC; 2011. Available at: http://www.cdc.gov/chronicdisease/resources/publications/aag/pdf/2011/Obesity_AAG_WEB_508.pdf. Retrieved May 17, 2013. ⇐

20. Baker JL, Gamborg M, Heitmann BL, Lissner L, Sorensen TI, Rasmussen KM. Breastfeeding reduces postpartum weight retention. Am J Clin Nutr 2008;88:1543–51. [PubMed] [Full Text] ⇐

21. Hatsu IE, McDougald DM, Anderson AK. Effect of infant feeding on maternal body composition. Int Breastfeed J 2008;3:18. [PubMed] [Full Text] ⇐

22. Harder T, Bergmann R, Kallischnigg G, Plagemann A. Duration of breastfeeding and risk of overweight: a meta-analysis. Am J Epidemiol 2005;162:397–403. [PubMed] [Full Text] ⇐

23. Centers for Disease Control and Prevention. National diabetes fact sheet, 2011. Atlanta (GA): CDC; 2011. Available at: http://www.cdc.gov/diabetes/pubs/pdf/ndfs_2011.pdf. Retrieved May 17, 2013. ⇐

24. Stuebe AM, Rich-Edwards JW, Willett WC, Manson JE, Michels KB. Duration of lactation and incidence of type 2 diabetes. JAMA 2005;294:2601–10. [PubMed] [Full Text] ⇐

25. Kurian AK, Cardarelli KM. Racial and ethnic differences in cardiovascular disease risk factors: a systematic review. Ethn Dis 2007;17:143–52. [PubMed] ⇐

26. Schwarz EB, Ray RM, Stuebe AM, Allison MA, Ness RB, Freiberg MS, et al. Duration of lactation and risk factors for maternal cardiovascular disease. Obstet Gynecol 2009;113:974–82. [PubMed] [Obstetrics & Gynecology] ⇐

27. Stuebe AM, Schwarz EB, Grewen K, Rich-Edwards JW, Michels KB, Foster EM, et al. Duration of lactation and incidence of maternal hypertension: a longitudinal cohort study. Am J Epidemiol 2011;174:1147–58. [PubMed] [Full Text] ⇐

28. Department of Health and Human Services. Healthy People 2020 topics and objectives: family planning. Available at: http://healthypeople.gov/2020/topicsobjectives2020/overview.aspx?topicid=13. Retrieved May 17, 2013. ⇐

29. Kennedy KI, Visness CM. Contraceptive efficacy of lactational amenorrhoea. Lancet 1992;339:227–30. [PubMed] ⇐

30. Weimer JP. The economic benefits of breastfeeding a review and analysis. Washington, DC: Department of Agriculture; 2001. Available at: http://www.ers.usda.gov/media/329098/fanrr13_1_.pdf. Retrieved May 17, 2013. ⇐

31. United States Breastfeeding Committee. Benefits of breastfeeding. Raleigh (NC): USBC; 2002. Available at: http://www.usbreastfeeding.org/LinkClick.aspx?link=Publications%2fBenefits-2002-USBC.pdf&tabid=70&mid=388. Retrieved May 17, 2013. ⇐

32. Wolfberg AJ, Michels KB, Shields W, O'Campo P, Bronner Y, Bienstock J. Dads as breastfeeding advocates: results from a randomized controlled trial of an educational intervention. Am J Obstet Gynecol 2004;191:708–12. [PubMed] [Full Text] ⇐

33. Watkins S, Meltzer-Brody S, Zolnoun D, Stuebe A. Early breastfeeding experiences and postpartum depression. Obstet Gynecol 2011;118:214–21. [PubMed] [Obstetrics & Gynecology] ⇐

34. Breastfeeding and the use of human milk. Section on Breastfeeding. Pediatrics 2012;129:e827–41. [PubMed] [Full Text] ⇐

35. Healthy Mothers, Healthy Babies National Coalition. Baby friendly hospital initiative feasibility study: final report. Washington, DC: HMHBNC; 1994. ⇐

36. Health Resources and Services Administration. Women's preventive services: required health plan coverage guidelines. Available at: http://hrsa.gov/womensguidelines. Retrieved May 17, 2013. ⇐

37. Kaiser Family Foundation. The Medicaid program at a glance. Washington, DC:KFF; 2013. Available at: http://kaiserfamilyfoundation.files.wordpress.com/2013/03/7235-061.pdf. Retrieved May 13, 2013. ⇐

38. Food and Nutrition Service, Department of Agriculture. WIC breastfeeding data local agency report. Washington, DC: USDA; 2012. Available at: http://www.fns.usda.gov/wic/fundingandprogramdata/FY2011-BFdata-localagency report.pdf. Retrieved May 17, 2013. ⇐

39. Whaley SE, Koleilat M, Whaley M, Gomez J, Meehan K, Saluja K. Impact of policy changes on infant feeding decisions among low-income women participating in the Special Supplemental Nutrition Program for Women, Infants, and Children. Am J Public Health 2012;102:2269–73. [PubMed] [Full Text] ⇐

Breastfeeding in underserved women: increasing initiation and continuation of breastfeeding. Committee Opinion No. 570. American College of Obstetricians and Gynecologists. Obstet Gynecol 2013; 122:423–8.